T0200175

ADVANCE PRAISE FOR

Office-Based Buprenorphine Treatment of Opioid Use Disorder
SECOND EDITION

"*Office Based Buprenorphine Treatment of Opioid Use Disorder*, 2nd Edition, is an invaluable guide to any provider licensed to prescribe this evidence-based medication-assisted treatment for opioid use disorder. Experts in the field provide detailed chapters on topics such as opioid use and rates of overdose deaths; efficacy and safety of buprenorphine; and clinical use in dosing involving special populations such as adolescents, pregnant women, and patients with pain; as well as sections on psychiatric and medical comorbidities. In addition to being an excellent guide for prescribers of buprenorphine, this text serves as an excellent learning tool for medical students, residents, fellows in addiction medicine or addiction psychiatry, and medical providers interested in treating this challenging, but potentially very rewarding population."

> *Lon R. Hays, M.D., M.B.A., Professor and Chairman, Department of Psychiatry, University of Kentucky*

"*Office-Based Buprenorphine Treatment of Opioid Use Disorder*, 2nd Edition, is the long-sought-after missing link to effective and comprehensive opioid treatment. This masterful manuscript provides expert clinical guidance that both novice and experienced practitioners will find to be immediately useful. The comprehensiveness of this book is unmatched and invaluable for those seeking to provide 'state of the art' competent opioid use disorder treatment."

> *Louis E. Baxter Sr., M.D., DFASAM, President and CEO, Professional Assistance Program New Jersey, Inc.; Past President of ASAM; Director of ABAM; and Codirector of Addiction Medicine Fellowship, Howard University Hospital*

"This book is the most up-to-date resource on the principal office-based treatment for opioid-dependent patients. Because it draws on the leadership of the addiction field and is comprehensive and clearly focused, both experienced physicians and those new to these patients can turn to it with great confidence."

Marc Galanter, M.D., *Professor of Psychiatry, NYU School of Medicine*

"Treatment for addictive disease must break through long-existing stigma to be incorporated into the fabric of the medical treatment community. Education is the key to breaking through stigma. Renner, Levounis, and LaRose and the chapter authors expertly educate by answering buprenorphine-related questions asked by both longstanding addiction practitioners and general practice clinicians. By adding historic perspective, the authors provide necessary context to help clinicians reduce morbidity and mortality in their patient population."

Stuart Gitlow, M.D., M.P.H., *Past President, American Society of Addiction Medicine*

Office-Based Buprenorphine Treatment

OF OPIOID USE DISORDER

SECOND EDITION

Office-Based Buprenorphine Treatment
OF OPIOID USE DISORDER

SECOND EDITION

Edited by

John A. Renner Jr., M.D.
Petros Levounis, M.D., M.A.
Anna T. LaRose, M.D.

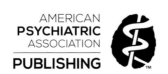

AMERICAN
PSYCHIATRIC
ASSOCIATION
PUBLISHING

Note: The authors have worked to ensure that all information in this book is accurate at the time of publication and consistent with general psychiatric and medical standards, and that information concerning drug dosages, schedules, and routes of administration is accurate at the time of publication and consistent with standards set by the U.S. Food and Drug Administration and the general medical community. As medical research and practice continue to advance, however, therapeutic standards may change. Moreover, specific situations may require a specific therapeutic response not included in this book. For these reasons and because human and mechanical errors sometimes occur, we recommend that readers follow the advice of physicians directly involved in their care or the care of a member of their family.

Books published by American Psychiatric Association Publishing represent the findings, conclusions, and views of the individual authors and do not necessarily represent the policies and opinions of American Psychiatric Association Publishing or the American Psychiatric Association.

If you wish to buy 50 or more copies of the same title, please go to www.appi.org/special discounts for more information.

Copyright © 2018 American Psychiatric Association Publishing

ALL RIGHTS RESERVED

Second Edition

Manufactured in the United States of America on acid-free paper
21   20   19   18   17   5   4   3   2   1

American Psychiatric Association Publishing
1000 Wilson Boulevard
Arlington, VA 22209-3901
www.appi.org

Library of Congress Cataloging-in-Publication Data
Names: Renner, John A., Jr., 1938– editor. | Levounis, Petros, editor. | LaRose, Anna T., 1979– editor.

Title: Office-based buprenorphine treatment of opioid use disorder / edited by John A. Renner Jr., Petros Levounis, Anna T. LaRose.

Other titles: Handbook of office-based buprenorphine treatment of opioid dependence.

Description: Second edition. | Arlington, Virginia : American Psychiatric Association Publishing, [2018] | Preceded by Handbook of office-based buprenorphine treatment of opioid dependence, edited by John A. Renner Jr., Petros Levounis, 1st. ed., 2011. | Includes bibliographic references and index. |

Identifiers: LCCN 2017039793 (print) | LCCN 2017040999 (ebook) | ISBN 9781615371709 (eb) | ISBN 9781615370832 (pb : alk. paper)

Subjects: | MESH: Opioid-Related Disorders—drug therapy |

  Buprenorphine—therapeutic use | Opiate Substitution Treatment

Classification: LCC RC568.O45 (ebook) | LCC RC568.O45 (print) | NLM WM 284 | DDC 615/.7822—dc23

LC record available at https://lccn.loc.gov/2017039793

British Library Cataloguing in Publication Data
A CIP record is available from the British Library

Contents

Contributors

Gregory Acampora, M.D.
Psychiatrist, MGH/Harvard Center for Addiction Medicine, MGH/Charlestown Community Health Center, Pain Management Center at MGH, Massachusetts General Hospital, Boston, Massachusetts

Daniel P. Alford, M.D., M.P.H., FACP, DFASAM
Professor of Medicine, Boston University School of Medicine, Boston Medical Center, Boston, Massachusetts

Elie Aoun, M.D.
Forensic Psychiatry Fellow, Columbia University, New York State Psychiatric Institute, New York, New York

Jonathan Avery, M.D.
Assistant Clinical Professor of Psychiatry and Assistant Dean of Student Affairs, Weill Cornell Medical Center, New York, New York

Jeffrey D. Baxter, M.D.
Associate Professor, Department of Family Medicine and Community Health, University of Massachusetts Medical School, and Chief Medical Officer, Spectrum Health Systems, Worcester, Massachusetts

Joseph H. Donroe, M.D.
Assistant Professor of Medicine, Yale University School of Medicine, New Haven, Connecticut

Beatrice A. Eld
Consultant and former Deputy Director of Education for Addiction Psychiatry, American Psychiatric Association, Arlington, Virginia

Saria El Haddad, M.D.
Instructor in Psychiatry, Harvard Medical School, and Director, Partial Hospitalization Program, Department of Psychiatry, Brigham and Women's Faulkner Hospital, Boston, Massachusetts

Gerard Iru I. Fernando, M.D.
Medical Director of Addiction Services, Truxtun Psychiatric Medical Group, Bakersfield, California

David A. Fiellin, M.D.
Professor of Medicine and Public Health, Yale University School of Medicine, New Haven, Connecticut

Lynn E. Fiellin, M.D.
Associate Professor of Medicine and the Child Study Center, Yale University School of Medicine, New Haven, Connecticut

Peter D. Friedmann, M.D., M.P.H., DFASAM, FACP
Chief Research Officer and Endowed Chair for Clinical Research, Baystate Health; Associate Dean for Research and Professor of Medicine, University of Massachusetts Medical School (UMMS)—Baystate; Professor of Quantitative Health Sciences, UMMS Office of Research, Springfield, Massachusetts

Hendrée E. Jones, Ph.D.
Executive Director, UNC Horizons, and Professor, Department of Obstetrics and Gynecology, University of North Carolina, Chapel Hill, North Carolina

Anna T. LaRose, M.D.
Instructor in Psychiatry, Boston University Medical School, and Staff Psychiatrist, VA Boston Healthcare System, Boston, Massachusetts

Petros Levounis, M.D., M.A.
Professor and Chair, Department of Psychiatry, Rutgers New Jersey Medical School, and Chief of Service, University Hospital, Newark, New Jersey

Sharon Levy, M.D., M.P.H.
Associate Professor of Pediatrics, Harvard Medical School, and Director, Adolescent Substance Abuse Program, Boston Children's Hospital, Boston Massachusetts

Elinore F. McCance-Katz, M.D., Ph.D.
Chief Medical Officer, Rhode Island Department of Behavioral Healthcare, Developmental Disabilities and Hospitals, and Professor of Psychiatry and Human Behavior, Alpert Medical School, Brown University, Providence, Rhode Island

Dong Chan Park, M.D.
Staff Psychiatrist, Department of Psychiatry, Edith Nourse Rogers Memorial Veterans Hospital, Bedford, Massachusetts

Tae Woo Park, M.D., MSc
Assistant Professor of Psychiatry, Boston University School of Medicine, Boston, Massachusetts

John T. Pichot, M.D.
Private practice of psychiatry, San Antonio, Texas

Mark T. Pichot, D.O.
Psychiatry Resident (PGY-1), University of Texas Health San Antonio—Long Medical School, San Antonio, Texas

John A. Renner Jr., M.D.
Professor of Psychiatry, Boston University School of Medicine, and Associate Chief of Psychiatry, VA Boston Healthcare System, Boston, Massachusetts

Ricardo Restrepo, M.D., M.P.H.
Substance Abuse Treatment Program-SATP/Buprenorphine Clinic Medical Director VA Long Beach Healthcare System and Associate Clinical Professor at University of California, Irvine, California

Claudia P. Rodriguez, M.D.
Director of Outpatient Addiction Recovery Program, Brigham and Women's Faulkner Hospital, and Instructor in Psychiatry, Harvard Medical School, Boston, Massachusetts

Ximena Sanchez-Samper, M.D.
Instructor, Harvard Medical School, Boston, Massachusetts, and Psychiatrist, McLean Hospital, Weston, Massachusetts

Brad W. Stankiewicz, M.D.
Addiction Psychiatry Fellow, Boston Medical Center/VA Boston Healthcare System, Boston, Massachusetts

Eric C. Strain, M.D.
Professor, Department of Psychiatry and Behavioral Sciences, Johns Hopkins University School of Medicine, Baltimore, Maryland

Joji Suzuki, M.D.
Director, Division of Addiction Psychiatry, Department of Psychiatry, Brigham and Women's Hospital, and Assistant Professor of Psychiatry, Harvard Medical School, Boston, Massachusetts

Jeanette M. Tetrault, M.D.
Associate Professor of Medicine, Yale University School of Medicine, New Haven, Connecticut

Erin Zerbo, M.D.
Assistant Professor, Department of Psychiatry, Rutgers New Jersey Medical School, Newark, New Jersey

Disclosure of Interests

The following contributors to this book have indicated a financial interest in or other affiliation with a commercial supporter, a manufacturer of a commercial product, a provider of a commercial service, a nongovernmental organization, and/or a government agency, as listed below:

Peter D. Friedmann, M.D., M.P.H., DFASAM, FACP.   *Honorarium and travel reimbursement*: Indivior Advisory Board Meeting 2015. *Training*: Braeburn. *Consultant*: Endo Pharmaceuticals. *Study drug-in-kind*: Alkermes

Anna T. LaRose, M.D.   *Travel grant*: AAAP, 2015

Elinore F. McCance-Katz, M.D., Ph.D.   *Consultant*: Indivior, 2015

John A. Renner Jr., M.D.   *Stockholder*: Johnson & Johnson, General Electric (both of which produce drugs but none that are relevant to addiction treatment). *Honoraria*: APA and AAP

Eric C. Strain, M.D.   *Grant support*: Alkermes. *Consultant*: Egalet Corporation, Indivior Pharmaceuticals.   *Advisory board*: The Oak Group, Pinney Associates

The following contributors have indicated that they have no financial interests or other affiliations that represent or could appear to represent a competing interest with their contributions to this book:

Gregory Acampora, M.D.; Daniel P. Alford, M.D., M.P.H., FACP, DFASAM; Elie Aoun, M.D.; Jonathan Avery, M.D.; Jeffrey D. Baxter, M.D.; Joseph H. Donroe, M.D.; Saria El Haddad, M.D.; Beatrice A. Eld; Gerard Iru I. Fernando, M.D.; David A. Fiellin, M.D.; Lynn E. Fiellin, M.D.; Hendrée E. Jones, Ph.D.; Petros Levounis, M.D., M.A.; Sharon Levy, M.D., M.P.H.; Dong Chan Park, M.D.; Tae Woo Park, M.D., M.Sc.; John T. Pichot, M.D.; Mark T. Pichot, D.O.; Ricardo Restrepo, M.D., M.P.H.; Claudia P. Rodriguez, M.D.; Ximena Sanchez-Samper, M.D.; Brad W. Stankiewicz, M.D.; Joji Suzuki, M.D.; Jeanette M. Tetrault, M.D.; Erin Zerbo, M.D.

Dedication

PEOPLE sometimes ask us, "Why do you do this work?" The assumption is that caring for addicts is frustrating and depressing; these patients do not get better and are manipulative, ungrateful, or worse. For those of us within the addiction treatment community, these ideas have always seemed strange and more than a little sad—and very foreign to our actual experience as clinicians.

The first edition of this book was conceived in the early years of buprenorphine treatment. We were very optimistic about the potential for this medication and hoped that it would be widely adopted. Looking back over the last decade, it is clear that buprenorphine has lived up to our clinical expectations. It has convincingly demonstrated that medication-assisted treatment is the most successful option for the treatment of opioid use disorder. Equally important, the availability of office-based treatment has expanded more than sevenfold the number of individuals in treatment.

Despite this success, the opioid misuse epidemic has grown even worse. It is critical that we learn from the experience of the past decade. Prescribers, patients, and especially adolescents and young adults must be better educated on the risks of opioid pharmaceuticals and about safe prescribing practices. Buprenorphine providers must understand the value of long-term treatment and the importance of careful patient management geared to minimizing diversion and abuse of the medication. A major disappointment has been the slow adoption of buprenorphine treatment into clinical practice, both in primary care and in general psychiatry. The expansion of waivered clinicians to include nurse practitioners and physician assistants and the focus on providing waiver education during residency training are encouraging developments that should help address this issue. This second edition of *Office-Based Buprenorphine Treatment for Opioid Use Disorder* was designed both to incorporate advances in our clinical knowledge and to provide a new option for obtaining the buprenorphine waiver, hopefully making it possible for even more clinicians to join the ranks of buprenorphine providers.

In 2005, I decided to start a buprenorphine therapy group for returning veterans as part of the addiction treatment program at the VA Boston Healthcare System. These young men easily bonded as combat veterans and as addicts in recovery, and buprenorphine very quickly enabled most of them to gain control over their opioid use problem. The core issue for the "BUP Group" became their struggle to regain self-respect and confidence for a meaningful future. How do you square your image as a tough combat veteran—responsible for the survival of your squad—with the conning, lies, and degradation of addictive behavior? What do you do with the terror and guilt that haunts your dreams when you know that opioids will provide instant relief?

The BUP Group taught me the meaning of true courage—honestly facing the worst in your past and finding the strength both to forgive yourself and to move forward. For some of these men, recovery came with little or no support or trust from family, friends, and even other members of 12-step groups. The unique bond within this remarkable group of combat veterans has been a powerful source of understanding, respect, and caring. It has been my good fortune to be a part of the buprenorphine story, to see recovery become possible where before there was little hope and much despair. I have learned that we do not cure addiction but we can manage it successfully and that recovery is real.

This book is dedicated to all the patients who have used buprenorphine to reclaim their hope and their lives, but most especially to the veterans in my BUP Group, with my love, respect, and admiration. It has been my privilege to share this road with you.

John A. Renner Jr., M.D.

Foreword

FOUR decades ago, Donald Jasinski, a researcher at the Intramural Research Program of the National Institute on Drug Abuse (NIDA), recognized the potential of a new injectable analgesic, buprenorphine, as a possible treatment for addiction to opioids. In 1978, Jasinski conducted the first study demonstrating the efficacy of buprenorphine. This became the foundation for a collaboration between NIDA and Reckitt Benckiser Pharmaceuticals, working first to create an easier-to-administer oral formulation and then, in the 1990s, to develop an abuse- and diversion-resistant formulation that incorporated the opioid receptor antagonist naloxone. In 2002, the U.S. Food and Drug Administration (FDA) approved buprenorphine and buprenorphine-naloxone (Suboxone) for treatment of opioid use disorders.

This was a milestone for the field. It meant that for the first time, someone with an illicit drug use disorder could receive a prescription from a regular health care provider to treat his or her addiction—a much-needed step toward the integration of addiction treatment into general health care.

The FDA approval of Suboxone could not have come soon enough, coinciding with the escalating opioid crisis that now claims more than 33,000 lives annually (Rudd et al. 2016). However, as we know, a medication can make an impact only if it reaches patients in need, and thus far buprenorphine is grossly underutilized. Only 21% of private sector specialty addiction treatment facilities offer buprenorphine treatment, and only 37% of opioid-addicted patients in those programs receive it (Knudsen et al. 2011).

Historical reluctance to use medications for addiction treatment, which is a legacy of older models of recovery rooted in 12-step programs, has resulted in inadequate buprenorphine dosing and/or inadequate treatment duration, leading to treatment failure and reinforcing doubt about buprenorphine's efficacy even among some addiction treatment providers (MacDonald et al. 2016; Mattick et al. 2014). But study after study has shown the efficacy of buprenorphine when it is used at an appropriate therapeutic dose for a sufficient duration. It improves engagement in treatment, reduces illicit opioid use, reduces overdose and relapse risk, reduces drug-related criminality and recidivism, reduces HIV and hepatitis C virus transmission, and improves quality of life.

Research is also revealing buprenorphine's promise for improving treatment engagement and health outcomes when initiated in emergency departments and in prisons prior to patients' discharge into the community (D'Onofrio et al. 2015; Zaller et al. 2013). This medication has great lifesaving potential. We must overcome outdated attitudinal barriers that limit the use of buprenorphine (and other medications) to treat opioid addiction, as well as address infrastructural impediments such as workforce shortages and preapproval requirements for insurance coverage.

Psychiatrists and other providers across diverse health care settings must take a more active role in helping end the opioid crisis, and increasing the use of buprenorphine is central to that goal. Research suggests that acceptance of medications for addiction treatment is linked to seeing them work (Mitchell et al. 2016). The more buprenorphine is used appropriately and with fidelity to the evidence base, the more patients with opioid use disorders will benefit, and the more providers will be ready to provide it to their patients. This updated single volume will be a very valuable resource to help guide clinicians in the use of buprenorphine for the management of opioid use disorders.

Nora D. Volkow, M.D.
Director, National Institute on Drug Abuse

References

D'Onofrio G, O'Connor PG, Pantalon MV, et al: Emergency department–initiated buprenorphine/naloxone treatment for opioid dependence: a randomized clinical trial. JAMA 313(16):1636–1644, 2015 25919527

Knudsen HK, Abraham AJ, Roman PM: Adoption and implementation of medications in addiction treatment programs. J Addict Med 5(1):21–27, 2011 21359109

MacDonald K, Lamb K, Thomas ML, Khentigan W: Buprenorphine maintenance treatment of opiate dependence: correlations between prescriber beliefs and practices. Subst Use Misuse 51(1):85–90, 2016 26771870

Mattick RP, Breen C, Kimber J, Davoli M: Buprenorphine maintenance versus placebo or methadone maintenance for opioid dependence. Cochrane Database of Systematic Reviews, 2014, Issue 2. Article No.: CD002207. DOI: 10.1002/14651858.CD002207.pub4

Mitchell SG, Willet J, Monico LB, et al. Community correctional agents' views of medication-assisted treatment: Examining their influence on treatment referrals and community supervision practices. Subst Abuse 37(1):127-133, 2016 26860334

Rudd RA, Seth P, David F, Scholl L: Increases in drug and opioid-involved overdose deaths — United States, 2010–2015. MMWR Morb Mortal Wkly Rep 65(5051):1445–1452, 2016 28033313

Zaller N, McKenzie M, Friedmann PD, et al: Initiation of buprenorphine during incarceration and retention in treatment upon release. J Subst Abuse Treat 45(2):222–226, 2013 23541303

Obtaining the Buprenorphine Waiver

Overview

This 8-hour activity and complementary online assessment meets the Federal training requirement of the Drug Addiction Treatment Act of 2000 (DATA 2000). Completion will allow qualified clinicians to apply for a waiver to their Drug Enforcement Administration (DEA) license and thus to provide office-based treatment of opioid use disorder with buprenorphine.

Development of this training was supported by the Center for Substance Abuse Treatment (CSAT), Substance Abuse and Mental Health Services, U.S. Department of Health and Human Services.

Educational Objectives

- Discuss the rationale and need for medication-assisted treatment of opioid use disorder.
- Apply the pharmacological characteristics of opioids in clinical practice.
- Describe buprenorphine protocols for all phases of treatment and for optimal patient-treatment matching.
- Describe the legislative and regulatory requirements of office-based opioid pharmacotherapy.
- Discuss treatment issues and management of opioid use disorder in adolescents, pregnant women, and patients with acute and/or chronic pain.

Target Audience

- Physicians interested in completing the training requirement for CSAT certification to qualify for the waiver authority from the requirements of the Controlled Substances Act

- Nurse practitioners and physician assistants interested in using this activity to satisfy 8 hours of their required training
- Physicians interested in learning more about office-based prescribing of buprenorphine for the treatment of opioid use disorder

Accreditation and Designation Information

The American Psychiatric Association (APA) is accredited by the Accreditation Council for Continuing Medical Education (ACCME) to provide continuing medical education for physicians.

The APA designates this enduring material for a maximum of 8 *AMA PRA Category 1 Credit™*. Physicians should claim only the credit commensurate with the extent of their participation in the activity.

The APA is one of the DATA 2000 organizations that can provide the 8-hour training for physicians, nurse practitioners, and physician assistants needed to obtain the waiver to prescribe buprenorphine. This book-based learning and complementary online assessment has been designed to meet these training requirements.

How to Earn Credit

Participants who wish to earn *AMA PRA Category 1 Credit™* or a certificate of participation may do so by completing all sections of the course, including the evaluation. A multiple-choice quiz is provided based on the content. A passing score of 80% must be achieved. Retakes are available for the test. After evaluating the program, course participants will be provided with an opportunity to claim hours of participation and print an official continuing medical education (CME) certificate (physicians) or certificate of participation (nonphysicians) showing the completion date and hours earned.

Instructions for Claiming CME Credit and Applying for a DEA Waiver

1. Visit www.psychiatry.org/buprenorphinetraining.
2. Click on the *Office-Based Buprenorphine Treatment of Opioid Use Disorder* "Credit Claim" link.
3. Enter the group ID from the inside cover of this book to unlock the activity in the APA Learning Center.

4. Complete the program requirements, including a 25-question online self-assessment. Participants must obtain a passing score of 80% or greater.
5. Complete the CME evaluation.
6. Print and retain your CME certificate.
7. Follow the instructions provided with the CME certificate to obtain a DEA waiver for buprenorphine prescribing.

1

Opioid Use Disorder in America

History and Overview

John A. Renner Jr., M.D.

OPIOID USE DISORDER (OUD) has been a serious problem in the United States since before the Civil War. In this chapter, I trace the evolution of this problem from the era of opium-laced patent medicines, through the problems with injectable morphine after the Civil War, to the heroin epidemics of the twentieth century, and finally to the current epidemic of opioid pharmaceutical misuse that began in the 1990s. I highlight the history of medical efforts to manage OUD and recurrent conflicts with a public policy approach that has emphasized criminal justice solutions to the problem. The introduction of office-based buprenorphine treatment is best understood as an effort to restore a medical treatment model and a more coherent public health approach to what has become an intractable medical, legal, and social problem.

Historical Overview

OPIOID USE DISORDER 1830–1899

In eighteenth-century America, opium extracts such as laudanum, which contained alcohol, and black drop opium, which contained no alcohol, were common ingredients in a wide range of prescriptions and patent medicines. These medications were used to treat food poisoning and other gastrointestinal problems and were valued for their sedating and calming effects.

The first apparent opioid problem in the United States occurred in the early nineteenth century, when patent medicines laced with tincture of opium were readily available from apothecaries or door-to-door peddlers. Because the drugs were cheap, individuals with mild OUD had no problem maintaining medication supplies and had relatively little functional disability. The typical misuser of opioids at that time was a white, middle-class farm housewife who became addicted while self-medicating a wide range of physical and psychological ailments. Although some individuals were more impaired by their OUD, there was no association with criminal behavior. At worst, the individual with OUD was perceived as "sickly" or neurasthenic (Musto 1999). Physicians and the public associated the risk of problems with the lower social classes. These risks were noted, but they were thought to be minimal and to be balanced by the medicinal benefits of opium. Some physicians even claimed that opiates could improve the functioning of strong-willed individuals (Wood 1856).

Advances in technology in the early nineteenth century permitted the isolation of specific alkaloids from crude opium and led to the identification of morphine as a potent agent with significant physiological and psychological effects. Commercial morphine production began in the United States in 1832. The invention of the hypodermic syringe permitted the direct injection of this powerful and habit-forming substance and opened the door to both more effective pain treatment and increased risks for OUD.

A second and more visible group of individuals with OUD were Civil War veterans who became physiologically dependent on intramuscular morphine after being treated for combat injuries. By 1870, some physicians began to recognize the habit-forming risk of morphine injections, although injectable morphine was thought to present less of a dependence risk than oral opium preparations (Allbutt 1870). In the decades following the Civil War, it became common medical practice for physicians to give patients morphine as long-term therapy to manage chronic pain. This morphine dependence syndrome was called *soldier's disease*, a reflection of the origin of the disorder, the relatively acceptable social status of the patient, and the medical paradigm that informed society's understanding of the condition. During the late nineteenth century, rates of morphine dependence in the United States far exceeded those of other

Western industrialized nations. Although this was commonly attributed to the aftermath of Civil War injuries, other major European nations also experienced wars and extensive use of morphine without having comparable rates of OUD (Musto 1999). The reasons for the high levels of U.S. opium consumption and the unique vulnerability to OUD in this country have never been adequately explained.

In the United States, social attitudes regarding the long-term use of opiates began to shift with the increased immigration of Chinese laborers and growing public concern about the devastating effects of opium misuse in China. This change in attitudes, along with the growth of the Temperance Movement, led to a fear of OUD as a dangerous, foreign, "un-American" problem that needed to be eradicated. These attitudes led to a decline in the per capita consumption of crude opium, which was first noted in 1887. By the end of the nineteenth century, the conceptual paradigm for OUD had shifted from a medical model to a moral and criminal justice model—a conceptual ambiguity that continued throughout the twentieth century. Although the medical value of morphine was not questioned, physicians gradually came to recognize the dangers associated with overprescription of this drug. There was a perception that the risks of addiction were most prevalent in immigrant groups such as the Chinese and in the lower social classes. It was presumed that the social deterioration associated with chronic opiate use was a reflection of the user's weak character and lack of morals. Very gradual dose reduction, or *detoxification*, was thought to be the cure, although it was recognized that successful treatment requires a high level of motivation. In Germany, there were reports of high relapse rates following attempts to wean patients from morphine, and it was hypothesized that regular use of morphine would induce predictable physiological changes that would make anyone an addict (Levinstein 1878). These observations contrasted with the dominant opinion in England and in the United States and supported the notion that the moral deterioration associated with OUD was a consequence of the disorder and not the cause.

OPIOID USE DISORDER 1900–1914:
MORPHINE MAINTENANCE CLINICS

By 1900, there were an estimated 250,000 individuals with OUD in the United States (Musto 1973, p. 5). In many cities, efforts to manage the problem medically shifted from the individual physician's office to a system of morphine clinics, where groups of individuals with OUD were given daily morphine injections. In some cities, these clinics were administered by law enforcement authorities, a further reflection of the confusion between the medical and criminal justice paradigms. OUD was lumped together with alcoholism and syphilis as vices—social afflictions that were difficult to cure; impacted predominantly the lower classes; and led to eventual physical, moral, and social deterioration. With the gradual development of modern treatments for many common medical conditions, the value of opiates as all-purpose medications for a wide range of physical and psychological conditions became identified with a form of backward and unscientific medical practice. This shift in practice made it much easier to support the need to closely regulate this aspect of medicine.

Beyond modest tariffs, no restrictions on the importation of opium and opium products existed during the nineteenth century. The unregulated use of inexpensive patent medicines, often with opiates or cocaine as their primary active ingredient, reached a peak in the late nineteenth century. Attempts by individual states to regulate the sale of opiate products were largely ineffective, although some states and cities began to require a physician's prescription for ordering morphine. There was no requirement for accurate labels on patent medicines involved in interstate commerce until the passage of the Pure Food and Drug Act in 1906. In 1909, the importation of smoking opium was prohibited. However, none of these measures was successful in eliminating the opiate misuse problem (or OUDs).

Opioid Use Disorder 1914–1960: Harrison Act and the Prohibition of Addiction Treatment

The control of opioid medications changed dramatically in 1914 with the passage of the Harrison Narcotics Tax Act, which established the U.S. Food and Drug Administration (FDA) and a federal system for the regulation of drug manufacturers, pharmacies, and physician prescribing. The Harrison Act made it illegal to prescribe opioids for the treatment of OUD. This led to the closing of the existing 44 morphine maintenance clinics and ultimately the jailing of more than 3,000 physicians who refused to stop prescribing opioids for their patients. After the Supreme Court upheld the Harrison Act in 1919, organized medicine abandoned all support for the treatment of these individuals, and management of the OUD problem effectively was shifted to the criminal justice system.

Ultimately, the criminal justice model proved unsuccessful as a strategy for handling the OUD problem. In the late nineteenth century, a process had been discovered for converting morphine into heroin (diacetylmorphine). The commercial availability of heroin in 1898 introduced a new, potent, and highly reinforcing opioid that ensured the perpetuation of the OUD problem. Regulation of patent medicine production and the elimination of any legitimate medical treatment for OUD ushered in the era of the heroin black market. Despite efforts to eliminate the problem, there were major heroin epidemics in the United States following World War I, World War II, and the

Vietnam War. Chronic heroin users were stigmatized as a deviant and criminal minority. For most of the twentieth century, the lifetime risk for heroin use disorder was assumed to be relatively low, ranging from 0.4% to 0.7% (Compton et al. 2007; Grant 1996; Kessler et al. 1994; Regier et al. 1990). At any one time, there were an estimated 1,000,000 individuals with heroin use disorder in the United States. The typical individual in this era was a white, urban, working class male; the largest and most visible segment of the addicted population was localized in New York City.

OPIOID USE DISORDER 1960–1995

Methadone Maintenance Treatment

In the 1960s, Vincent Dole, an internist at The Rockefeller Institute (now The Rockefeller University), was approached by New York law enforcement authorities and was asked to explore a medical approach for managing OUD. In 1965, Dole and his wife, Marie Nyswander, published their landmark paper on the efficacy of methadone maintenance (Dole and Nyswander 1965). In 1972, the FDA issued the initial federal methadone regulations (Department of Health, Education, and Welfare, Food and Drug Administration 1972), which reversed elements of the Harrison Act and legalized methadone maintenance treatment. Although this change reflected the failure of the prohibitionist criminal justice model, the FDA regulations established a heavily regulated methadone clinic system that typically operated outside mainstream medical practice.

Dole and Nyswander (1965) stressed the importance of adequate methadone doses to block the euphoria caused by heroin; the need for long-term, if not indefinite, maintenance treatment; and the importance of counseling and other ancillary psychosocial services. Over the next 30 years, there were rarely more than 100,000 individuals in methadone maintenance treatment at any one time—generally less than 10% of the population in need of treatment. The requirement for daily clinic attendance was a strong barrier to patient acceptance. Despite evidence of efficacy (Ball and Ross 1991), methadone maintenance treatment was never welcomed by the majority of individuals with OUD or by most communities.

Nonpharmacological Treatments

There is little evidence of efficacy for the nonpharmacological treatments available for OUD. Short-term medication withdrawal treatment, even when followed by intensive outpatient counseling, is generally associated with a 95% relapse rate. Although the therapeutic community movement attracted some measure of public support, therapeutic community programs have never been particularly effective in retaining participants. Rarely do more than 10% of voluntarily admitted participants complete treatment. However, among those individuals who complete a 9- to 18-month therapeutic community program, about 80% achieve long-term recovery (Hubbard et al. 1997). Today, most of these programs primarily work with court-referred individuals, although retention in treatment still remains a problem.

Opioid Use Disorder: Long-Term Course

The most comprehensive review of the long-term course of OUD is the work of Hser et al. (2001), who conducted a 33-year follow-up of 581 men with heroin use disorder treated in the California Civil Addict Program from 1962 to 1964 (Figure 1–1). By 1996–1997, at the time of the 33-year follow-up, 284 individuals (48% of the original sample) had died. Among the 242 surviving subjects who were interviewed, 40.5% had used heroin within the past year, 20.7% tested positive for heroin, 9.5% refused to be tested, and 4% were incarcerated. In addition, 22.1% were daily alcohol drinkers, and many others reported other illicit drug use (35.5%, marijuana; 19.4%, cocaine; 10.3%, crack; and 11.6%, amphetamines). Only 22% were abstinent, and another 6% were in methadone maintenance treatment. Overall, this study demonstrated the lethality of OUD in individuals who use intravenous heroin; the relatively low rate of recovery, even with enforced treatment; and the long-term stable pattern of heroin use for the majority of people with OUD. OUD was demonstrated to be a chronic lifetime disorder with severe health and social consequences (Hser et al. 2001). In a comparable 3-year follow-up study of heroin users, the Starting Treatment with Agonist Replacement Therapies (START) study (NIDA CTN-0027), a randomized, open-label, 24-week comparison of methadone and buprenorphine-naloxone, both medications were shown to have comparable efficacy at the 36-month end point (Hser et al. 2016).

HEROIN MISUSE IN THE POST–WORLD WAR II/ VIETNAM ERA

From World War II to the early 1990s, heroin misuse was the predominant opioid problem in the United States. Annual estimates of drug use have been available from the Monitoring the Future survey since 1975 and from the National Survey on Drug Use and Health (NSDUH; formerly called the National Household Survey on Drug Abuse) since the early 1990s, but information on drug use disorders has rarely been collected. Data from the 2006 NSDUH indicate that the annual number of new users of heroin ranged from 28,000 to 80,000 between 1984 and 1994. This increased to an average of 100,000 from 1995 to 2001 but then declined slightly to 91,000 in 2006 (Substance Abuse and Mental Health

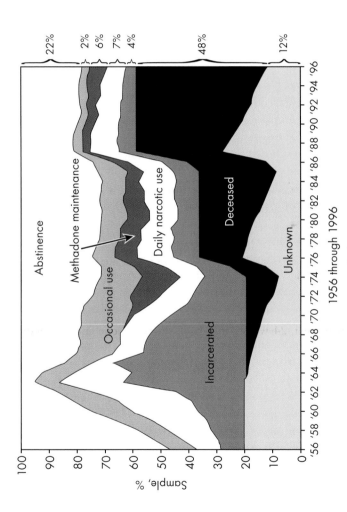

FIGURE 1–1. **The natural history of narcotics addiction among a male sample (*N*=581) [follow-up of the California Civil Addict Program].**

Source. Reprinted from Hser YI, Hoffman V, Grella CE, et al: "A 33-Year Follow-Up of Narcotic Addicts." *Archives of General Psychiatry* 58:503–508, 2001. Copyright ©2001 American Medical Association. All rights reserved.

Services Administration 2007). NSDUH 2006 data estimated that 3.79 million Americans had used heroin at least once in their lifetime; of that group, 323,000, or less than 10%, were classified with OUD (Substance Abuse and Mental Health Services Administration 2007). That number has continued to grow and reached a peak of 591,000 heroin users who met criteria for OUD in 2015 (Lipari et al. 2016; Substance Abuse and Mental Health Services Administration, Center for Behavioral Health Statistics and Quality 2016).

OPIOID USE DISORDER 1995 TO TODAY: CHANGING PATTERNS OF OPIOID MISUSE

Even though the number of individuals who misuse opioids has been growing steadily since 1995, the 2006 NSDUH data were consistent with earlier studies that estimated that 10%–15% of individuals who use licit or illicit opioids are at risk for developing OUD. The risk was presumed to be significantly higher in individuals with co-occurring psychiatric disorders, particularly depressive disorder. Another major national survey on substance use disorders, the 2001–2002 National Epidemiologic Survey on Alcohol and Related Conditions (NESARC), collected specific data on the use and misuse of both illicit drugs and prescribed medications according to DSM IV-TR (American Psychiatric Association 2000) definitions. This was the first national survey that separated data on opioids from data on other drugs of abuse and the first to separate data on heroin from data on the misuse of prescription pain relievers. NESARC data indicated that prevalence rates of 12-month and lifetime drug dependence (severe substance use disorder) were 0.6% and 2.6%, respectively; the corresponding rates for drug abuse were 1.4% and 7.7% (Compton et al. 2007). Higher rates of abuse and dependence were reported in men versus women and in American Indians versus whites. The mean age of onset for opioid dependence or abuse was 22.8 years. Data for the nonmedical use of prescription opioids indicated a 4.7% lifetime prevalence of use, compared with a lifetime prevalence of 1.4% for nonmedical OUD (Huang et al. 2006). These findings suggest that among users of prescription pain relievers there is at least a 30% risk for developing an OUD, which is between two and three times the risk reported for the development of drug use disorders among users of heroin. This rate is higher than the estimates based on the 2006 NSDUH data. This may reflect the greater risk for developing OUD associated with the misuse of high-potency pain relievers, as compared with heroin (see the next section).

More recent data from the NESARC-III (2012–2013) showed that nonmedical opioid drug use continues to increase. Rates for 12-month and lifetime DSM-5 (American Psychiatric Association 2013) nonmedical OUDs were 0.9% and 4.7%, respectively, and 12-month and lifetime nonmedical opioid use were 4.1% and 11.3%, respectively (Saha et al. 2016). A retrospective analysis of long-term opioid use for more than 215,000 Medicare beneficiaries showed marked differences in physician prescribing practices and suggested that the overuse of opioids in this older population may be driven not as much by patient characteristics as by the clinical practice patterns of "high-intensity opioid prescribers" (Barnett et al. 2017).

The New Epidemic of Misuse of Pain Relievers

For most of the twentieth century, the illicit use of pain relievers was assumed to be a relatively small part of the U.S. drug problem. Physicians thought that there was minimal risk for OUD among individuals treated for acute or chronic pain. The introduction of pentazocine (Talwin) in the 1960s was associated with a brief period of misuse after some individuals discovered that they could induce a potent sense of euphoria by injecting a combination of Talwin and amphetamines ("Ts and blues"). This problem was resolved after the FDA ordered a reformulation of the drug as a combination tablet of Talwin and naloxone (Talwin Nx). The misuse of opioid pharmaceuticals remained at a low level until more potent pain medications were introduced to the U.S. market in the 1990s. From 1970 to 1995, the annual number of new nonmedical users of pain relievers was reported to range from 700,000 to 1,000,000 (Substance Abuse and Mental Health Services Administration 2005b).

As the medical community became comfortable with the use of these new opioid pharmaceuticals for the treatment of severe pain, there was interest in the development of more potent medications with low abuse potential and a longer duration of action that would permit patients with pain to sleep through the night. Although oxycodone showed promise because of its potency, the sustained-release technology that had been successful in the development of a long-acting formulation of morphine, morphine sulfate (MS Contin), could not be successfully adapted for oxycodone. In 1996, Purdue Pharma resolved this problem with the introduction of OxyContin, an acrylic-coated formulation of oxycodone that dissolved slowly and provided 12 hours of pain relief. Doses ranging from 10 mg to 160 mg could be delivered with this formulation, far exceeding the 30-mg maximum dose of oxycodone tablets. Neither the FDA nor Purdue anticipated a significant misuse problem with such a slow-release formulation, and Purdue was permitted to market OxyContin as a first-line medication for the treatment of nonmalignant pain with less misuse potential than other comparable pain relievers. The drug proved highly successful and rapidly gained a significant share of the U.S. market for pain medications (Meier 2003).

Within 2–3 years of the introduction of OxyContin, physicians in rural Maine and Virginia reported that young adults were crushing the tablets and injecting or snorting the drug. With these methods of ingestion, users were exposed to very high doses of oxycodone. The experience was extremely euphoric and reinforcing, and many of the users rapidly developed an OUD. Correspondingly, the number of opioid overdose deaths reported nationally began to increase dramatically. It gradually became apparent that the reports of OUD and the growing number of overdose deaths did not involve just individuals using the drug illicitly. Physicians began to report that patients being treated for legitimate pain problems were developing an OUD related to OxyContin and that some of them were finding it impossible to stop using the drug (Meier 2003). Over the next few years, NSDUH data showed a dramatic increase in the number of nonmedical users of opioid pharmaceuticals. Physicians eventually realized that very little data existed to support the notion that there is a minimal risk for iatrogenic OUD when opioids are used to treat chronic pain. Most of the published reports describing a low risk for iatrogenic OUD dealt only with the treatment of acute pain. There was no credible published research on the risks for OUD associated with newer, long-acting, and high-potency drugs such as OxyContin when prescribed for either acute or chronic pain.

Rapid Growth of Misuse of Pain Relievers

By 2000, the number of new individuals who were misusing pain relievers tripled to 2,500,000 (Figure 1–2) (Substance Abuse and Mental Health Services Administration 2003). This change corresponded with the introduction of OxyContin to the U.S. market, and it also reflected the widespread misuse of such drugs as hydrocodone-acetaminophen (Vicodin) and oxycodone-acetaminophen (Percocet). During this same period, there was a growing emphasis in medical practice in the United States on the provision of more complete control of pain and more generous prescribing of opioids. These events marked a significant shift from the misuse of heroin to the misuse of opioid pharmaceuticals as the dominant opioid misuse problem in the United States. In 2007, 5.2 million Americans—2.1% of individuals age 12 years and older—reported using prescription pain relievers nonmedically in the previous month. Of note is the decline in new initiates of OxyContin abuse from 615,000 in 2004 to 478,000 in 2008 (Substance Abuse and Mental Health Services Administration 2009). The mean age for first use among new initiates to the abuse of pain relievers in 2007 was 21.2 years (Substance Abuse and Mental Health Services Administration 2008). This new group of drug abusers tended to be younger, better educated, and less antisocial than the typical heroin addict (Table 1–1). They initially used the drug orally or snorted it and were much less likely to use drugs intravenously. They were also more likely to have psychiatric problems such as depression or anxiety.

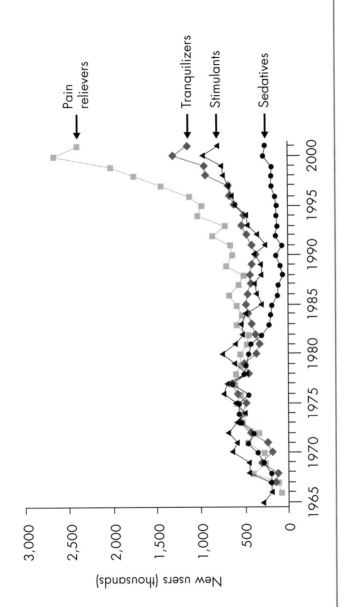

FIGURE 1–2.   **Annual numbers of new nonmedical users of psychotherapeutics: 1965–2001.**

Source.   Substance Abuse and Mental Health Services Administration 2003.

TABLE 1–1.   **Comparison of heroin users with abusers of pain relievers**

Characteristics	Pre-1995	Post-1995
Drug of choice	Heroin	Prescription pain relievers
Age	Older	Younger
Drug source	Dealer	Free from friends
Use pattern	Intravenous	Oral/snorting
Medical problems	Hepatitis C; HIV infection	None or pain issues
Legal problems	Common	Rare
Education	High school dropouts	Some college

The NSDUH 2015 survey reported that 2,038,000 individuals age 12 years and older met criteria for "pain reliever use disorder" in the past year, up from 1.7 million in 2008 and 1.9 million in 2014 (Hughes et al. 2016; Substance Abuse and Mental Health Services Administration 2009). Despite the growing number of individuals with OUD, fewer than one-third of individuals in this group have ever received treatment. NESARC wave I data showed a lag of 3.4 years between the mean age of onset of an OUD (22.8 years) and the mean age of first treatment (26.2 years) (Compton et al. 2007). More recent NESARC wave II (2004–2005) data showed that the lifetime probability of treatment seeking was 42%, and there was a mean lag of 3.83 years between onset and first treatment for prescription OUD (Blanco et al. 2013).

Reduced Opioid Misuse Among Younger Individuals: Possible Response to Control Efforts

There was some suggestion in the 2015 NSDUH data that the number of users of pain relievers and heroin had stabilized or begun to drop. This may be related to the introduction of abuse-deterrent formulations of some pain relievers and greater awareness among the public and physicians about the risk of opioid pain relievers. The 2015 NSDUH questionnaire was redesigned to improve data quality, but the change made direct comparison with earlier data difficult. The most recent data from the NSDUH show that in 2015, the nonmedical prescription opioid misuse for individuals older than 12 years were 3,775,000 for past month use and 12,462,000 for the past year. OxyContin misuse in the past year was found to be 1,748,000 (Substance Abuse and Mental Health Services Administration, Center for Behavioral Health Statistics and Quality 2016, Tables 1.1A and 1.139A). Heroin use in the past year was 828,000, and heroin use in the past month for individuals 12 years and older dropped from 0.2% of the population in 2014 to 0.1% of the population in 2015 (Substance Abuse and Mental Health Services Administration, Center for Behavioral Health Statistics and Quality 2016, Figures 8 and 9).

New Drugs, New Users, and New Supply Patterns

More than 53.7% of people age 12 years and older who abuse pain relievers are given their drugs for free or buy or take them from friends or relatives (40.5% get them for free and another 9.4% buy them), whereas 4.9% purchase their drugs from a dealer or stranger (Figure 1–3) (Hughes et al. 2016). Another 34% report they get the drug from just one physician. Although many in this group are able to control their use and remain occasional social users, a significant number become dependent. It has been estimated that 10%–30% of individuals exposed to licit and illicit opioids may develop symptoms of an OUD. Rates may be significantly higher in individuals with a family history of drug or alcohol use disorders or in individuals with co-occurring psychiatric disorders, particularly individuals with attention-deficit/hyperactivity disorder or those exposed to combat trauma or sexual abuse.

As users' habits progress, they start purchasing drugs from illicit sources and often switch to heroin once they recognize that it is less expensive than pain relievers. At this point, some, but not all, users also switch from snorting to injecting heroin or other opioids. This transition is often associated with a rapid deterioration in social functioning and an increase in antisocial behavior. Data from the 2015 NSDUH showed that 20,810,000 individuals older than 12 years (7.8% of the population) met criteria for a substance use disorder (SUD) in the past year (Substance Abuse and Mental Health Services Administration, Center for Behavioral Health Statistics and Quality 2016, Table 5.4A). There has been an increase in the number of individuals misusing pain relievers, which now rank second to marijuana among significant illicit drugs of misuse in the United States (see Figure 1–4). The current prevalence of nonmedical OUDs is almost three times the level of prior estimates of heroin use disorders. In 2015, the incidence of past year OUD for pain relievers in persons 12 years and older was 2,038,000, and the incidence of OUD for heroin was 591,000 (Substance Abuse and Mental Health Services Administration, Center for Behavioral Health Statistics and Quality 2016, Table 5.2A). These data from the 2015 NSDUH suggest that misuse of both prescription pain relievers and heroin has begun to drop, but it is premature to conclude that this change is permanent.

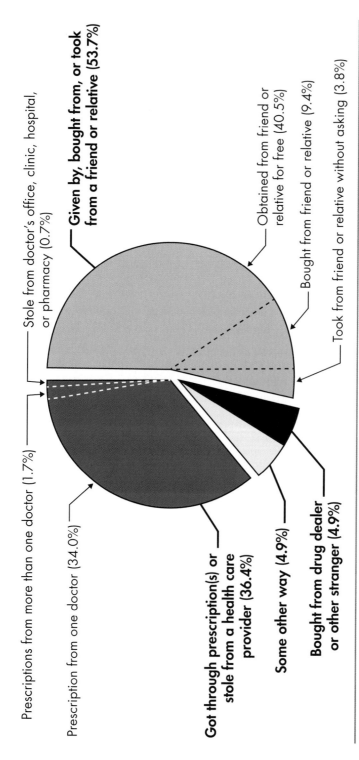

FIGURE 1–3.   **Source where pain relievers were obtained for most recent misuse among people age 12 years and older who misused prescription pain relievers (total 12.5 million) in the past year (2015).**

Source.   Hughes et al. 2016, Figure 24.

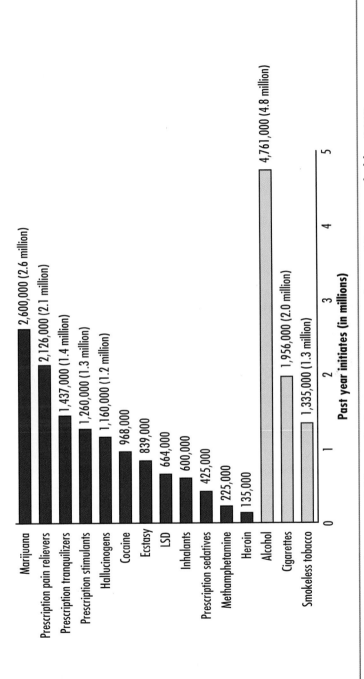

FIGURE 1–4. **Numbers of past year initiates of substances among people ages 12 years and older, 2015.**

LSD=lysergic acid diethylamide.

Source. Lipari et al. 2016, Figure 10.

Unfortunately, there has been no drop in the number of individuals who meet criteria for OUD or in the number of treatment admissions or opioid-related overdose deaths. Instead, the number of opioid-related overdose deaths has been rising steadily since 2000. Deaths involving fentanyl more than doubled from 2012 through 2014. It is estimated that fentanyl was involved in 41% of heroin-related deaths during this period (see Figure 1–5) (Frank and Pollack 2017; Gladden et al. 2016). It is clear that OUD remains a major public health threat.

NSDUH data estimated that 23.2 million persons ages 12 years and older needed treatment for an illicit drug or alcohol problem in 2007, of whom only 2.4 million received treatment at a specialty substance abuse treatment facility (Substance Abuse and Mental Health Services Administration 2008). Data from the Substance Abuse and Mental Health Services Administration (SAMHSA) Treatment Episode Data Set showed a steady increase in the number of individuals seeking treatment for OUD from 2007 through 2013 (see Figure 1–6). By 2014, the number of admissions reached almost 500,000 per year: the number related to the misuse of prescription pain relievers dropped to 132,000, but the number related to heroin increased to more than 357,000 (Substance Abuse and Mental Health Services Administration, Center for Behavioral Health Statistics and Quality 2016). Admissions for alcohol, cocaine, and marijuana dropped during this same period.

The Buprenorphine Story

BUPRENORPHINE AND THE RETURN TO OFFICE-BASED TREATMENT

Concerns about the legal and clinical constraints mandated for methadone maintenance treatment and its relatively low level of appeal to most individuals with OUDs led to a search for safer yet effective alternative treatments. This led to research on the effectiveness of sublingual buprenorphine and extended-release intramuscular naltrexone (XR-NTX) for the treatment of OUD. The problem became even more acute in the mid-1990s when the rapid increase in the number of individuals misusing opioid pharmaceuticals far outstripped the capacity of the SUD treatment system. Buprenorphine was identified as a target medication for treating OUD after early studies suggested clinical efficacy, a strong safety profile, and less misuse potential than methadone (see Chapter 3, "Efficacy and Safety of Buprenorphine"). Its very favorable safety profile suggested that buprenorphine could be prescribed safely in office-based clinical settings, thus avoiding the legal constraints of the methadone clinic system that were felt to discourage patients from participating in treatment. Indeed, individuals with heroin use disorder typically delay participation in methadone main-

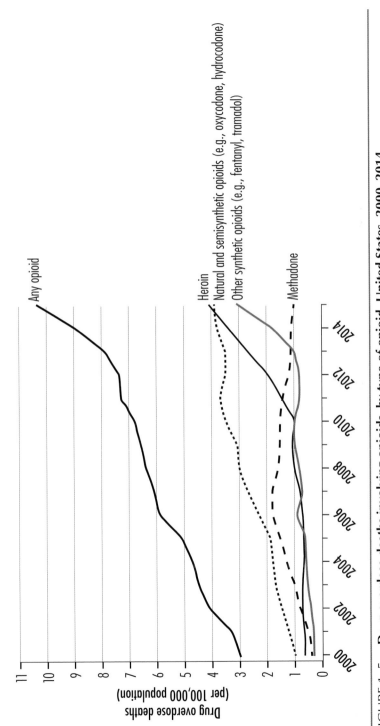

FIGURE 1–5. **Drug overdose deaths involving opioids, by type of opioid, United States, 2000–2014.**

Source. Data from Frank and Pollack 2017; Rudd et al. 2016.

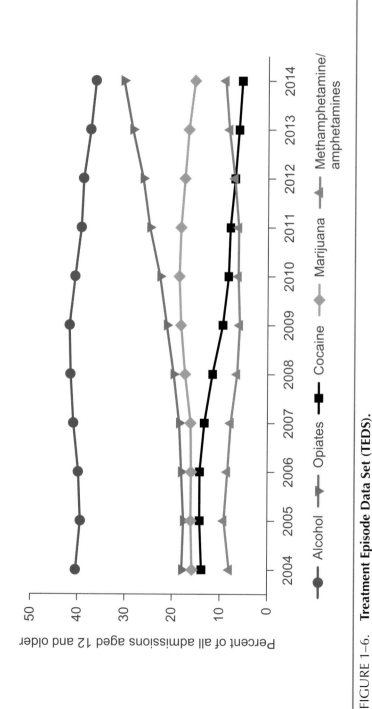

FIGURE 1–6.   **Treatment Episode Data Set (TEDS).**

Source.   Substance Abuse and Mental Health Services Administration, Center for Behavioral Health Statistics and Quality: Treatment Episode Data Set (TEDS): 2004–2015. National Admissions to Substance Abuse Treatment Services. BHSIS Series S-84, HHS Publication No. (SMA) 16-4986. Rockville, MD, Substance Abuse and Mental Health Services Administration, 2016.

tenance treatment for 4–5 years beyond the point when treatment is warranted. This delay translates into more severe social, behavioral, and medical deterioration, thus guaranteeing a more treatment-resistant and complicated condition.

Before 2002, only methadone and levo-α-acetylmethadol (LAAM) were approved as opioid agonist treatments, and both medications could be dispensed only in heavily regulated opioid treatment programs (OTPs). When buprenorphine was approved by the FDA in 2002 for the treatment of OUD in office-based settings, it was estimated that fewer than 1 in 10 individuals with heroin use disorder were receiving any type of effective treatment. Medication withdrawal treatment was still the most common form of treatment provided, despite little evidence of efficacy. Because of buprenorphine's wider availability in less stigmatized office-based settings, it was hoped that this new treatment option would both fill the gap in treatment resources and lead to earlier participation in treatment. The primary goal was to expand treatment options by returning OUD treatment to mainstream medical practice and to train a much larger group of physicians to care for these patients effectively. It was hoped that better-educated physicians would encourage patients to shift to more effective long-term treatment models and avoid repeated episodes of short-term medication withdrawal treatment. (For a more detailed discussion of the role of XR-NTX in the treatment of OUD, see Chapter 9, "Methadone, Naltrexone, and Naloxone.")

Drug Addiction Treatment Act of 2000

Implementing the change to office-based treatment required an amendment to the federal Controlled Substances Act, the Drug Addiction Treatment Act of 2000 (DATA 2000). This law authorized practitioners to prescribe FDA-approved narcotic drugs in Schedules III, IV, and V, or combinations of such drugs, for "maintenance or detoxification treatment of opioid dependence." The law placed no limit on the quantities of drugs that could be prescribed for unsupervised use unless the drugs have been subject to an adverse determination. In essence, this meant that clinicians could prescribe up to a month's supply of medication, with refills, as deemed appropriate. DATA 2000 specified that the drugs used and the prescribing physicians (practitioners) must meet certain requirements. Practitioners had to be deemed "qualifying physicians," which was defined as having the capacity to refer patients for appropriate counseling and ancillary services. There was no legal requirement that the clinician personally provide drug counseling or other ancillary services. The intent of the law was to require that the physician provide the more traditional and relatively limited medical role of monitoring medication use. It was hoped that this would encourage physicians who were not specialists in addiction psychiatry or addiction medicine to expand their practice to include the management of opioid agonist treatment.

Qualifying Physicians and Providers

Qualifying physicians were initially limited to no more than 30 buprenorphine patients at one time for an individual practice or a group practice; only patients with an active prescription were counted toward the 30-patient limit. The 30-patient limit was intended to avoid the development of large buprenorphine practices, similar to the "methadone mills" seen in the 1970s, and to thus ensure more individualized and appropriate care for all patients. It was quickly realized that limiting group practices (which in many cases meant very large health care systems) to 30 patients was unrealistic and defeated the purpose of expanding access to OUD treatment. In 2006, DATA 2000 was amended to eliminate the 30-patient limit for group practices and to permit individual physicians to request approval to expand their practice to 100 patients after 1 year of experience prescribing buprenorphine. In 2016, the U.S. Department of Health and Human Services (DHHS) issued regulations permitting certain waivered physicians to request authorization to treat up to 275 patients, and the U.S. Congress passed the Comprehensive Addiction and Recovery Act, permitting nurse practitioners and physician assistants to apply for a waiver to prescribe buprenorphine to treat OUD (see below).

DATA 2000 defined seven possible routes through which a licensed physician could be recognized as qualifying under the requirements of the legislation:

1. Being board-certified in addiction psychiatry by the American Board of Psychiatry and Neurology
2. Being certified in addiction medicine by the American Society of Addiction Medicine (now the American Board of Addiction Medicine)
3. Being certified in addiction medicine by the American Osteopathic Association
4. Having experience as an investigator in buprenorphine clinical trials
5. Completing 8 hours of training provided by the American Psychiatric Association, American Academy of Addiction Psychiatry, American Society of Addiction Medicine, American Medical Association, American Osteopathic Association, or other organizations that may be designated by the secretary of DHHS
6. Having training or experience as determined by a state medical licensing board
7. Fulfilling other criteria as established by the secretary of DHHS

Resident physicians are eligible to obtain the waiver as long as the resident is able to obtain his or her own federal U.S. Drug Enforcement Administration (DEA) license.

Required Buprenorphine Provider Training

The required 8 hours of training are offered either in person, online, or "half and half" (i.e., 4 hours of online training and 4 hours of in-person training). In

2017, DHHS/SAMHSA added the American Nurses Credentialing Center, the American Association of Nurse Practitioners, and the American Academy of Physicians Assistants to the group of organizations authorized under DATA 2000 to provide the training required to qualify for the waiver to prescribe buprenorphine. The American Medical Association has chosen not to offer buprenorphine addiction treatment training courses. No state medical licensing board has designated other specific training or experience as required for prescribing buprenorphine.

To obtain the waiver necessary to prescribe buprenorphine, a practitioner must notify the secretary of DHHS online at http://www.samhsa.gov/medication-assisted-treatment/buprenorphine-waiver-management/apply-for-physician-waiver and complete the buprenorphine waiver notification, giving his or her name and DEA registration number, identifying the category under which he or she meets the criteria to become a qualifying practitioner (of the seven listed above), and certifying that he or she will comply with the requirements of the law. DHHS has 45 days to review the practitioner's application to determine whether the practitioner meets the requirements of DATA 2000. With the current online system, DHHS has been responding to most applicants within 2–3 weeks. Once a positive determination is made, DHHS notifies the DEA, which then assigns a new DEA identification number to the practitioner. This number comprises the practitioner's original DEA number but with the first letter substituted by an X. The DEA is also required to issue this X number if DHHS has not completed its review within the 45-day period.

Once the practitioner has received his or her X number, the practitioner may begin to prescribe buprenorphine for the treatment of OUD. Whenever practitioners write a prescription under the requirements of DATA 2000, they must list both their primary DEA number and their X number on the prescription. Should a practitioner decide to prescribe sublingual buprenorphine for an unapproved indication—for a condition other than OUD, such as for pain—he or she should *not* use the X number. Despite the fact that the X number is to be used only when prescribing buprenorphine for the treatment of opioid dependence, it is important that practitioners recognize that any violation of federal or state prescribing regulations or narcotics laws puts both their X number *and* their primary DEA number at risk. The most common circumstance that has led to revocation of DEA registration is violation of the 30/100/275 patient limit.

Buprenorphine Treatment Locator

The buprenorphine waiver notification also asks whether the applicant wants to be listed as a provider of buprenorphine treatment on the buprenorphine treatment physician locator page of SAMHSA's Web site (http://www.samhsa.gov/medication-assisted-treatment/physician-program-data/treatment-physician-locator). If the applicant indicates his or her willingness to be listed, his or her name, address, and telephone number are posted on the Web site. Because prospective patients use this information to contact providers, it is important that office contact information and not home numbers be provided. Practitioners can choose to be listed on the physician locator page at any time and also can request that their information be removed at any time.

FDA Approval of Buprenorphine

The second principal element of DATA 2000 is the specification that the authorization to treat OUD in an office-based setting applies only to narcotic drugs that have been approved by the FDA for the "maintenance or detoxification treatment" of OUD. The law applies to drugs, or combinations of drugs, in Schedules III, IV, or V. Sublingual buprenorphine; the combination sublingual formulation of buprenorphine-naloxone; and Probuphine, a subdermal buprenorphine implant (approved by the FDA on May 26, 2016) are the only drugs currently approved by the FDA for this purpose under DATA 2000. When the FDA initially approved the two sublingual formulations of buprenorphine, all of the available formulations of buprenorphine were rescheduled to Schedule III. Previously, the only FDA-approved formulations of buprenorphine were the intramuscular and intravenous formulations, marketed as Buprenex. In July 2010, the FDA also approved a new extended-release transdermal buprenorphine patch, Butrans, for the treatment of severe pain. Buprenex and Butrans are approved only for the treatment of pain. Before the approval of sublingual buprenorphine, many hospitals had been using Buprenex outside of its approved labeling, for the medication withdrawal treatment of OUD. It is important to understand that the DEA considers such off-label use of Buprenex or Butrans to be illegal and that practitioners risk sanctions if they continue this practice.

Exemptions to Buprenorphine Waiver Regulations

There are two circumstances in which nonwaivered clinicians can dispense (not prescribe) a narcotic drug, either methadone or buprenorphine, for the treatment of an OUD. If an individual with an OUD is admitted for inpatient treatment of a medical or psychiatric condition other than OUD (in situations in which OUD is the secondary, not the primary, admitting diagnosis), then federal regulations permit a narcotic drug to be dispensed without a buprenorphine waiver or registration as a narcotic treatment program for either maintenance or withdrawal treatment as long as required to stabilize the patient during hospitalization (U.S. Department of Justice, Drug Enforcement Administration 2005). Prescriptions cannot be provided at discharge, and the patient must be referred to a methadone program or a waivered clinician. If the primary admitting diagnosis is OUD, then a narcotic drug cannot be dispensed unless the clinician has a waiver or the program is separately registered with the DEA as a narcotics treatment program.

These regulations also include an exception to the narcotic dispensing regulations known as the "3-day rule." This permits any DEA-registered practitioner to administer or dispense (but not prescribe) narcotic drugs to a patient for the purpose of relieving acute withdrawal symptoms while arranging for the patient's referral for treatment under the following conditions: 1) not more than 1 day's medication may be administered or given to the patient at one time, 2) the treatment may not be carried out for more than 72 hours, and 3) the 72-hour treatment cannot be renewed or extended. The intent of this regulation is to give the clinician flexibility in emergency situations while he or she arranges for maintenance or withdrawal treatment. In this circumstance, the law provides for the *dispensing* of single doses, not a prescription. The buprenorphine waiver under DATA 2000 applies only to *outpatient* settings where the waivered clinician provides a *prescription* to a patient to treat an OUD. XR-NTX is approved by the FDA for the treatment of OUD, but it is not classified as a controlled substance and is not covered under the provisions of DATA 2000.

Providing Buprenorphine in an Opioid Treatment Program

DATA 2000 also permits the dispensing of sublingual buprenorphine in OTPs that are registered as a methadone program. There is no limit on the number of buprenorphine patients who can be treated in the OTP setting. In 2009, the secretary of DHHS instituted a modification of OTP regulations to remove the restrictions on take-home use for buprenorphine dispensed in the OTP setting (Health and Human Services Department 2009), permitting the same flexibility in medication treatment available in the office-based practice setting. Although this change has expanded the use of buprenorphine in OTPs, there are still relatively few buprenorphine patients treated in this setting. In addition to providing closer supervision and monitoring than office-based treatment, the OTP setting also has the advantage of providing a higher level of onsite ancillary services. OTPs are a more appropriate setting for the treatment of complicated patients who require close monitoring and high levels of counseling and other services. OTPs are particularly appropriate for patients at high risk for diversion or for unstable individuals who are not at the stage where they can successfully comply with the requirements of office-based treatment.

Clinical Resources

SAMHSA was mandated by DATA 2000 to publish a treatment improvement protocol (TIP) that provides clinical guidance for the use of buprenorphine. This protocol, TIP 40, "Clinical Guidelines for the Use of Buprenorphine in the Treatment of Opioid Addiction," was published in 2004. The TIP series has been an invaluable resource for clinicians treating patients with alcohol- and drug-related problems. Of particular interest are TIP 42, "Substance Abuse Treatment for Persons With Co-occurring Disorders," and TIP 43, "Medication-Assisted Treatment for Opioid Addiction in Opioid Treatment Programs." All of the TIPs are available free of charge at SAMHSA's Web site, https://store.samhsa.gov/list/series?name=TIP-Series-Treatment-Improvement-Protocols-TIPS. TIPs 40 and 43 are currently under revision, and updated versions are scheduled for publication in 2017. Other useful sources of information and support are the Federation of State Medical Boards Web site (www.fsmb.org/policy/advocacy-policy/policy-documents) and the National Alliance of Advocates for Buprenorphine Treatment (www.naabt.org).

Two other particularly useful free resources are the Providers' Clinical Support System for Medication Assisted Treatment (PCSS-MAT; www.pcssmat.org) and the Providers' Clinical Support System for Opioid Therapies (PCSS-O; www.pcss-o.org). Both PCSS-MAT and PCSS-O are administered by the American Academy of Addiction Psychiatry under a contract from SAMHSA's Center for Substance Abuse Treatment and in cooperation with other DATA 2000–approved training organizations (the American Psychiatric Association, American Society of Addiction Medicine, and American Osteopathic Association). Any clinician with the buprenorphine waiver is eligible to join PCSS-MAT. He or she is then assigned to a buprenorphine expert clinician in the clinician's area, who acts as an ongoing mentor and supervisor. Mentors are readily available by telephone and e-mail and also are willing to have their mentees visit their offices for direct observation of patient care. A variety of other training opportunities are provided to augment the 8-hour waiver course. All services are provided without charge. The PCSS-O is a partnership of the DATA 2000 organizations and a wide group of medical and nursing subspecialty organizations that provides free training resources that focus on the appropriate use of opioids in the treatment of chronic pain and the assessment and treatment of OUD. Both PCSS-MAT and PCSS-O have proved to be particularly valuable resources for clinicians with little prior experience treating OUD and patients with chronic pain.

Evaluation of DATA 2000

DATA 2000 required an evaluation of the results of this legislation during the first 3 years following FDA approval of buprenorphine. DHHS was mandated to assess the clinical efficacy of the drug, including whether the treatment was effective in the office setting, whether access to treatment improved, and whether there were any adverse consequences for the public health. The DEA was mandated to evaluate safety issues, including the extent of violations of the 30-patient limit, clinician record-keeping and security measures related to on-site drug storage, data related to emergency department drug mentions, and the risks of overdose (Substance Abuse and Mental Health Services Administration 2006b). In compliance with this mandate, the DEA inspected two buprenorphine practitioners in each DEA district every 18 months. On the basis of these evaluations, DHHS and the DEA could decide whether the provisions of DATA 2000 should remain in effect. The law would cease to be in effect 60 days after an adverse evaluation was published; thus, additional legislative action was not required to repeal the law. Should difficulties such as significant misuse or drug diversion become a major problem, it would be relatively easy for these government agencies to terminate office-based treatment for OUD with buprenorphine.

In March 2006, the secretary of DHHS issued a formal determinations report on the evaluation of DATA 2000 that indicated that the buprenorphine waiver program had expanded access to treatment and had produced effective treatment outcomes without producing negative public health issues (Substance Abuse and Mental Health Services Administration 2006a). As of May 2010, it was estimated that 1–2 million patients in the United States had been treated with buprenorphine. Regarding accessibility of treatment, DHHS determined that 31% of patients taking buprenorphine were new to any type of substance abuse treatment, and 60% were new to medication-assisted treatment. Only 9% were transferred from methadone to buprenorphine treatment.

Of equal importance was the finding that 60% of buprenorphine patients had been treated for OUD related to non-heroin opioids, a population that has historically avoided participation in methadone treatment (Substance Abuse and Mental Health Services Administration 2005a). Indeed, patients treated under the buprenorphine waiver have much more accurately reflected the population of illicit drug users in the community, as compared with patients in methadone treatment. In community samples of individuals misusing opioids, only 4% of the population were using heroin, whereas 96% were misusing non-heroin opioids. Patients entering methadone treatment for OUD were primarily using heroin (83% vs. 17% who used non-heroin opioids or the combination of heroin and non-heroin opioids), whereas those who entered buprenorphine treatment had higher rates of OUD with non-heroin opioids (40%; Substance Abuse and Mental Health Services Administration 2005a).

There also were significant demographic differences between methadone and buprenorphine patients. Buprenorphine treatment populations had higher percentages of women than did methadone treatment populations as well as higher percentages of whites and employed individuals and more than three times as many individuals with some postsecondary education (Figure 1–7) (Stanton et al. 2006; Substance Abuse and Mental Health Services Administration 2005a). A retrospective review of long-term retention in office-based buprenorphine treatment reviewed data on 1,237 patients treated in a large urban safety-net primary care practice. A majority of patients (53.7%) had at least one ≥1-year period in treatment. Better retention was associated with female

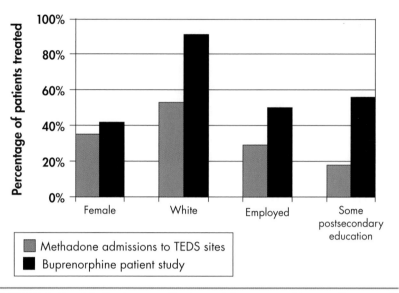

FIGURE 1–7. **Methadone patients and buprenorphine patient study sample: demographic differences.**
The Treatment Episode Data Set (TEDS) reports primarily on admissions to facilities receiving public funding. Admissions to private facilities are underrepresented.
Source. Substance Abuse and Mental Health Services Administration 2005a.

gender, older age, or having a psychiatric diagnosis; lower retention rates were associated with unemployment, being black or Hispanic, or having a diagnosis of hepatitis C (Weinstein et al. 2017). In another review of treatment retention, data on 3,151 patients admitted to buprenorphine treatment within the Veterans Health Administration in fiscal year 2012 were analyzed. There was a mean duration of treatment of 1.68 years, with 61.6% retained for more than a year and 31.83% retained for more than 3 years. Black race and emergency room visits were correlated with treatment discontinuation (Manhapra et al. 2017).

TRENDS IN BUPRENORPHINE USE SINCE 2003

After the original approval of buprenorphine for the treatment of OUD in 2002, there was an initial spurt of buprenorphine use; another spurt occurred in 2008 after the increase in the waiver number to 100. Initially, psychiatrists accounted for the majority of treatment visits; by 2013, psychiatrists accounted for 32.8% of visits, internists accounted for 32.2%, osteopaths accounted for 13.9%, and family physicians accounted for 14.2% (Turner et al. 2015). In 2016, more than 2,000 waivered physicians applied for the increase in the prescribing limit to 275. It is not yet clear how this regulatory change will impact the number of patients in treatment. Buprenorphine has been increasingly used in outpatient treatment centers, with the number of outpatient visits increasing about fifteenfold from 0.16 to 2.1 million visits; visits quadrupled from 2005 to 2013 (Figure 1–8). Data on patients using buprenorphine for pain management or other nonopioid dependence diagnosis were excluded. Data were derived from the IMS Health National Disease and Therapeutic Index (NDTI) from 2003 through 2013.

Comprehensive Addiction and Recovery Act

LEGISLATIVE AND REGULATORY CHANGES AS OF 2016

The number of individuals in medication-assisted treatment for OUD has more than quadrupled since the introduction of sublingual buprenorphine in 2002. Despite this success, the number of individuals with OUD and the number of opioid-related overdoses have grown at alarming rates. Efforts to educate physicians and the public about the dangers of opioid pain relievers and the introduction of abuse-deterrent formulations began to show some effect in 2014 and 2015 with a drop in the number of individuals misusing these drugs (Guy et al. 2017). A comparable drop in the use of heroin was also noted (Center for Behavioral Health Statistics and Quality 2016). However, the number of individuals seeking treatment for OUD has continued to rise. This suggests a drop in new initiates to misuse and in the incidence of more casual misuse, while individuals with OUD have been unable to stop using and continue to swell the numbers seeking admission to treatment (see Figure 1–6). One disappointing aspect of the development of office-based buprenorphine treatment has been the relatively low number of physicians who have obtained the waiver (mainly addiction medicine and addiction psychiatry specialists) and the relatively low number of patients treated by each practitioner (typically five or fewer) (Neilson 2014). Less than 30% of the providers trained under DATA 2000 have gone on to prescribe buprenorphine, and less than 60% of the buprenorphine treatment capacity is utilized (Arfken et al. 2010; Hutchinson et al. 2014; Kunins et al. 2013).

EXPANDING PROVIDERS AND PRACTICE LIMITS

In 2016, concerns about the increasing number of people seeking treatment for OUD led to proposals to increase the number of patients treated under the buprenorphine waiver and to authorize prescribing by nurse practitioners and physician assistants. In response, Congress passed by overwhelming majorities the Comprehensive Addiction and Recovery Act of 2016 (CARA), which stressed

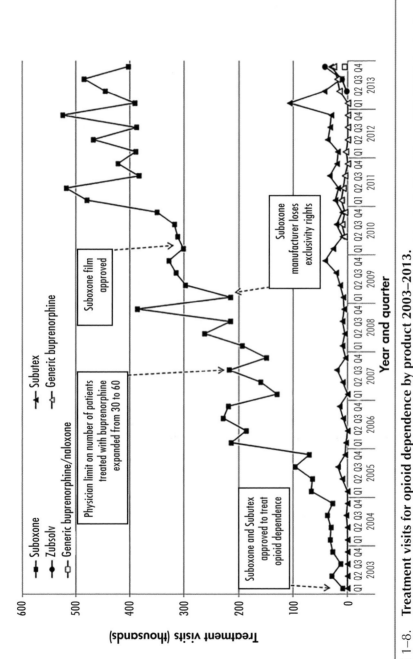

FIGURE 1–8.   **Treatment visits for opioid dependence by product 2003–2013.**

Source. Turner L, Kruszewski SP, Alexander G: "Trends in the use of buprenorphine by office-based physicians in the United States, 2003–2013." *American Journal on Addictions* 24(1):24–29, 2015. Used with permission.

the importance of evidence-based treatment interventions for OUD (mainly medication-assisted treatment), access to behavioral health services, individualized treatment plans, diversion control plans, and use of prescription drug monitoring programs. CARA added nurse practitioners and physician assistants to the group of practitioners eligible to apply for the buprenorphine waiver and specified the requirement of 24 hours' training in addiction treatment for these new groups. The training covers the following topics: opioid maintenance and medically supervised withdrawal, clinical use of all FDA-approved drugs for medication-assisted treatment, patient assessment, treatment planning, psychosocial services, staff roles, and diversion control. Nurse practitioners and physician assistants can fulfill 8 of the 24 required hours by completing the same buprenorphine-naloxone (BUP/NX) waiver course that is completed by physicians. The remaining 16 hours of training are completed through other options, such as online courses available from PCSS-MAT or other SAMHSA-approved organizations. Beginning in 2017, nurse practitioners and physician assistants who have completed the required training can apply to prescribe BUP/NX for up to 30 patients. If required by state law, approved nurse practitioners and physician assistants must be supervised by or work in collaboration with a qualifying physician (http://www.asam.org/quality-practice/practice-resources/nurse-practitioners-and-physician-assistants-prescribing-buprenorphine).

Earlier in 2016, the White House Office of National Drug Control Policy issued a statement identifying medication-assisted treatment as the recommended first-line treatment for OUD, and SAMHSA specifically required that all criminal justice programs that received federal funding ensure that clients have access to it (Knopf 2015). Shortly after this announcement, DHHS issued new regulations permitting clinicians holding the buprenorphine waiver to treat 100 patients to apply to increase their practice limit to 275 patients. Clinicians are required to have been at the 100-patient limit for 1 year and to be board certified in either addiction medicine or addiction psychiatry or to practice in a "qualified practice setting." A qualified practice setting is defined as a practice that provides 24-hour emergency coverage and case management and related services; uses health information technology; is registered with the State Prescription Monitoring Program; accepts third-party payment for some services; and uses established practice guidelines for the management of OUD (Department of Health and Human Services 2016). This was a clear action on the part of DHHS to expand buprenorphine treatment services, to ensure high-quality services, and to discourage the development of buprenorphine pill mills. These actions by the Office of National Drug Control Policy, DHHS, and Congress have reinforced the position of medication-assisted treatment as the primary evidence-based treatment for OUD. By early 2017, more than 25,000 providers had the waiver to prescribe for up to 30 patients, more than 9,000 had the waiver for up to 100 patients, and more than 3,000 had the waiver for up to 275 patients (Substance Abuse and Mental Health Services Administration 2017).

Conclusion

OUD has been a long-standing problem in the United States. Although medical management of OUD was common practice in the nineteenth century, it was made illegal under the Harrison Narcotics Tax Act in 1914, and most contemporary physicians have no experience treating these patients. Heroin misuse remained endemic throughout the twentieth century despite ongoing efforts to eliminate supplies and incarcerate users. A new epidemic of misuse of pain relievers began in the mid-1990s, and opioid pharmaceuticals quickly replaced heroin as the dominant opioid problem among young adults, almost surpassing the prevalence of marijuana abuse in this population. As compared with heroin misuse, the misuse of these more potent opioid pharmaceuticals is associated with a higher risk of OUD, even among legitimate pain treatment patients, and a more rapid progression of the addiction syndrome. This new population with OUD is younger, better educated, and less antisocial than typical individuals with heroin use disorder, although there is a high incidence of co-occurring depressive and anxiety disorders.

The legalization of methadone maintenance treatment in 1972 represented a return to a medical management model, but few individuals with OUD were willing to attend heavily regulated methadone clinics, and this approach had minimal impact on the incidence of heroin misuse. The limitations of the methadone clinic system led authorities to consider other medications that might be safely used in more general medical practice settings.

Buprenorphine, a partial opioid agonist, was identified as both an effective and a safe medication for use in office-based settings. With the approval of sublingual buprenorphine in 2002, there has been a significant increase in available treatment options. By 2016, it was estimated that 450,000 individuals were currently in buprenorphine treatment, compared with an estimated 300,000 individuals in methadone treatment. Although the misuse of both heroin and opioid pharmaceuticals continues to be a major problem, office-based buprenorphine treatment has been proven to be an effective public health approach to containing the epidemic (Sullivan et al. 2005). Although recent drops in the nonmedical use of prescription pain relievers among young people ages 12 years and older is promising, it is premature to assume that buprenorphine treatment has effectively curbed the OUD problem in the United States. It is clear, however, that large numbers of individuals have found life-saving treatment and have been able to become functioning and contributing members of society. For the first time, an effective medical treatment has had a significant impact on this chronic public health problem.

References

Allbutt TC: On the abuse of hypodermic injections of morphia. Practitioner 5:327–331, 1870

American Psychiatric Association: Diagnostic and Statistical Manual of Mental Disorders, 4th Edition, Text Revision. Arlington, VA, American Psychiatric Association, 2000

American Psychiatric Association: Diagnostic and Statistical Manual of Mental Disorders, 5th Edition. Arlington, VA, American Psychiatric Association, 2013

Arfken CL, Johanson CE, di Menza S, et al: Expanding treatment capacity for opioid dependence with office-based treatment with buprenorphine: National surveys of physicians. J Subst Abuse Treat 39(2):96–104, 2010 20598829

Ball JC, Ross A: The Effectiveness of Methadone Maintenance Treatment: Patients, Programs, Services, and Outcome. New York, Springer-Verlag, 1991

Barnett ML, Olenski AR, Jena AB: Opioid-prescribing patterns of emergency physicians and risk of long-term use. N Engl J Med 376(7):663–673, 2017 28199807

Blanco C, Iza M, Schwartz RP, et al: Probability and predictors of treatment-seeking for prescription opioid use disorders: a national study. Drug Alcohol Depend 131(1–2):143–148, 2013 23306097

Center for Behavioral Health Statistics and Quality: Key substance use and mental health indicators in the United States: Results from the 2015 National Survey on Drug Use and Health (HHS Publ No SMA 16-4984, NSDUH Series H-51). Rockville, MD, Substance Abuse and Mental Health Services Administration, 2016. Available at: www.samhsa.gov/data/. Accessed August 16, 2017.

Compton WM, Thomas YF, Stinson FS, et al: Prevalence, correlates, disability, and comorbidity of DSM-IV drug abuse and dependence in the United States: results from the national epidemiologic survey on alcohol and related conditions. Arch Gen Psychiatry 64(5):566–576, 2007 17485608

Department of Health, Education, and Welfare, Food and Drug Administration: Methadone: listing as new drug with special requirements and opportunity for hearing. Fed Regist 37(242):26,790–26,807, December 15, 1972

Department of Health and Human Services: 42 CFR part 8: medication assisted treatment for opioid use disorders; final rule. Fed Regist 81(131), 2016

Dole VP, Nyswander M: A medical treatment for diacetylmorphine (heroin) addiction: a clinical trial with methadone hydrochloride. JAMA 193:646–650, 1965 14321530

Drug Addiction Treatment Act of 2000, Pub. L. No. 106-310. Available at: www.congress.gov/bill/106th-congress/house-bill/4365. Accessed August 16, 2017.

Frank RG, Pollack HA: Addressing the fentanyl threat to public health. N Engl J Med 376(7):605–607, 2017 28199808

Gladden RM, Martinez P, Seth P: Fentanyl law enforcement submissions and increases in synthetic opioid-involved overdose deaths—27 states, 2013–2014. MMWR Morb Mortal Wkly Rep 65(33):837–843, 2016 27560775

Grant BF: Prevalence and correlates of drug use and DSM-IV drug dependence in the United States: results of the National Longitudinal Alcohol Epidemiologic Survey. J Subst Abuse 8(2):195–210, 1996 8880660

Guy GP Jr, Zhang K, Bohm MK, et al: Vital signs: changes in opioid prescribing in the United States, 2006–2015. MMWR Morb Mortal Wkly Rep 66(26):697–704, 2017 28683056

Health and Human Services Department: Proposed rule: opioid drugs in maintenance and detoxification treatment of opiate addiction; buprenorphine and buprenorphine combination; approved opioid treatment medications use. 42 CFR Part 8, RIN 0930-AA14. Fed Regist 74(117):29153–29158, Friday, June 19, 2009

Health and Human Services Department: Proposed rule: medication assisted treatment for opioid use disorders. 42 CFR Part 8, RIN 0930-AA22. Fed Regist 81(61):17,639–17,662, March 30, 2016

Hser YI, Hoffman V, Grella CE, et al: A 33-year follow-up of narcotics addicts. Arch Gen Psychiatry 58(5):503–508, 2001 11343531

Hser YI, Evans E, Huang D, et al: Long-term outcomes after randomization to buprenorphine/naloxone versus methadone in a multi-site trial. Addiction 111(4):695–705, 2016 26599131

Huang B, Dawson DA, Stinson FS, et al: Prevalence, correlates, and comorbidity of nonmedical prescription drug use and drug use disorders in the United States: results of the National Epidemiologic Survey on Alcohol and Related Conditions. J Clin Psychiatry 67(7):1062–1073, 2006 16889449

Hubbard RL, Craddock SG, Flynn PM, et al: Overview of 1-year follow-up outcomes in the Drug Abuse Treatment Outcome Study (DATOS). Psychol Addict Behav 11(4):261–278, 1997

Hughes A, Williams MR, Lipari RN, et al: Prescription drug use and misuse in the United States: results from the 2015 National Survey on Drug Use and Health. NSDUH Data Review, September 2016. Available at: https://www.samhsa.gov/data/sites/default/files/NSDUH-FFR2-2015/NSDUH-FFR2-2015.htm. Accessed February 10, 2017.

Hutchinson E, Catlin M, Andrilla CH, et al: Barriers to primary care physicians prescribing buprenorphine. Ann Fam Med 12(2):128–133, 2014 24615308

Kessler RC, McGonagle KA, Zhao S, et al: Lifetime and 12-month prevalence of DSM-III-R psychiatric disorders in the United States. Results from the National Comorbidity Survey. Arch Gen Psychiatry 51(1):8–19, 1994 8279933

Knopf A: SAMHSA bans drug court grantees from ordering participants off MAT. Alcoholism Drug Abuse Weekly, February 16, 2015. Available at: http://alcoholismdrugabuseweekly.com/m-article-detail/samhsa-bans-drug-court-grantees-from-ordering-participants-off-mat.aspx. Accessed February 27, 2017.

Kunins HV, Sohler NL, Giovanniello A, et al: A buprenorphine education and training program for primary care residents: implementation and evaluation. Subst Abus 34(3):242–247, 2013 23844954

Levinstein E: Morbid Craving for Morphia. Translated by Harrer C. London, Smith, Elder, 1878

Lipari RN, Williams MR, Copello EA, et al: Risk and protective factors and estimates of substance use initiation: results from the 2015 National Survey on Drug Use and Health. NSDUH Data Review, October 2016. Available at: www.samhsa.gov/data/sites/default/files/NSDUH-PreventionandInit-2015/NSDUH-PreventionandInit-2015.htm. Accessed February 10, 2017.

Manhapra A, Petrakis I, Rosenheck R: Three-year retention in buprenorphine treatment for opioid use disorder nationally in the Veterans Health Administration. Am J Addict May 4, 2017 [Epub ahead of print] 28472543

Meier B: Pain Killer: A "Wonder" Drug's Trail of Addiction and Death. Emmaus, PA, Rodale, 2003

Musto DF: The American Disease. New Haven, Yale University Press, 1973

Musto DF: The American Disease: Origins of Narcotic Control, 3rd Edition. New York, Oxford University Press, 1999

Neilson A: Buprenorphine treatment capacity: agent-based modeling for policy analysis. Substance Abuse and Mental Health Services Administration (SAMHSA), Center for Substances Abuse Treatment (CSAT) and the National Institute on Drug Abuse (NIDA), Report of Proceedings 2014 Buprenorphine Summit, September 22–23, 2014.

Regier DA, Farmer ME, Rae DS, et al: Comorbidity of mental disorders with alcohol and other drug abuse. Results from the Epidemiologic Catchment Area (ECA) Study. JAMA 264(19):2511–2518, 1990 2232018

Rudd RA, Aleshire JD, Zibbell JE, et al: Increases in drug and opioid overdose deaths—United States, 2000–2014. MMWR Morb Mortal Wkly Rep 64(50):1378–1382, 2016

Saha TD, Kerridge BT, Goldstein RB, et al: Nonmedical prescription opioid use and DSM-5 nonmedical prescription opioid use disorder in the United States. J Clin Psychiatry 77(6):772–780, 2016 27337416

Stanton A, McLeod C, Luckey B, et al: SAMHSA/CSAT evaluation of the buprenorphine waiver program. Paper presented at the annual meeting of the American Society of Addiction Medicine, San Diego, CA, May 2006

Substance Abuse and Mental Health Services Administration: Results From the 2002 National Survey on Drug Use and Health: National Findings (Office of Applied Studies, NHSDA Series H-22, DHHS Publ No SMA 03-3836). Rockville, MD, Substance Abuse and Mental Health Services Administration, 2003. Available at: http://www.oas.samhsa.gov/nhsda/2k2nsduh/results/2k2Results.htm. Accessed April 29, 2010.

Substance Abuse and Mental Health Services Administration: Evaluation of the Buprenorphine Waiver Program: Results From SAMHSA/CSAT's Evaluation of the Buprenorphine Waiver Program, June 20, 2005a. Available at: http://www.buprenorphine.samhsa.gov/findings.pdf. Accessed May 31, 2010.

Substance Abuse and Mental Health Services Administration: Results From the 2004 National Survey on Drug Use and Health: National Findings (Office of Applied Studies, NSDUH Series H-28, DHHS Publ No SMA 05-4062). Rockville, MD, Substance Abuse and Mental Health Services Administration, 2005b. Available at: http://www.oas.samhsa.gov/NSDUH/2k4NSDUH/2k4results/2k4results.htm. Accessed April 29, 2010.

Substance Abuse and Mental Health Services Administration: The Determinations Report: A Report on the Physician Waiver Program Established by the Drug Addiction Treatment Act of 2000 ("DATA"), March 30, 2006a. Available at http://www.buprenorphine.samhsa.gov/SAMHSA_Determinations_Report.pdf. Accessed April 29, 2010.

Substance Abuse and Mental Health Services Administration: The SAMHSA Evaluation of the Impact of the DATA Waiver Program: Summary Report, Task Order 277-00-6111, March 30, 2006b. Available at: http://www.buprenorphine.samhsa.gov/FOR_FINAL_summaryreport_colorized.pdf. Accessed April 29, 2010.

Substance Abuse and Mental Health Services Administration: Results From the 2006 National Survey on Drug Use and Health: National Findings (Office of Applied Studies, NSDUH Series H-32, DHHS Publ No SMA 07-4293). Rockville, MD, Substance Abuse and Mental Health Services Administration, 2007. Available at: http://www.oas.samhsa.gov/NSDUH/2k6NSDUH/2k6results.cfm. Accessed June 29, 2008.

Substance Abuse and Mental Health Services Administration: Results From the 2007 National Survey on Drug Use and Health: National Findings (Office of Applied Studies, NSDUH Series H-34, DHHS Publ No SMA 087-4343). Rockville, MD, Substance Abuse and Mental Health Services Administration, 2008. Available at: http://www.oas.samhsa.gov/NSDUH/2k7NSDUH/2k7results.cfm. Accessed November 14, 2008.

Substance Abuse and Mental Health Services Administration: Results From the 2008 National Survey on Drug Use and Health: National Findings (Office of Applied Studies, NSDUH Series H-36, DHHS Publ No SMA 09-4434). Rockville, MD, Substance Abuse and Mental Health Services Administration, 2009. Available at: http://www.oas.samhsa.gov/nsduh/2k8nsduh/2k8Results.cfm. Accessed April 29, 2010.

Substance Abuse and Mental Health Services Administration, Center for Behavioral Health Statistics and Quality: Treatment Episode Data Set (TEDS): 2004–2015. National Admissions to Substance Abuse Treatment Services. BHSIS Series S-84, HHS Publication No (SMA) 16-4986. Rockville, MD, Substance Abuse and Mental Health Services Administration, 2016.

Substance Abuse and Mental Health Services Administration: Physician and Program Data, 2017. Available at: http://www.samhsa.gov/programs-campaigns/medication-assisted-treatment/physician-program-data. Accessed May 26, 2017.

Sullivan LE, Chawarski M, O'Connor PG, et al: The practice of office-based buprenorphine treatment of opioid dependence: is it associated with new patients entering into treatment? Drug Alcohol Depend 79(1):113–116, 2005 15943950

Turner L, Kruszewski SP, Alexander GC: Trends in the use of buprenorphine by office-based physicians in the United States, 2003–2013. Am J Addict 24(1):24–29, 2015 25823632

U.S. Department of Justice, Drug Enforcement Administration: Title 21 Code of Federal Regulations, Part 1306—Prescriptions: General Information. Sect 1306.07 Administering or dispensing of narcotic drugs (39 FR 37986, Oct. 25, 1974, as amended at 70 FR 36344, June 23, 2005). Available at: https://www.deadiversion.usdoj.gov/21cfr/cfr/1306/1306_07.htm. Accessed March 15, 2017.

Weinstein ZM, Kim HW, Cheng DM, et al: Long-term retention in office based opioid treatment with buprenorphine. J Subst Abuse Treat 74:65–70, 2017 28132702

Wood GB: A Treatise on Therapeutics, and Pharmacology, or Materia Medica, 3rd Edition. Philadelphia, PA, JB Lippincott, 1856

2

General Opioid Pharmacology

John T. Pichot, M.D.
Mark T. Pichot, D.O.

OPIOIDS have played a significant role in the human experience for more than five millennia. Evidence found at Neolithic period dig sites located in present-day Switzerland indicates cultivation of *Papaver somniferum* seeds and pods and suggests that the first organized human farming included the intentional growing of the opium poppy (Booth 1999). The earliest historical record began with the Sumerian civilization located along the banks of the Tigris-Euphrates river system of lower Mesopotamia in what is now southern Iraq. Clay tablets from around 3400 B.C. include the oldest-known medical writings and represent the opium poppy with the ideograms *hul* and *gil*, which translate to "joy plant" (Booth 1999).

For thousands of years, opioids have been used to control coughing, diarrhea, and pain and to induce euphoria, primarily by oral ingestion of opium. In the 1600s, opium smoking also became prevalent and spread around the world from Asia to Europe and the American colonies, primarily through British-controlled trade routes (Booth 1999). In the nineteenth century, a number of scientific and technical developments set the stage for the modern era of opioid use and misuse. In 1806, a German publication described the first isolation of a component of opium, named *morphium* after Morpheus, the Greek god of dreams and sleep. By the 1820s, morphine was commercially available around the world. The development of the syringe in the mid-1800s, perfected by Dr. Alexander Wood of Edinburgh in 1853, allowed efficient parenteral delivery of morphine. The first semisynthetic opioid, heroin, was discovered in 1874 by pharmacist C.R. Wright in London's St. Mary's Hospital. The first completely synthetic opioid was designed as a replacement for morphine by German scientists during World War II when the Allied blockade prevented access to opium (Booth 1999).

In this chapter, we review key features of the opioids and their interactions with opioid receptors. We then focus on buprenorphine interactions with opioid receptors. Finally, we turn our attention to pharmacological issues with clinical relevance for using buprenorphine in the treatment of opioid addiction, including the treatment of withdrawal and its use as a maintenance medication for opioid use disorder (OUD).

Key Features of Opioids

Opioid is the broad term for the entire group of compounds that have agonist effects on the μ opioid receptors. The term opioid includes three basic subgroups (Booth 1999):

- Opiates—these are the naturally occurring substances present within raw opium. Examples of these naturally occurring compounds isolated from raw opium include morphine, codeine, and thebaine.
- Semisynthetic opioids—these do not occur in nature but are derived by modification of a naturally occurring opiate. Examples of semisynthetic opioids include heroin, developed from the opiate morphine; oxycodone and buprenorphine, each developed from the opiate thebaine; and hydrocodone, developed from codeine.
- Synthetic opioids—these neither occur in nature nor are developed from opiates but are fully synthetic compounds designed to act as opioid receptor agonists. Methadone and fentanyl are examples of synthetic opioids, as are many of the other opioid prescription medications in common clinical use.

There are several pharmacological characteristics of drugs that increase abuse potential as demonstrated in animal experimental models and in human behavior. Three primary factors that all result in a more rapid onset of opioid pharmacological effects are relevant to this increase in abuse potential: 1) drugs with a *faster route of administration* have greater abuse potential—that is, injecting and smoking a drug give it greater abuse potential than oral ingestion; 2) drugs with a *shorter half-life*, such as short-acting heroin versus long-acting methadone, have greater abuse

TABLE 2–1. **Opioid agonist effects**

Acute use effects	Chronic use effects	Overdose effects
Euphoria	Physical dependence	Nonresponsive
Emesis	Psychological dependence	Pinpoint pupils or "blown"
Constricted pupils	Variable energy changes	pupils
Slowed respirations	Constipation	Bradycardia
Drowsiness		Hypotension
Analgesia		Skin cyanotic
Decreased awareness		Muscles flaccid
Altered consciousness		Pulmonary edema
		Slowed respirations

Source. American Psychiatric Association 2013; Center for Substance Abuse Treatment 2004.

potential; and 3) drugs with *greater lipophilic properties*, which allow for more rapid transport across the blood-brain barrier, are associated with greater abuse potential. For example, heroin (diacetylmorphine) rapidly crosses the blood-brain barrier, even faster than morphine, because of the presence of two extra acetyl groups. These factors help explain why heroin is so euphorigenic; is so addictive; and is at the center of a multibillion dollar, worldwide illegal market—and has been for many decades (Booth 1999; Center for Substance Abuse Treatment 2004).

OPIOID RECEPTORS

There are three main types of opioid receptors: μ, κ, and δ receptors. The μ opioid receptor is the primary receptor relevant to the use of buprenorphine in the treatment of patients with severe OUD, and therefore it is the focus of the rest of this clinically oriented chapter. For those interested in a more thorough discussion of buprenorphine's potential interactions with other receptors, Cowan published a paper focusing on this topic (Cowan 2007). The μ opioid receptor was named *mu* specifically because it was found to be the binding site for morphine. Mu receptors are widely distributed throughout the human nervous system. Agonist binding and activation of these receptors result in the actions listed in Table 2–1.

After a substance binds to the μ opioid receptor, its action can be very different depending on some key pharmacological properties. These differences are demonstrated in Figure 2–1 (Center for Substance Abuse Treatment 2004). In this figure, moving up the vertical axis represents an increasing opioid effect and moving to the right on the horizontal axis represents an increasing dose of the medication.

Full agonists of the μ receptor include morphine, heroin, and methadone, as well as most of the prescription opioids. Full agonist binding is highly reinforc-

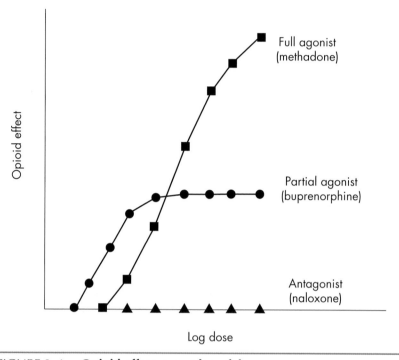

FIGURE 2–1.   **Opioid effect versus log of dose.**
Conceptual representation only; not to be used for dosing purposes.
Source.   Center for Substance Abuse Treatment 2004.

ing in animal models of addiction and in human beings; full agonists are clearly the most widely misused type of opioid. This is demonstrated in Figure 2–1 by the squares labeled "Full agonist (methadone)." The illustration demonstrates how the level of opioid effect steadily increases (vertical axis) as the dose of the full agonist increases (horizontal axis). If the full agonist dose is too high, then the opioid effect may become too great and the individual is at risk of dying from respiratory depression.

Partial agonists of the μ receptor bind to the receptors but have a ceiling to the level of agonist activity that results from the receptor binding. Buprenorphine is an example of a partial agonist of the μ receptor. When it binds to the μ receptor, opioid agonist effects as listed in Table 2–1 may be experienced, or if the person is in opioid withdrawal, withdrawal symptoms may be relieved, but these effects are limited in degree. It is clear that buprenorphine's ability to induce euphoria and respiratory depression has a ceiling effect even at high doses. This is demonstrated in Figure 2–1 by the circles labeled "Partial agonist (buprenorphine)." As the dose of the partial agonist increases (horizontal axis), the level of opioid effect steadily increases (vertical axis) until a ceiling is reached and no additional opioid effect is added even if the dose continues to increase. Even if the dose is very high, the opioid effect is limited and the risk of opioid overdose is minimal.

Antagonists of the μ receptor are also shown in Figure 2–1, represented by the triangles labeled "Antagonist (naloxone)," demonstrating that they, too, bind to the receptor, but they provide no opioid effect at all, regardless of the dose. Two examples of opioid antagonists are naltrexone and naloxone. Naltrexone is an oral medication with a half-life of sufficient duration to allow for once-daily dosing, or even alternate-day dosing, that is approved by the U.S. Food and Drug Administration (FDA) as a treatment for OUD. It works primarily by blocking agonists from binding to the μ receptor (Center for Substance Abuse Treatment 2004). Naloxone is also an antagonist medication, but it must be given parenterally. Its primary clinical role has been to treat acute opioid overdose emergently by reversing the opioid effects, including respiratory depression, by displacing opioid agonists off the μ receptors. Naloxone triggers a full opioid withdrawal disorder in individuals who are physically tolerant and dependent. Naloxone also has a clinical role in preventing diversion of buprenorphine as an integrated component of one sublingual product that combines buprenorphine and naloxone in a single tablet. This product is discussed in greater detail later in this chapter (see the subsection "Clinical Use Issues").

In summary, buprenorphine functions as a partial agonist with a ceiling effect for both opioid-induced euphoria and opioid-induced respiratory depression and therefore clearly has an improved safety margin over all full opioid agonists. This is the primary reason that buprenorphine has been proven to be a clinically effective and safe treatment for OUD and has FDA approval for use in office-based settings in sublingual and implant forms (Center for Substance Abuse Treatment 2004; U.S. Food and Drug Administration 2016).

Opioid Withdrawal Issues

When opioids are repeatedly dosed within a relatively short period of time, physical tolerance develops. Tolerance manifests as either a need for increased amounts of opioids to obtain the desired effect or a markedly diminished effect with continued use of the same amount of opioid (American Psychiatric Association 2013). Once physical tolerance and physical dependence on opioids have been established, opioid withdrawal is often experienced. Opioid withdrawal is a specific mental disorder defined in the current version of the *Diagnostic and Statistical Manual of Mental Disorders* (DSM-5; American Psychiatric Association 2013); criteria include the following key signs and symptoms: 1) dysphoric mood; 2) nausea or vomiting; 3) muscle aches; 4) lacrimation or rhinorrhea; 5) pupillary dilation, piloerection, or sweating; 6) diarrhea; 7) yawning; 8) fever; and 9) insomnia. This DSM-5 definition also accounts for the two main types of opioid withdrawal that are important to understand in the clinical use of buprenorphine: spontaneous withdrawal and precipitated withdrawal.

- *Spontaneous withdrawal* occurs when the usual opioid dosage is significantly reduced or when opioids are suddenly discontinued. For patients who are tolerant of short-acting opioids, such as hydrocodone or heroin, the onset of spontaneous withdrawal occurs within 24 hours of stopping opioid use and often begins within 8 hours after last use. In the case of long-acting opioids, such as methadone, spontaneous withdrawal does not develop for 24 hours or more after opioid use has ended.
- *Precipitated withdrawal* occurs when full agonists are displaced from the μ opioid receptor by substances that have greater affinity for receptor binding and that have less agonist action; therefore, displacement by either an antagonist or a partial agonist rapidly reduces the level of agonist effect. If the person is opioid tolerant, this will likely trigger opioid withdrawal, often suddenly and with a strong intensity.

Affinity and dissociation are two characteristics of μ opioid receptor binding that are important for understanding buprenorphine's pharmacological actions. The *affinity* for a receptor refers to the strength with which the substance binds to the receptor regardless of its action once bound. Buprenorphine has very strong affinity for the μ receptor, so much so that it displaces any full agonist that may be occupying the μ receptor. The patient must wait until all full opioid agonists are off the receptors before taking buprenorphine so that buprenorphine will not displace the full agonists and precipitate opioid withdrawal. Clinically this is indicated by the patient presenting with opioid withdrawal symptoms. Naloxone and naltrexone also have strong μ receptor affinity and displace full agonists and trigger full opioid withdrawal disorder (Center for Substance Abuse Treatment 2004).

Figure 2–2 illustrates the concept of precipitated withdrawal by the downward arrow representing the clinically significant sudden displacement of full agonists from the μ receptor by buprenorphine and the resultant decrease in the full agonist opioid effect in the central nervous system to a much reduced level, represented by the ceiling effect of the partial agonist. This rapid relative reduction to the partial agonist ceiling level results in opioid withdrawal symptoms even though some opioid agonist effect is still present from the binding of buprenorphine. If an antagonist is given and displaces the full agonist from the μ receptors, the point of the arrow will drop all the way to the horizontal axis, where no opioid agonist effect is present, and full opioid withdrawal disorder will be experienced.

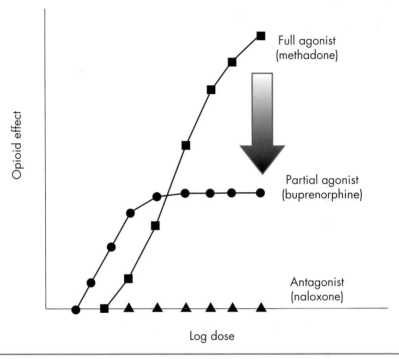

FIGURE 2–2.   **Precipitated withdrawal if buprenorphine displaces full opioid agonist.**
Conceptual representation only; not to be used for dosing purposes.
Source.   Center for Substance Abuse Treatment 2004.

Dissociation from a receptor refers to how easily the drug uncouples from the receptor when it is already bound. Buprenorphine dissociates very slowly from the μ receptor and, once bound, stays tightly attached—so tightly that full opioid agonists given after buprenorphine has attached to the μ receptors cannot displace it. This has two important clinical implications:

- If the physician accidentally precipitates withdrawal in a patient by displacing full agonists with buprenorphine, that patient should *not* then be given full agonists to treat the precipitated opioid withdrawal because the agonists will not displace the buprenorphine.
- Once buprenorphine has been inducted successfully and the patient continues to take it, taking another opioid will not produce any additional opioid effects, and most likely the person will feel no effect. Even the injection of heroin will not displace buprenorphine off the μ receptors. Thus, the slow dissociation of buprenorphine from the receptors has an added therapeutic advantage. This also has potential implications for giving opioids for analge-

sia if a buprenorphine patient needs acute pain management, but there are several options to address pain management in these circumstances (see Chapter 12, "Acute and Chronic Pain").

The specifics of spontaneous and precipitated withdrawal are relevant for buprenorphine induction and in explaining to patients the importance of having stopped taking all opioids prior to induction, how long they must wait for initial buprenorphine dosing, and that they must be experiencing opioid withdrawal before the first dose of buprenorphine may be given. The details of induction are covered in Chapter 5 ("Clinical Use of Buprenorphine").

Buprenorphine

PHARMACOKINETICS

Buprenorphine is approximately 96% protein bound in the plasma and undergoes *N*-dealkylation via the cytochrome P450 (CYP) 3A4 enzyme system to produce an active metabolite, norbuprenorphine. Both buprenorphine and norbuprenorphine also undergo glucuronidation in the liver. Thirty percent of the drug is eliminated in urine and 70% in feces. Buprenorphine has a mean elimination half-life from plasma of 37 hours (Braeburn Pharmaceuticals 2016a; Center for Substance Abuse Treatment 2004; Reckitt Benckiser Healthcare 2006).

Buprenorphine's metabolism by the CYP3A4 enzyme means that inhibitors of 3A4 or other substrates metabolized by the 3A4 enzyme could raise buprenorphine levels and that 3A4 inducers could lower buprenorphine levels. Table 2–2 shows a partial list of medications interacting with the CYP3A4 enzyme system. With the exception of interactions with some antiretroviral medications, it appears that most of these interactions are not clinically significant (see also Chapter 5, section "Drug-Drug Interactions," and Chapter 10, "Psychiatric Comorbidity," section "Drug Interactions With Buprenorphine").

Buprenorphine use may impair the mental or physical abilities required for the performance of potentially dangerous tasks such as driving a car or operating machinery, especially for the first 24–48 hours of use. Once tolerance to buprenorphine develops, there is no significant mental or physical impairment associated with its use. Deaths have been associated with injecting buprenorphine along with benzodiazepines and/or other central nervous system depressants (U.S. Food and Drug Administration 2016). Therefore, the use or misuse of sedative-hypnotics (e.g., benzodiazepines, barbiturates) is a relative contraindication to treatment with buprenorphine because the combination of buprenorphine and sedative-hypnotics may increase depression of the central nervous system. If treatment with buprenorphine and sedative hypnotics is necessary,

TABLE 2–2.   **Partial list of clinically relevant cytochrome P450 3A4 interactions**

Inhibitors	Substrates		Inducers
Amiodarone	Alfentanyl	Nifedipine	Carbamazepine
Buprenorphine	Alprazolam	Nisoldipine	Efavirenz
Cimetidine	Amlodipine	Nitrendipine	Nevirapine
Clarithromycin	Aripiprazole	Pimozide	Phenobarbital
Diltiazem	Astemizole	Prednisone	Phenytoin
Erythromycin	Atorvastatin	Progestins	Pioglitazone
Fluvoxamine	Boceprevir	Quinine	Rifabutin
Grapefruit juice	Buspirone	Quinidine	Rifampin
Indinavir	Carbamazepine	Ritonavir	St. John's wort
Itraconazole	Chlorpheniramine	Saquinavir	Troglitazone
Ketoconazole	Cisapride	Sildenafil	
Nefazodone	Clarithromycin	Simvastatin	
Nelfinavir	Cyclosporine	Sirolimus	
Ritonavir	Diazepam	Tacrolimus	
Troleandomycin	Diltiazem	Tadalafil	
Verapamil	Erythromycin	Tamoxifen	
Voriconazole	Felodipine	Telaprevir	
	Gleevec	Trazodone	
	Haloperidol	Triazolam	
	Indinavir	Vardenafil	
	Lovastatin	Verapamil	
	Midazolam	Vincristine	
	Nevirapine		

Note.   Reviewed December 2016 from an updated cytochrome P450 (CYP) drug interactions list, available at http://medicine.iupui.edu/CLINPHARM/ddis/clinical-table. An updated table of all CYP drug interactions can be found at http://medicine.iupui.edu/CLINPHARM/ddis/main-table.

the doses of both medications may need to be lowered (Center for Substance Abuse Treatment 2004; U.S. Food and Drug Administration 2016). Buprenorphine also can cause severe respiratory depression in children who are accidentally exposed, and there have been child fatalities. Instruct patients to keep buprenorphine away from others, especially children, and to not consume alcohol while taking this medication (U.S. Food and Drug Administration 2016).

Side effects of buprenorphine can include constipation, nausea, and emesis, but the frequency and intensity of these side effects are lower than with full opioid agonists. Patients maintained with buprenorphine show no clinically significant disruption in cognitive and psychomotor performance on formal testing. Orthostatic hypotension and elevated cerebrospinal fluid pressure may occur, and therefore, buprenorphine should be used with caution in patients with head injury, intracranial lesions, and other circumstances in which cerebrospinal pressure may be increased. Furthermore, buprenorphine can produce miosis and changes in the level of consciousness that may interfere with the evaluation of a patient with an acute central nervous system disease process. Buprenorphine has also been shown to increase intracholedochal pressure, as do other opioids, and thus should be administered with caution to a patient with known biliary tract dysfunction. Buprenorphine may obscure the diagnosis or clinical course of patients with acute abdominal conditions (Center for Substance Abuse Treatment 2004; U.S. Food and Drug Administration 2016; Walsh et al. 1994).

Neonatal abstinence syndrome is an expected and treatable outcome of prolonged use of opioids by the mother, including any form of buprenorphine during pregnancy. Neonatal abstinence syndrome may be life-threatening if not recognized and treated; therefore, it is important to advise pregnant women receiving buprenorphine treatment of the risk of neonatal opioid withdrawal syndrome and to help ensure that appropriate treatment will be available. This risk must be balanced against the risk of untreated opioid addiction, which often results in continued or relapsing illicit opioid use and is associated with poor pregnancy outcomes (U.S. Food and Drug Administration 2016).

Saxon and Bisaga (2014) summarized the issue of buprenorphine and hepatotoxicity as follows:

> in summary, data from large and diverse cohort of patients provide reassurance to providers regarding the safety of buprenorphine-naloxone in their patients. These studies suggest that liver injury from buprenorphine occurs rarely, however patients with hepatitis C are at higher risk to experience elevations in transaminases and reversible hepatic injury. Most of the evidence suggests that these elevations are related to underlying liver disease and not to the buprenorphine exposure. Serious hepatic injury appears to be quite rare considering that many hundreds of thousands of individuals have been treated with buprenorphine around the world. Moreover, maintenance on buprenorphine may have

indirect beneficial effect on liver health via reduction of illicit opioid use as it may minimize the toxic impact of adulterants found in heroin or acetaminophen found in prescription analgesics.

Adrenal insufficiency has been reported with opioid use, more often following greater than 1 month of use. Adrenal insufficiency syndrome includes nausea, vomiting, anorexia, fatigue, weakness, dizziness, and low blood pressure. If adrenal insufficiency is suspected, diagnostic testing to confirm should be done as soon as possible. Treatment is physiological replacement doses of corticosteroids with tapering off of opioids to allow adrenal function to recover and continued corticosteroid treatment until adrenal function recovers. Other opioids may be tried, as it has been reported that use of a different opioid in the same individual may be successful without an adrenal insufficiency response. The information available does not identify any particular opioids as being more likely to be associated with adrenal insufficiency (U.S. Food and Drug Administration 2016).

CLINICAL USE ISSUES

Buprenorphine has a primary clinical action of acting as a partial agonist at the μ opioid receptor. A parenteral formulation of buprenorphine was approved by the FDA in 1981 for the treatment of pain. In 2002, the FDA approved two sublingual tablet formulations for the treatment of OUD, and in 2010, sublingual film formulations were also approved for OUD treatment. Three other transmucosal formulations and a transdermal patch have subsequently been approved by the FDA for pain treatment.

Parenteral Analgesic

Parenteral buprenorphine hydrochloride (HCl) is a formulation available in the United States since the early 1980s for use as an analgesic. Parenteral buprenorphine HCl is available in a solution with a concentration of 0.3 mg/mL, and recommended dosing for moderate to severe pain is 0.3 mg intramuscularly or intravenously. This initial dose may be repeated once after 30–60 minutes, then every 6–8 hours as needed for pain control (Reckitt Benckiser Pharmaceuticals 2007). It is important to understand that it is against U.S. federal laws for any prescriptions to be written for parenteral buprenorphine for the treatment of either opioid withdrawal or OUD. It is not just beyond the FDA-approved uses to prescribe parenteral buprenorphine HCl for these opioid disorders; it is against federal law and puts the physician at risk for federal prosecution and punishment.

Sublingual Forms

Sublingual buprenorphine is available in the United States in two basic forms. One form, referred to as the *combo product,* combines buprenorphine and naloxone to prevent diversion for parenteral use; the other, referred to as the *mono product,* contains only buprenorphine. Both are FDA approved for the treatment of OUD. In 2012, 9.3 million buprenorphine prescriptions were dispensed in the United States, and from January to March 2013, 2.5 million buprenorphine prescriptions were dispensed (U.S. Drug Enforcement Administration 2013).

The combo sublingual product combining buprenorphine and naloxone is now available in a number of generic versions and dosing sizes, all of which follow essentially a 4-to-1 ratio of buprenorphine to naloxone. This combo form should be used for all patients being treated as outpatients for OUD to minimize diversion for misuse by inhaling or injection. The mono product contains only buprenorphine, and its use is generally clinically limited to patients in controlled environments where it is dispensed in a controlled manner or on an outpatient basis to pregnant patients.

The target clinical dosage range for both the combo and mono product is 5.7–16 mg/day of buprenorphine depending on the specific generic form being prescribed. With an increasing number of generic versions, in 2016 the FDA stated that equivalent doses include 8 mg generic buprenorphine tablets; 8 mg generic buprenorphine/2 mg generic naloxone tablets; Zubsolv tablets with 5.7 mg buprenorphine and 0.71 naloxone; and Bunavail buccal film with 4.2 mg buprenorphine and 0.7 mg naloxone. Suboxone film (8 mg buprenorphine/2 mg naloxone) delivers a somewhat higher exposure to buprenorphine than buprenorphine-naloxone tablets at the same dose. Suboxone and Subutex branded tablets are no longer marketed, but the film versions remain available (U.S. Food and Drug Administration 2016).

The sublingual formulation has poor intravenous and intramuscular bioavailability but good sublingual bioavailability (Table 2–3). Dissolving buprenorphine tablets sublingually, as designed, allows the buprenorphine to be absorbed and to be clinically effective. In the case of the combo product, the buprenorphine is absorbed when dissolved sublingually, but the naloxone is not significantly absorbed and has no clinical effect. However, if the combo product is dissolved into solution and injected, then the naloxone is clinically active and binds to the µ receptors, and its antagonist effect predominates, blocking much of the opioid effect. Naloxone also triggers opioid withdrawal if the individual who injects it is opioid dependent. When the mono product is injected, buprenorphine can produce significant levels of euphoria; as a result, it clearly can be misused for its euphoric effect and is subject to diversion for misuse. The only reason naloxone is an added component of the combo tablet is to prevent dissolving and injecting the tablet for euphoric effect, thus minimizing the risk of diversion (Center for Substance Abuse Treatment 2004; Stoller et al. 2001).

TABLE 2–3. **Bioavailability of buprenorphine**

| Route of administration | Buprenorphine bioavailability relative to route of administration | | |
	Intravenous	Intramuscular	Sublingual solution
Intravenous	100%	—	—
Intramuscular	70%	100%	—
Sublingual solution	49%	70%	100%
Sublingual tablet	29%	42%	50%–70%

Source. Brewster et al. 1981; Kuhlman et al. 1996; Lloyd-Jones et al. 1980; Nath et al. 1999; Schuh and Johanson 1999; Strain and Stitzer 1999; Weinberg et al. 1988. Adapted from Center for Substance Abuse Treatment 2004.

Buprenorphine Implant

Probuphine is a long-acting buprenorphine implant injected subdermally to provide a long-term constant dose of buprenorphine (Volkow 2016). It is a rod-shaped implant that is designed to provide sustained delivery of buprenorphine for up to 6 months when four rods are inserted. Implanting Probuphine is a maintenance treatment for patients with OUD who are clinically stable on a low dose of sublingual buprenorphine (equivalent to 8 mg/day or less of buprenorphine combo product). Pharmacokinetic comparisons in two clinical pharmacology studies (TTP-400-02-01 and PRO-810) of the implants, conducted by Titan Pharmaceuticals and reported in an FDA committee report, demonstrated that steady-state buprenorphine exposures obtained with four implants (80 mg of buprenorphine each, 320 mg total) were approximately 0.72–0.83 ng/mL, which were approximately half the trough concentrations observed with 16 mg/day sublingual buprenorphine at steady state (1.6±0.6 ng/mL; Psychopharmacologic Drugs Advisory Committee 2016).

Additionally, the literature confirms that the relationship between buprenorphine plasma levels and the effects of opioid blockade are different from the relationship between buprenorphine levels and withdrawal suppression. Greenwald, Comer, and Fiellin reviewed the scientific data on buprenorphine (BUP)-induced changes in µ opioid receptor (µOR) availability, pharmacokinetics, and clinical efficacy (Greenwald et al. 2014). They concluded that

> opioid withdrawal suppression appears to require ≤50% µOR availability, associated with BUP plasma concentrations ≥1 ng/mL; for most patients, this may require single daily BUP doses of 4 mg to defend against trough levels, or lower

divided doses.... Blockade of typical doses of abused opioids...probably requires <20% μOR availability, associated with BUP trough plasma concentrations ≥3 ng/mL; for most individuals, this may require single daily BUP doses
>16 mg. (pp. 13–14)

To the extent that blockade of exogenous opioids plays a role in efficacy for
addiction treatment, it must be noted that Probuphine is not expected to provide this effect. However, lower plasma levels are required to provide relief of
withdrawal symptoms. The exposure provided by Probuphine may be sufficient
for this purpose in some patients.

In addition to the side effects associated with sublingual forms noted earlier, implants are associated with the added risk of implant infection, migration,
protrusion, or expulsion and nerve damage resulting from the surgical procedure. There is also risk of accidental overdose or misuse if an implant comes out
or protrudes from the skin or is removed by the patient (U.S. Food and Drug
Administration 2016). The Probuphine Risk Evaluation and Mitigation Strategy (REMS) was created by Braeburn Pharmaceuticals (2016b) and the FDA
and require providers who want to prescribe, insert, or remove buprenorphine
implants to participate in a live training and be formally certified as providers.

Conclusion

Humans have used opiates for medicinal and euphorigenic purposes for thousands of years. The recent development of opioid antagonists and partial agonists has expanded our therapeutic options and, with buprenorphine, has added
a unique agent for the treatment of OUD. Because of its high affinity for opioid
receptors, its long duration of action, and the ceiling effect on respiratory depression, buprenorphine has proved to be an unusually safe and effective medication for managing OUD. Dosing is relatively straightforward, but clinicians
must be careful to avoid precipitating opioid withdrawal when initiating buprenorphine treatment in individuals who have recently used other opioids.
The presence of naloxone in the buprenorphine combo tablet is an added safety
feature that reduces the potential for misuse and diversion and further enhances
the drug's clinical utility.

Clinical Pearls

- Opioids are more likely to be misused if they have a faster route of
administration; have a shorter half-life; or are more lipophilic,
which allows them to pass through the blood-brain barrier more
easily.

- Buprenorphine, a μ opioid receptor partial agonist, binds tightly to opioid receptors but only partially activates them. Thus, buprenorphine's ability to produce euphoria and respiratory depression is limited, even at high doses.

- Patients who are physically dependent on opioids can develop a precipitated withdrawal with buprenorphine; therefore, patients need to be in opioid withdrawal before receiving the initial dose of buprenorphine.

- Buprenorphine is metabolized by the CYP3A4 system, but most drug-drug interactions do not appear to be clinically significant.

- Buprenorphine is available in a number of generic sublingual forms, and for patients who have demonstrated stability with sublingual use, an implant form is now an option.

- The buprenorphine-naloxone combination is the preferred sublingual form of the medication in order to diminish the likelihood of diversion to injected use.

References

American Psychiatric Association: Diagnostic and Statistical Manual of Mental Disorders, 5th Edition. Arlington, VA, American Psychiatric Association, 2013

Booth M: Opium: A History. New York, St Martin's Griffin, 1999

Braeburn Pharmaceuticals: Medication Guide: Probuphine, 2016a. Available at: http://probuphinerems.com/wp-content/uploads/2016/02/medguide-clean.pdf. Accessed August 4, 2017.

Braeburn Pharmaceuticals: Probuphine Risk Evaluation and Mitigation Strategy (REMS) Program, 2016b. Available at: http://probuphinerems.com. Accessed August 4, 2017.

Center for Substance Abuse Treatment: Clinical Guidelines for the Use of Buprenorphine in the Treatment of Opioid Addiction. Treatment Improvement Protocol (TIP) Series 40. DHHS Publ No (SMA) 04-3939. Rockville, MD, Substance Abuse and Mental Health Services Administration, 2004. Available at: www.ncbi.nlm.nih.gov/books/NBK64245/. Accessed August 16, 2016.

Cowan A: Buprenorphine: the basic pharmacology revisited. J Addict Med 1(2):68–72, 2007 21768937

Greenwald MK, Comer SD, Fiellin DA: Buprenorphine maintenance and mu-opioid receptor availability in the treatment of opioid use disorder: implications for clinical use and policy. Drug Alcohol Depend 144:1–11, 2014 25179217

Psychopharmacologic Drugs Advisory Committee: Probuphine (Buprenorphine Hydrochloride Subdermal Implant) for Opioid Dependence. Silver Spring, MD, Food and Drug Administration Center for Drug Evaluation and Research, January 12, 2016. Available at: www.fda.gov/downloads/AdvisoryCommittees/Committees MeetingMaterials/Drugs/PsychopharmacologicDrugs AdvisoryCommittee/UCM480732.pdf. Accessed August 4, 2017.

Reckitt Benckiser Healthcare: Buprenorphine Hydrochloride and Naloxone Hydrochloride Dihydrate Sublingual Tablets (Suboxone) and Buprenorphine Hydrochloride Sublingual Tablets (Subutex): Prescribing Information. Hull, UK, Reckitt Benckiser Healthcare, September 2006

Reckitt Benckiser Pharmaceuticals: Buprenex injectable solution prescribing information. Richmond, VA, Reckitt Benckiser Pharmaceuticals, 2007. Available at: www.naabt.org/documents/buprenex_PI.pdf. Accessed August 4, 2017.

Saxon A, Bisaga A: Monitoring of Liver Function Tests and Hepatitis in Patients Receiving Buprenorphine (With or Without Naloxone). Providence, RI, Providers' Clinical Support System for Medication Assisted Treatment, 2014

Stoller KB, Bigelow GE, Walsh SL, et al: Effects of buprenorphine/naloxone in opioid-dependent humans. Psychopharmacology (Berl) 154(3):230–242, 2001 11351930

U.S. Drug Enforcement Administration: Buprenorphine. Springfield, VA, U.S. Drug Enforcement Administration, July 2013. Available at: www.deadiversion.usdoj.gov/drug_chem_info/buprenorphine.pdf#search=2012%20buprenorphine%20prescriptions. Accessed August 4, 2017.

U.S. Food and Drug Administration: Full Prescribing Information for Probuphine Implant. Silver Spring, MD, U.S. Food and Drug Administration, May 2016

Volkow N: Probuphine: A Game-Changer in Fighting Opioid Dependence. National Institute on Drug Addiction Advancing Addiction Science, May 26, 2016. Available at: www.drugabuse.gov/about-nida/noras-blog/2016/05/probuphine-game-changer-in-fighting-opioid-dependence. Accessed August 4, 2017.

Walsh SL, Preston KL, Stitzer ML, et al: Clinical pharmacology of buprenorphine: ceiling effects at high doses. Clin Pharmacol Ther 55(5):569–580, 1994 8181201

3

Efficacy and Safety of Buprenorphine

Eric C. Strain, M.D.
Gerard Iru I. Fernando, M.D.

History and Rationale for the Development of Buprenorphine for the Treatment of Opioid Use Disorder

Buprenorphine was first synthesized in the late 1960s and initially was developed and marketed throughout the world as an analgesic. In the United States, it was sold under the brand name Buprenex, and outside the United States, it was sold as Temgesic. In the United States, it was available only in a parenteral form for the treatment of pain. However, a sublingual analgesic form was marketed in other countries (e.g., New Zealand).

Although the initial marketed indication of buprenorphine was for the treatment of pain, it was quickly recognized that buprenorphine might have value as a medication that could be used for the treatment of opioid use disorder (OUD). In a 1978 paper published in the *Archives of General Psychiatry*, Jasinski and coauthors described the pharmacological profile of buprenorphine in humans under a variety of experimental conditions and concluded that the medication had characteristics that might make it particularly useful and effective for the treatment of OUD (Jasinski et al. 1978).

PHARMACOLOGICAL FEATURES

Of the pharmacological characteristics described by Jasinski et al. (1978), there are three primary features of buprenorphine that are particularly relevant to its use as a treatment medication for OUD. Two of these may be seen as advantageous, whereas the third is a relatively minor detriment to its use. Although addressing all three characteristics in detail is beyond the scope of this chapter, they have direct clinical implications that will be reviewed briefly here.

The first feature is that buprenorphine acts as an agonist at the μ opioid receptor. It has been long recognized that buprenorphine is a *partial* agonist at the μ receptor. Partial agonist medications produce effects that are very similar to *full* agonist medications at the lower end of a dose-response curve, but as the dose of a partial agonist increases, the effect of the medication plateaus, such that there is less of a maximal effect compared with a full agonist medication. The common medications that are contrasted to buprenorphine are full μ agonist opioids such as methadone, heroin, and morphine, which generally have the capacity to produce greater effects than buprenorphine at higher doses. Notably, the relative degree of maximal effect of a partial agonist relative to a full agonist can vary as a function of the outcome measure being considered (e.g., in the case of opioids, respiratory depression versus gastrointestinal motility versus analgesia).

The fact that buprenorphine acts at the μ opioid receptor is important for several reasons. Agonism at the μ receptor means that buprenorphine can suppress spontaneous opioid withdrawal, ensuring that a patient who is in opioid withdrawal at the time he or she receives the first dose of buprenorphine will experience suppression of those withdrawal symptoms. In addition, occupancy at the μ receptor provides blockade (or cross-tolerance), so a subsequently administered dose of another μ agonist opioid (such as heroin) is not experienced to the same degree as occurs if no buprenorphine is present. Finally, opioids that act at the μ receptor generally decrease craving for illicit opioids in persons physically dependent on opioids.

The second pharmacological feature of buprenorphine is that its dose-response curve is bell-shaped. That is, as the dose of buprenorphine increases, there is an increase in a measured effect (e.g., analgesia, respiratory depression), a maximal effect is achieved, and then the measured effect decreases at even higher doses. Notably, this bell-shaped dose-response curve has been shown only in animal models (i.e., no human studies to date have shown it). However, in animals, buprenorphine's bell-shaped curve has been shown for a number of measures, including analgesia, gastrointestinal motility (i.e., constipation), and respiratory depression.

The reason for the decrease in effects at higher doses was originally thought to be related to a second opioid receptor effect of buprenorphine: antagonism at the κ receptor. This combination of partial agonism at the μ receptor and antagonism at the κ receptor is the reason buprenorphine was originally called an *opioid mixed agonist-antagonist*. There are several other marketed opioid mixed agonist-antagonist analgesics, such as pentazocine and butorphanol. However, preclinical data now suggest that the descending limb of buprenorphine's dose-response curve can be attributed to an alternative pharmacological action of this medication at the opiate receptor–like 1 (ORL-1) receptor. That is, buprenorphine acts as an agonist at the ORL-1 receptor. Animal studies suggest that when ORL-1 receptors are not present, buprenorphine produces effects that look like a full agonist opioid (i.e., no descending limb to the dose-response curve).

These two pharmacological effects translate to clinical advantages. The μ agonism means that buprenorphine suppresses withdrawal, blocks the effects of other opioids, and decreases opioid craving. The bell-shaped dose-response curve, combined with the lower maximal effect of buprenorphine as a partial μ agonist, means that there is a lower risk of respiratory depression associated with an overdose of the drug.

The third feature of buprenorphine is that it has poor oral bioavailability. Although this feature of the drug is not a particularly advantageous characteristic, it is not a marked disadvantage, either. The most common delivery route for any medication taken on an outpatient basis is by swallowing, and although other routes can be used (e.g., injection of insulin, topical administration of nicotine with a patch), these are less common routes of administration. Buprenorphine has fair sublingual bioavailability, and a sublingual form was developed for the treatment of OUD. This route of administration is relatively uncommon for medications that are self-administered (although there are other buccally administered medications, such as the antipsychotic drug asenapine), but it has been accepted by patients. Because a sublingual tablet must be water soluble, a concern with this formulation was that it could be relatively easy to dissolve it in water and inject it. Given that the sublingual bioavailability is only fair compared with parenteral bioavailability, sublingual doses are relatively high compared with typical parenteral analgesic doses (8–16 mg vs. 0.2–0.3 mg, respectively). Thus, dissolving and injecting the sublingual tablet delivers a relatively higher dose of the drug.

These aspects of administration route and relative bioavailability could impact the risk of diversion and parenteral misuse of a sublingual buprenorphine tablet. To address this potential, tablets that contain naloxone were developed. Although a full description of the scientific basis for a buprenorphine-naloxone (BUP/NX) tablet will not be provided here, the logic of this combination is based on three observations. First, naloxone has very poor sublingual bioavailability. Second, injected naloxone will precipitate opioid withdrawal in persons with OUD. Third, opioid withdrawal is distressing but rarely life-threatening. Thus, when a combined BUP/NX tablet is taken via the intended therapeutic route (sublingually), the desired therapeutic effect is achieved. However, if the tablet is dissolved and injected by an opioid-dependent person, a naloxone effect occurs, and the person experiences distressing opioid withdrawal. (Note that this would be the case only for a person who is physiologically opioid dependent.) Although this withdrawal is distressing, it is generally tolerable and not a medical emergency. The addition of naloxone was not meant to produce some beneficial effect, such as additional opioid blockade, when the BUP/NX combination is taken sublingually. The combination of buprenorphine and naloxone does appear to have less intranasal (Jones et al. 2015) and intravenous (Comer et al. 2010) abuse potential compared with buprenorphine alone.

The pharmacological features of buprenorphine suggested that it could be a useful agent for the treatment of OUD and, furthermore, that it would be pharmacologically different from traditional full μ agonist opioid medication treatments (i.e., methadone and levo-α-acetylmethadol [LAAM]). As these features came to be appreciated, there was recognition that it might be possible for buprenorphine to be used safely outside the traditional methadone clinic delivery system. In order to understand this aspect of buprenorphine's development, the context of medication development and, in particular, the approval and use of LAAM in the United States can be useful from a historical perspective.

APPROVAL AND USE OF LAAM IN THE UNITED STATES AND ITS IMPACT ON DEVELOPMENT OF BUPRENORPHINE

During the 1990s, when buprenorphine was being studied intensively as a potential treatment for OUD, another opioid treatment medication also was being studied and eventually was approved for use in the United States—LAAM. Although LAAM had been identified as a possible treatment for OUD in the 1970s, it had languished for years until the National Institute on Drug Abuse (NIDA) took the initiative to obtain U.S. Food and Drug Administration (FDA) approval for this medication in 1993.

However, LAAM needed to be provided through the opioid treatment program (OTP) system—that is, methadone clinics. Despite the availability of this new, alternative medication that had good efficacy, there was very limited use of LAAM and essentially no expansion of the treatment system associated with its availability. Although subsequent concerns arose regarding potential cardiac effects of LAAM, its eventual withdrawal from the U.S. market was due to low sales rather than the cardiac effects.

The experience with LAAM impacted planning for the eventual approval and use of buprenorphine. LAAM could be provided only through the OTP system, and its treatment capacity had not been expanded. In order to avoid a similar experience with buprenorphine, federal legislative changes in the United States were enacted that permitted the use of certain types of medications in office-based practices for the treatment of OUD. The Drug Addiction Treatment Act of 2000 (Pub. L. No. 106-310) identified potential medications for office-based treatment as being Schedule III, IV, or V (i.e., having less abuse potential than Schedule II medications, such as methadone). Although this legislation did not specify buprenorphine, it was clearly designed with buprenorphine in mind. Because buprenorphine was approved as a Schedule III medication (on the basis of its pharmacological characteristics suggesting it has a lower abuse potential), it could be used in office-based practices. This increased the likelihood that buprenorphine would not be another LAAM.

HISTORY AND RATIONALE FOR DEVELOPMENT OF BUPRENORPHINE

It is interesting that although buprenorphine was initially developed for use as an analgesic, its major clinical impact has occurred as a treatment for OUD. As has been noted repeatedly over the years, the pharmacological effects of buprenorphine are unique, and these unique features—such as its partial agonist effects and the bell-shaped dose-response curve—make it particularly suited for the treatment of OUD. These features also made buprenorphine well positioned to be used outside of the traditional OTP system, which in turn has helped to expand the treatment of OUD.

Controlled Trials Assessing Efficacy of Buprenorphine for Maintenance Treatment of Opioid Use Disorder

Clinical studies testing the efficacy of buprenorphine have included both inpatient (or residential) human laboratory studies and outpatient clinical trials. The former have tended to be smaller, within-subject design studies (i.e., studies in which volunteers serve as their own control over the course of the study). There have been an extensive number of these studies, and reviewing all of them is beyond the scope of this chapter. The results from these studies provided critical information about buprenorphine, although direct translation to clinical use of this medication was not always the purpose of the studies. Outpatient clinical trials, on the other hand, provided important data that are more representative of and relevant to clinical use. Generally, these trials were group comparison studies that tested the efficacy of buprenorphine compared with placebo, methadone, and/or naltrexone. Although most of these studies were conducted in the 1990s, prior to buprenorphine's approval in the United States, there continue to be outpatient clinical trials testing the efficacy of this medication.

HUMAN LABORATORY STUDIES OF SUBLINGUAL BUPRENORPHINE

Multiple human laboratory studies have tested the blockade efficacy of buprenorphine under different experimental conditions. In general, these studies enrolled volunteers who were physically dependent on opioids, maintained the subjects on buprenorphine or BUP/NX (either buprenorphine solution or, in later studies, the tablet form), and then tested whether opioid agonist–like effects were produced when subjects received a prototypical μ agonist opioid such as morphine, heroin, or hydromorphone. To determine if the relative reinforcing effects of the μ agonist opioid were diminished when the subject was treated with buprenorphine, the subject either was challenged directly with the drug (Bickel et al. 1988; Strain et al. 1997, 2002) or was allowed to self-administer the drug (Comer et al. 2001, 2005; Mello and Mendelson 1980).

One difficulty with these human laboratory studies is that the ideal control condition—a period of time when the subject is maintained on placebo and challenged with an opioid or allowed to self-administer an opioid—was not included in the studies. A placebo maintenance period would permit the efficacy of buprenorphine to be more accurately characterized. However, it is not practical to conduct such a study, even under the controlled conditions of an inpatient ward as is typical for these projects. Participants would need to be fully withdrawn off opioids, making blinding of buprenorphine versus placebo maintenance conditions problematic. Alternatively, a separate group of subjects who do not have active OUD could be used as a comparison group, although groups need to be matched to ensure that other factors do not account for differences that might be noted. Given these qualifications, studies have typically compared the relative efficacy of different doses of buprenorphine, with the idea that greater attenuation of opioid effect or less self-administration while treated with a higher dose of buprenorphine (versus a lower dose) provides evidence of efficacy.

When buprenorphine is studied in the human laboratory, in general, dose-related blockade is demonstrated. That is, volunteers maintained on buprenorphine (or BUP/NX) report fewer opioid agonist–like effects for higher maintenance doses of buprenorphine and self-administer less of a μ agonist opioid at these higher doses. Doses of either 2 mg/day or 4 mg/day of buprenorphine (or the equivalent of BUP/NX) produce significantly less blockade to opioid effects and greater self-administration of an opioid compared with doses of 8–32 mg/day of buprenorphine (or the equivalent of BUP/NX). These effects have been shown with both direct challenge sessions and self-administration studies. There is some evidence that suggests that 16 mg may be more effective than 8 mg of daily buprenorphine, although not all studies have shown a distinction. However, this should not be interpreted to mean that doses of more than 8 mg/day of buprenorphine are not more effective than 8 mg/day of buprenorphine, and clearly there are some subjects in studies (and some patients in practices) who have better outcomes for doses greater than 8 mg/day. There can be considerable variability in responses between individuals in a human laboratory study.

Results from these studies also show that there is often incomplete blockade or suppression of self-administration of a μ agonist opioid when a person is maintained on buprenorphine—especially if a sufficiently high dose of the μ agonist opioid is employed in the study. Although these studies provide critical data relevant to the demonstration of buprenorphine's efficacy, they also highlight that the medication alone is not a magic bullet that fully addresses all of the factors that can lead to use of illicit opioids by a person with opioid addiction. Maintenance on buprenorphine—probably at least 8 mg/day for most patients—can be very effective at decreasing the subjective effects of opioids and the likelihood of self-administering opioids, but optimal outcomes are achieved when buprenorphine is taken by a motivated patient who is engaged in other treatment services that concurrently address drug use.

OUTPATIENT GROUP COMPARISON CLINICAL TRIALS WITH SUBLINGUAL BUPRENORPHINE

Human laboratory studies provide data from highly controlled experimental conditions that allow characterization of buprenorphine's efficacy when confounding factors (e.g., other drug use, presence of a comorbid condition) are controlled or excluded from study participants. Outpatient clinical trials, on the other hand, provide data that can be viewed as more "real life" like. Such studies, although closer than residential studies to clinical practice, often employ design features (e.g., double-blind dosing, random assignment to treatment conditions, intensive collection of standard outcome measures, careful control of counseling services provided) that distinguish these trials as significantly different from routine care. It is worth noting that the goal of a controlled clinical trial is not to model exactly how a medication will be used by clinicians but to provide a scientific basis for answering specific questions about the efficacy and/or safety of the medication under particular experimental conditions. There are advantages to both outpatient clinical trial and inpatient/residential laboratory approaches, and both approaches should be seen as complementary and relevant to the drug development process. In the following subsections, we describe findings from outpatient clinical trials of buprenorphine compared with placebo, methadone, and naltrexone.

Sublingual Buprenorphine Compared With Placebo

Relatively few studies have tested the efficacy of buprenorphine compared with a true placebo condition. In part, this is related to the inherent difficulty in blinding placebo medication for a person who is physically dependent on opioids. It is very likely that the blind would be immediately broken if an opioid-dependent person is directly started on placebo because the lack of withdrawal suppression and subjective opioid agonist effects and the resulting classic opioid withdrawal symptoms would be readily detected by the person. However, there have been strategies employed to provide placebo control conditions, and probably the most common approach has been to have participants assigned to a placebo condition undergo a period of active treatment medication that includes gradual withdrawal and transfer on to placebo doses of buprenorphine. In addition to this approach, one study also used a low-dose buprenorphine condition as a placebo-like control (Ling et al. 1998), and another used a novel choice procedure that allowed volunteers to switch from two different doses of medication, including (potentially) from placebo to active buprenorphine (Johnson et al. 1995).

Controlled outpatient clinical trials that have tested the efficacy of buprenorphine compared with placebo have consistently shown that buprenorphine is more effective than placebo for primary outcome measures of treatment retention and illicit opioid use (Fudala et al. 2003; Johnson et al. 1995; Kakko et al. 2003; Krook et al. 2002; Ling et al. 1998). Cross-study comparisons are somewhat difficult, given the use of different doses of buprenorphine, different durations of treatment, and different outcome assessments. However, in general, doses of 8–16 mg/day of sublingual buprenorphine (or BUP/NX) have typically been compared with either 0 mg (or in one case a 1-mg placebo-like control condition) and shown to be superior. Although doses greater than 16 mg/day have been tested, the relative efficacy of such higher doses compared with 8–16 mg/day has not been a primary outcome. Such higher doses (up to 32 mg/day) may be clinically indicated for some patients, and there is clearly variability in the optimal dose needed for some patients.

Although it is difficult to compare outcomes from these studies, it is worth noting that retention for buprenorphine-treated patients is consistently superior to that for patients treated with placebo. Indeed, placebo-treated participants in these studies generally dropped out. For example, after 16 weeks of treatment in one study, the retention rate for patients treated with 16 mg of daily buprenorphine was 61% versus 40% for the 1 mg (placebo-like) condition (Ling et al. 1998). In another study, 75% of participants treated with 16 mg daily sublingual buprenorphine remained in treatment at 1 year, compared with none of those who underwent a double-blind buprenorphine withdrawal followed by placebo treatment (Kakko et al. 2003).

In summary, these rigorously conducted controlled clinical trials showed that daily sublingual buprenorphine is superior to placebo in the outpatient treatment of OUD. A final point regarding these studies, and the clinical trials comparing buprenorphine with methadone that are summarized in the next subsection, is worth noting. The goal of these studies was to test the efficacy of buprenorphine. However, optimal clinical outcomes for the treatment of OUD (and other substance use disorders) occur when pharmacotherapies are combined with nonpharmacological treatments (Amato et al. 2011). Thus, if an interested clinician reviews these papers and studies, it is important to keep in mind that it is likely that the reported outcomes can be considerably improved when buprenorphine is used outside the constraints of a clinical trial and with the concurrent care of a committed clinician.

Sublingual Buprenorphine Compared With Methadone

Although there have been a relatively small number of studies testing buprenorphine's efficacy compared with placebo, there have been many more outpatient studies that have compared buprenorphine with methadone treatment (Mattick et al. 2014). The general conclusions drawn here are based on well-conducted clinical trials. Studies that were not double-blind, did not randomly assign participants to dose conditions, or had other methodological features that make interpretation of findings problematic are generally not factored in when considering buprenorphine's efficacy relative to methadone in this subsection. (Such studies can provide supportive evidence, but confounds in design or execution make interpretation of findings problematic.) Despite the use of good clinical trial methods, there are features of these studies that can differ considerably between clinical trials—for example, in the doses of buprenorphine and methadone used, the frequency of buprenorphine dosing, whether the doses of each medication were fixed or flexible, and the primary outcome assessments and the frequency of collection for these primary outcome assessments.

Despite these differences, several general conclusions can be made regarding buprenorphine's efficacy compared with methadone. Outcomes with buprenorphine treatment are generally similar to those achieved with methadone for methadone doses of up to about 60 mg/day. For doses greater than 60 mg of daily methadone, it appears that methadone has better outcomes (typically, treatment retention and some measure of illicit opioid use—self-reported use and/or urine results—are used as primary outcome measures in most studies). However, it is worth noting that most clinical trials have been conservative with buprenorphine dosing (despite the apparent safety of this medication at high doses); no studies have tested the efficacy of doses greater than 32 mg/day of sublingual buprenorphine, and few have tested doses even this high.

It is useful to elaborate on this point for a moment. Recall that buprenorphine has a bell-shaped dose-response curve. Theoretically, it is possible that at higher doses, a decrease in some effects might occur, but greater degrees of opioid blockade still might be achieved. Thus, it is interesting that despite the apparent safety of high doses of buprenorphine, there have been no controlled clinical trials testing doses greater than 32 mg/day. Indeed, there has been little research in humans that has examined the effects of doses greater than 32 mg under any experimental conditions, including human laboratory studies.

It appears that doses of about 8–24 mg/day of buprenorphine produce outcomes similar to those seen with moderate doses of methadone (i.e., doses of up to 60 mg/day). Most of the studies that compared buprenorphine with methadone were conducted in methadone treatment clinics (OTPs), and it is important to note that the circumstances under which buprenorphine is used in the United States, and often elsewhere as well—an office-based setting with a physician—are very different from the treatment provided at an OTP. Research looking at the efficacy of buprenorphine in office-based settings (Fiellin et al. 2006; Fudala et al. 2003) has shown good outcomes that appear to be maintained over sustained periods (Parran et al. 2010). When comparing office-based buprenorphine with traditional OTP-delivered methadone treatment, it has been shown that both treatments are effective but each program serves different populations. For example, one study found that buprenorphine-treated patients were less likely to abuse benzodiazepines and more likely to have health insurance, be employed, be male, abuse prescription opioids, and be HIV positive compared with methadone-treated patients (Fingerhood et al. 2014). In that study, methadone-treated patients ultimately had slightly better treatment outcomes, with a higher mean number of opioid-negative months and mean number of months in treatment.

Although findings from controlled clinical trials comparing daily sublingual buprenorphine with methadone suggest that outcomes achieved with methadone may be better at higher doses of methadone, this should not be interpreted to suggest that buprenorphine is not a treatment option for patients with higher levels of opioid physical dependence. There can be considerable variability in the responses of different patients to a medication. Indeed, it has been shown that the bioavailability of buprenorphine can vary twofold between different subjects treated with the same dose of this medication, suggesting that conclusions based on dose delivered may obscure differences related to blood levels (Strain et al. 2004). In addition, the impact of nonpharmacological aspects of treatment (e.g., intensity of counseling services), the particular circumstances of the patient (e.g., his or her level of motivation), and the features of the setting of treatment (e.g., ready access to office-based treatment) can impact the efficacy of buprenorphine. Perhaps the most important conclusions that can be drawn from the controlled clinical trials comparing buprenorphine with methadone are that both medications are effective and that a patient who is not responding well to one medication when all aspects of the treatment have been optimized (e.g., dose, level of counseling, involvement of significant others) should be considered for treatment with the other. Both are excellent options for the treatment of OUD.

Sublingual Buprenorphine Compared With Naltrexone

Naltrexone is another medication used to treat OUD. Because naltrexone acts as an antagonist at the μ opioid receptor and is not a controlled substance, some medical professionals may feel more comfortable prescribing naltrexone as opposed to methadone or buprenorphine. There are currently two formulations of naltrexone available: an oral formulation that is usually taken daily and an intramuscular injection that is given monthly.

In a randomized controlled trial that compared oral naltrexone with sublingual buprenorphine, buprenorphine was superior to oral naltrexone, with better treatment retention and a higher number of opioid-negative urine tests (Mokri et al. 2016). A second study also found buprenorphine superior to naltrexone; differences between naltrexone and placebo in that study were not significant (Schottenfeld et al. 2008).

Extended-release naltrexone, on the other hand, appears to be superior to placebo in treating OUD (Krupitsky et al. 2011). However, there are no data comparing buprenorphine with extended-release naltrexone, although there is a study currently being conducted comparing these two medications (Kunøe et al. 2016).

STUDIES OF LONG-ACTING FORMS OF BUPRENORPHINE

In addition to sublingual buprenorphine formulations, a buprenorphine implant indicated for maintenance treatment of OUD is now available (Rosenthal et al. 2016). One limitation to this product is that it is indicated for patients who have achieved and sustained prolonged clinical stability on low-to-moderate doses (8 mg/day or less) of transmucosal buprenorphine. Implantation occurs subdermally; four implants are inserted in the upper arm, remain for 6 months, and then are removed by the end of the sixth month. Complications, including nerve damage and migration resulting in embolism and death, can occur from insertion and removal, although these are rare side effects. When buprenorphine implants were compared with sublingual buprenorphine, patients with the implants had slightly higher (14%) illicit opioid-free urine samples (Rosenthal et al. 2016).

A 7-day transdermal patch of buprenorphine is also available for management of pain. Studies with this product have not tested its use as a treatment for patients with OUD. Two forms of a buprenorphine depot formulation (one for 7 days and two that are for a month duration) are currently in active development by the companies Indivior Pharmaceuticals and Braeburn Pharmaceuticals/Camurus and have been submitted to the FDA for review in 2017. These forms have been shown to block the reinforcing efficacy and subjective effects of hydromorphone (Nasser et al. 2016; Walsh et al. 2017).

Controlled Trials Assessing Efficacy of Buprenorphine for Opioid Withdrawal Treatment

OVERVIEW OF THE USE OF BUPRENORPHINE FOR OPIOID WITHDRAWAL

When buprenorphine first became available for the treatment of OUD in the United States, a considerable proportion of its use was for the treatment of opioid withdrawal. Indeed, prior to the approval of the sublingual tablet, it was very common for clinicians to report that they used the parenteral form of buprenorphine to treat opioid withdrawal. The current relative proportion of buprenorphine use for withdrawal versus maintenance treatment is not known, but it appears that the growth of buprenorphine use in the United States has been greater for maintenance than for withdrawal treatment.

Prior to the use of buprenorphine for the treatment of opioid withdrawal, a common pharmacological treatment used to alleviate opioid withdrawal, especially for inpatient settings, was clonidine. An early study that directly compared buprenorphine with clonidine found that buprenorphine had an overall better profile of efficacy and safety than did clonidine (Cheskin et al. 1994), and subsequent studies have found similar results (Gowing et al. 2017; Hussain et al. 2015; Ling et al. 2005; Ziaaddini et al. 2012; Ziedonis et al. 2009). Although one can imagine situations in which clonidine would be preferred for treatment of a particular patient or in which it might be a useful adjunct treatment (e.g., in the transition from buprenorphine to naltrexone), in general, clonidine is no longer a first-line agent for opioid withdrawal—especially on an inpatient basis, when dosing of buprenorphine can be supervised and risk of diversion or misuse is quite low.

On an outpatient basis, either methadone or buprenorphine may be used to treat opioid withdrawal. Studies that directly compare buprenorphine with methadone for the outpatient treatment of withdrawal are uncommon, and those that have done so tended to consist of small samples or special groups such as adolescents or subjects who were treated concurrently with other medications, making interpretation of findings more difficult (Ebner et al. 2004;

Gowing et al. 2017; Seifert et al. 2002). Studying the efficacy of buprenorphine compared with methadone in the outpatient treatment of opioid withdrawal in the United States is further confounded by the two very different mechanisms under which each medication can be provided. Virtually all methadone treatment in the United States is provided through OTPs, a centralized and regulated system of care that has limited availability and often has strict rules that emphasize treatment adherence in a very standardized form for patients at a particular clinic. This is a markedly different system of care compared with treatment with buprenorphine, which is available via office-based practices, where treatment is decentralized, can be more individualized, has a higher degree of medical involvement, and may involve fewer counseling services and behavioral interventions compared with an OTP.

Some general conclusions regarding the use of buprenorphine for the treatment of opioid withdrawal can be made. First, longer periods of withdrawal (at least 30 days) are probably more effective than shorter withdrawal periods (Amass et al. 1994; Katz et al. 2009). Second, buprenorphine is superior to clonidine (and buprenorphine is approved for the treatment of OUD in the United States, whereas clonidine is not) and should be the medication of choice when considering which of these two medications to use. This is also the case in the adolescent population (Marsch et al. 2005). It is worth noting here that lofexidine, an α_2 adrenergic agonist like clonidine, is available for use in opioid withdrawal in the United Kingdom but is not available in the United States. There have been a few studies comparing buprenorphine with lofexidine for the treatment of opioid withdrawal, but firm conclusions about relative efficacy of the two medications is probably premature at this time. Finally, the efficacy of buprenorphine compared with methadone for withdrawal has not been well characterized, and this is a topic area that needs to be addressed—both with respect to office-based methadone (versus buprenorphine) treatment and with respect to OTP-delivered buprenorphine (versus methadone) treatment.

EFFICACY OF BUPRENORPHINE FOR OPIOID WITHDRAWAL COMPARED WITH MAINTENANCE TREATMENT OF OUD

Buprenorphine has an overall better profile of efficacy and safety compared with clonidine when used to treat opioid withdrawal. However, if buprenorphine is used simply as a tool to manage withdrawal symptoms and patients are not maintained on it afterward, the outcomes are quite poor (Kakko et al. 2003). For example, in a study that had a 4-week buprenorphine taper, less than 10% of patients had minimal or no opioid use after the buprenorphine taper, whereas nearly 50% had positive outcomes while being maintained with buprenorphine (Weiss et al. 2011). Another interesting finding from this study was that counseling did not have any significant impact on outcomes. For many patients, buprenorphine maintenance is a more effective approach than withdrawal—although it is also worth noting that there are often patients who prefer medically supervised withdrawal rather than maintenance treatment.

Safety and Side Effects of Buprenorphine

Buprenorphine is a safe medication with a relatively unremarkable side effect profile. There have been several areas of potential concern identified in recent years for medications used to treat OUD, and each of these topics will be addressed in this section as it relates to buprenorphine, followed by a summary of the side effects associated with buprenorphine treatment. However, in general, it is important to stress that buprenorphine is safe and effective for the overwhelming majority of patients who take it.

BUPRENORPHINE AND LIVER FUNCTION

A few case reports have shown that very high doses of buprenorphine delivered by intravenous injection can produce an acute increase in serum liver function tests. Prior to buprenorphine's approval in the United States, a retrospective evaluation found slight increases in liver function tests (serum transaminases) when patients with a history of hepatitis C were treated with sublingual buprenorphine (Petry et al. 2000). Subsequently, the FDA-approved label for buprenorphine included a caution regarding liver function. However, clinical experience has generally not supported a particular concern with this potential adverse event. The NIDA Clinical Trials Network conducted a large study looking at buprenorphine's possible effects on liver function and found no evidence of liver damage (Saxon et al. 2013). This suggests that physicians can prescribe buprenorphine without significant concerns of liver injury.

BUPRENORPHINE AND CARDIAC CONDUCTION

The opioid agonist medication LAAM was briefly marketed in the United States and Europe for the treatment of OUD. However, it was withdrawn from the European market because of concerns about cardiac conduction effects, especially prolongation of the QTc interval and the risk of torsades de pointes (a potentially fatal arrhythmia). It was also withdrawn from the U.S. market but at the initiative of the manufacturer, apparently because of poor sales. These experiences with LAAM led to a reappraisal of the potential cardiac effects of other μ agonist opioids. Various reports have examined both methadone and buprenorphine to see if there is evidence of QTc prolongation associated with either of these medications. This is a controversial topic with respect to methadone, with some reports suggesting there may be QTc prolongation with very high doses (although the full clinical meaning of such prolongation is debated). However, of more relevance to this chapter, assessments of buprenorphine have not found evidence that it is associated with prolongation of the QTc interval (Fanoe et al. 2007; Fareed et al. 2013; Kao et al. 2015; Wedam et al. 2007).

PRECIPITATED WITHDRAWAL

A potential adverse effect of sublingual buprenorphine is precipitated opioid withdrawal associated with the first dose. Buprenorphine's partial agonist effects at the μ receptor, as reviewed earlier in this chapter, may produce less effect than is produced by a full agonist opioid. Under the right circumstances, an acute dose of buprenorphine can precipitate an opioid withdrawal syndrome. It is important to note that this is an effect produced by buprenorphine itself, and this phenomenon differs from the precipitated withdrawal produced by naloxone when a BUP/NX tablet is injected (Stoller et al. 2001). Buprenorphine-related precipitated withdrawal can occur in opioid-dependent persons and is associated with the first sublingual dose of the medication. It generally increases in likelihood if the first dose of buprenorphine is high (e.g., 8 mg or greater of sublingual buprenorphine), if the patient has a high level of physical dependence on opioids (e.g., the equivalent of 60 mg or more of daily oral methadone), and/or if there is a short time interval between the last dose of full agonist opioid and the first dose of buprenorphine (e.g., 2 hours since the last dose of the full agonist). Thus, longer time intervals since the last dose of the agonist, lower first doses of buprenorphine, and lower levels of physical dependence decrease the risk of buprenorphine-related precipitated withdrawal. For patients who are thought to be at higher risk for buprenorphine-related precipitated withdrawal (e.g., a patient maintained on 100 mg/day of oral methadone), it may be useful to give small (e.g., 2 mg) repeated doses of buprenorphine every 2 hours rather than a single larger first dose (Rosado et al. 2007). Ideally, the patient should show evidence of early spontaneous opioid withdrawal prior to the first dose of buprenorphine to minimize the risk of precipitating withdrawal. Finally, the risk of buprenorphine-related precipitated withdrawal occurs with the first dose of the medication; once the patient is regularly taking buprenorphine, there is no risk of buprenorphine precipitating withdrawal.

OVERDOSE AND BUPRENORPHINE

Although patients have overdosed on buprenorphine, there does not appear to be the same risk of respiratory depression as seen with overdoses of full agonist opioids (e.g., heroin). The exception to this is when a patient overdoses on bu-prenorphine along with a sedative such as a benzodiazepine. Shortly after bu-prenorphine became available in France, there were reports of patient deaths associated with injection of buprenorphine tablets along with a benzodiazepine such as flunitrazepam, an injectable sedative-hypnotic not available in the United States (Reynaud et al. 1998; Tracqui et al. 1998). However, overdose of buprenorphine alone does not seem to carry the same risk of death. The U.S. label for buprenorphine notes that caution should be used when buprenorphine is used concurrently with a benzodiazepine. This should be viewed as a relative rather than an absolute contraindication because oral benzodiazepines were used with buprenorphine by many patients enrolled in clinical trials prior to ap-proval of buprenorphine, and there were no deaths noted in these studies. The risk for death associated with a buprenorphine-benzodiazepine combination may be greatest when higher doses of both medications are injected or when these medications are combined with alcohol or other sedative-hypnotics.

OTHER SIDE EFFECTS

In addition to the safety and side effect points noted above, there are four other topics that should be addressed briefly when considering buprenorphine: head-ache, constipation, erectile dysfunction, and cognitive functioning/perfor-mance. According to the FDA-approved label for buprenorphine, in a 4-week study that compared buprenorphine with placebo, the most common side effect noted by patients treated with buprenorphine was headache, and the rate of headaches was higher in the BUP/NX (36.4%) and buprenorphine (29.1%) treated groups compared with a placebo group (22.4%). Similarly, rates of re-ported constipation were higher for BUP/NX (12.1%) and buprenorphine (7.8%) treated groups compared with the placebo group (2.8%). However, for both headache and constipation, comparisons with placebo tell only part of the story; it would be helpful to know how buprenorphine compares with another opioid treatment medication such as methadone. There are limited data report-ing on such comparisons, although it appears that differences between bu-prenorphine and methadone for these side effects generally are not markedly different (Lofwall et al. 2005).

Some evidence suggests that there may be higher rates of erectile dysfunc-tion in patients treated with methadone versus buprenorphine (Hallinan et al. 2008; Quaglio et al. 2008). However, it is important to note that studies to date have been based on patients in treatment who have been on nonblind doses of medications, and there are potential confounding features to such analyses that make interpretation of findings somewhat difficult.

Finally, studies of buprenorphine suggest that the doses typically used in the treatment of OUD do not produce impairment in cognitive functioning or performance (Mintzer et al. 2004; Soyka et al. 2001). However, there is some evidence that patients with OUD may fare less well than control subjects on such measures (Soyka et al. 2008).

SUMMARY OF THE SAFETY AND SIDE EFFECTS OF BUPRENORPHINE

On the basis of studies and reports published to date, buprenorphine appears to be a safe medication with no significant or critical side effects. Initial concerns regarding liver impairment with buprenorphine, which resulted in a warning in its label, generally have not been supported. Other effects, such as constipation and headache, are not uncommon for patients treated with opioids and do not appear to be severe. There are notable areas for which there appears to be a lack of effects, including on measures of cognition and performance, on erectile dysfunction, and on measures of cardiac conduction. Although other side effects may yet be identified, the extensive use of buprenorphine to date suggests that if major adverse effects or significant side effects were to occur, they should have been noted by now. The conscientious clinician should remain aware of possible effects noted in this section but should also be reassured that buprenorphine has an overall mild side effect profile.

Future Directions for Buprenorphine Treatment of Opioid Use Disorder

Buprenorphine has been a highly successful addition to the interventions clinicians can use for the treatment of OUD. There are a few future directions related to buprenorphine that will be mentioned briefly here. The first future direction related to buprenorphine is the use of higher doses. At present, studies have generally tested maximum daily doses of 32 mg. Given the dose-response curve for buprenorphine and its safety at higher doses, it is somewhat surprising that the efficacy and safety of doses higher than 32 mg/day have not been tested. Another future direction is the transition off of buprenorphine. There is evidence that outcomes are poor after a shorter course of buprenorphine; however, a prolonged taper over several months has yet to be well addressed. Given the success of this medication, it is probable that there is some proportion of patients maintained on buprenorphine who could transition off of it (e.g., on to the sustained release form of naltrexone). How this can be done optimally needs to be determined, especially for the clinician in an office-based practice. The use of higher doses and the transition off of buprenorphine should be areas of research as this medication continues to become established in clinical use.

Conclusion

Buprenorphine is a novel opioid. Its unique profile of effects makes it very well suited for the treatment of OUD, and research supporting this has been confirmed in its clinical use for the treatment of OUD. Studies have demonstrated its efficacy, showing that it is superior to placebo treatment and comparable to moderate doses of methadone (with the qualification that higher doses of buprenorphine have not been systematically tested for efficacy and safety). In addition to demonstrated efficacy, buprenorphine is also a safe medication with no substantial adverse or significant side effects. This profile of effects makes it well suited for use in office-based treatment, where it has been able to make a substantial impact.

Clinical Pearls

- Buprenorphine is superior to placebo treatment and comparable to moderate doses of methadone for treatment of OUD.

- Buprenorphine is superior to clonidine in managing opioid withdrawal.

- There does not seem to be a significant concern of liver injury or QTc prolongation with buprenorphine.

- For patients who are thought to be at higher risk for buprenorphine-related precipitated withdrawal at the time of medication initiation, it may be useful to give small (e.g., 2 mg) repeated doses of buprenorphine every 2 hours rather than a single larger first dose.

- Buprenorphine does not appear to have the same risk of respiratory depression as seen with overdoses of full agonist opioids; however, there is an increased risk when a patient combines it with a sedative such as a benzodiazepine.

References

Amass L, Bickel WK, Higgins ST, et al: A preliminary investigation of outcome following gradual or rapid buprenorphine detoxification. J Addict Dis 13(3):33–45, 1994 7734458

Amato L, Minozzi S, Davoli M, Vecchi S: Psychosocial and pharmacological treatments versus pharmacological treatments for opioid detoxification. Cochrane Database of Systematic Reviews 2011, Issue 9, Art. No.: CD005031. DOI: 10.1002/14651858.CD005031.pub4

Bickel WK, Stitzer ML, Bigelow GE, et al: Buprenorphine: dose-related blockade of opioid challenge effects in opioid dependent humans. J Pharmacol Exp Ther 247(1):47–53, 1988 2459370

Cheskin LJ, Fudala PJ, Johnson RE: A controlled comparison of buprenorphine and clonidine for acute detoxification from opioids. Drug Alcohol Depend 36(2):115–121, 1994 7851278

Comer SD, Collins ED, Fischman MW: Buprenorphine sublingual tablets: effects on iv heroin self-administration by humans. Psychopharmacology (Berl) 154(1):28–37, 2001 11292003

Comer SD, Walker EA, Collins ED: Buprenorphine/naloxone reduces the reinforcing and subjective effects of heroin in heroin-dependent volunteers. Psychopharmacology (Berl) 181(4):664–675, 2005 16025322

Comer SD, Sullivan MA, Vosburg SK, et al: Abuse liability of intravenous buprenorphine/naloxone and buprenorphine alone in buprenorphine-maintained intravenous heroin abusers. Addiction 105(4):709–718, 2010 20403021

Ebner R, Schreiber W, Zierer C: Buprenorphine or methadone for detoxification of young opioid addicts? [in German]. Psychiatr Prax 31 (suppl 1):S108–S110, 2004 15570521

Fanoe S, Hvidt C, Ege P, et al: Syncope and QT prolongation among patients treated with methadone for heroin dependence in the city of Copenhagen. Heart 93(9):1051–1055, 2007 17344330

Fareed A, Patil D, Scheinberg K, et al: Comparison of QTc interval prolongation for patients in methadone versus buprenorphine maintenance treatment: a 5-year follow-up. J Addict Dis 32(3):244–251, 2013 24074190

Fiellin DA, Pantalon MV, Chawarski MC, et al: Counseling plus buprenorphine-naloxone maintenance therapy for opioid dependence. N Engl J Med 355(4):365–374, 2006 16870915

Fingerhood MI, King VL, Brooner RK, et al: A comparison of characteristics and outcomes of opioid-dependent patients initiating office-based buprenorphine or methadone maintenance treatment. Subst Abus 35(2):122–126, 2014 24821346

Fudala PJ, Bridge TP, Herbert S, et al: Office-based treatment of opiate addiction with a sublingual-tablet formulation of buprenorphine and naloxone. N Engl J Med 349(10):949–958, 2003 12954743

Gowing L, Ali R, White J, Mbewe D: Buprenorphine for the management of opioid withdrawal. Cochrane Database of Systematic Reviews 2017, Issue 2, Art. No.: CD002025. DOI: 10.1002/14651858.CD002025.pub5

Hallinan R, Byrne A, Agho K, et al: Erectile dysfunction in men receiving methadone and buprenorphine maintenance treatment. J Sex Med 5(3):684–692, 2008 18093096

Hussain SS, Farhat S, Rather YH, et al: Comparative trial to study the effectiveness of clonidine hydrochloride and buprenorphine-naloxone in opioid withdrawal—a hospital based study. J Clin Diagn Res 9(1):FC01–FC04, 2015 25738001

Jasinski DR, Pevnick JS, Griffith JD: Human pharmacology and abuse potential of the analgesic buprenorphine: a potential agent for treating narcotic addiction. Arch Gen Psychiatry 35(4):501–516, 1978 215096

Johnson RE, Eissenberg T, Stitzer ML, et al: A placebo controlled clinical trial of buprenorphine as a treatment for opioid dependence. Drug Alcohol Depend 40(1):17–25, 1995 8746920

Jones JD, Sullivan MA, Vosburg SK, et al: Abuse potential of intranasal buprenorphine versus buprenorphine/naloxone in buprenorphine-maintained heroin users. Addict Biol 20(4):784–798, 2015 25060839

Kakko J, Svanborg KD, Kreek MJ, et al: 1-year retention and social function after buprenorphine-assisted relapse prevention treatment for heroin dependence in Sweden: a randomised, placebo-controlled trial. Lancet 361(9358):662–668, 2003 12606177

Kao DP, Haigney MC, Mehler PS, et al: Arrhythmia associated with buprenorphine and methadone reported to the Food and Drug Administration. Addiction 110(9):1468–1475, 2015 26075588

Katz EC, Schwartz RP, King S, et al: Brief vs. extended buprenorphine detoxification in a community treatment program: engagement and short-term outcomes. Am J Drug Alcohol Abuse 35(2):63–67, 2009 19199166

Krook AL, Brørs O, Dahlberg J, et al: A placebo-controlled study of high dose buprenorphine in opiate dependents waiting for medication-assisted rehabilitation in Oslo, Norway. Addiction 97(5):533–542, 2002 12033654

Krupitsky E, Nunes EV, Ling W, et al: Injectable extended-release naltrexone for opioid dependence: a double-blind, placebo-controlled, multicentre randomised trial. Lancet 377(9776):1506–1513, 2011 21529928

Kunøe N, Opheim A, Solli KK, et al: Design of a randomized controlled trial of extended-release naltrexone versus daily buprenorphine-naloxone for opioid dependence in Norway (NTX-SBX). BMC Pharmacol Toxicol 17(1):18, 2016 27121539

Ling W, Charuvastra C, Collins JF, et al: Buprenorphine maintenance treatment of opiate dependence: a multicenter, randomized clinical trial. Addiction 93(4):475–486, 1998 9684386

Ling W, Amass L, Shoptaw S, et al: A multi-center randomized trial of buprenorphine-naloxone versus clonidine for opioid detoxification: findings from the National Institute on Drug Abuse Clinical Trials Network. Addiction 100(8):1090–1100, 2005 16042639

Lofwall MR, Stitzer ML, Bigelow GE, Strain EC: Comparative safety and side effect profiles of buprenorphine and methadone in the outpatient treatment of opioid dependence. Addict Disord Their Treat 4(2):49–64, 2005

Marsch LA, Bickel WK, Badger GJ, et al: Comparison of pharmacological treatments for opioid-dependent adolescents: a randomized controlled trial. Arch Gen Psychiatry 62(10):1157–1164, 2005 16203961

Mattick RP, Breen C, Kimber J, Davoli M: Buprenorphine maintenance versus placebo or methadone maintenance for opioid dependence. Cochrane Database of Systematic Reviews 2014, Issue 2, Art. No.: CD002207. DOI: 10.1002/14651858.CD002207.pub4

Mello NK, Mendelson JH: Buprenorphine suppresses heroin use by heroin addicts. Science 207(4431):657–659, 1980 7352279

Mintzer MZ, Correia CJ, Strain EC: A dose-effect study of repeated administration of buprenorphine/naloxone on performance in opioid-dependent volunteers. Drug Alcohol Depend 74(2):205–209, 2004 15099664

Mokri A, Chawarski MC, Taherinakhost H, et al: Medical treatments for opioid use disorder in Iran: a randomized, double-blind placebo-controlled comparison of buprenorphine/naloxone and naltrexone maintenance treatment. Addiction 111(5):874–882, 2016 26639678

Nasser AF, Greenwald MK, Vince B, et al: Sustained-release buprenorphine (RBP-6000) blocks the effects of opioid challenge with hydromorphone in subjects with opioid use disorder. J Clin Psychopharmacol 36(1):18–26, 2016 26650971

Parran TV, Adelman CA, Merkin B, et al: Long-term outcomes of office-based buprenorphine/naloxone maintenance therapy. Drug Alcohol Depend 106(1):56–60, 2010 19717249

Petry NM, Bickel WK, Piasecki D, et al: Elevated liver enzyme levels in opioid-dependent patients with hepatitis treated with buprenorphine. Am J Addict 9(3):265–269, 2000 11000922

Quaglio G, Lugoboni F, Pattaro C, et al: Erectile dysfunction in male heroin users, receiving methadone and buprenorphine maintenance treatment. Drug Alcohol Depend 94(1–3):12–18, 2008 18083312

Reynaud M, Petit G, Potard D, et al: Six deaths linked to concomitant use of buprenorphine and benzodiazepines. Addiction 93(9):1385–1392, 1998 9926544

Rosado J, Walsh SL, Bigelow GE, et al: Sublingual buprenorphine/naloxone precipitated withdrawal in subjects maintained on 100mg of daily methadone. Drug Alcohol Depend 90(2–3):261–269, 2007 17517480

Rosenthal RN, Lofwall MR, Kim S, et al: Effect of buprenorphine implants on illicit opioid use among abstinent adults with opioid dependence treated with sublingual buprenorphine: a randomized clinical trial. JAMA 316(3):282–290, 2016 27434441

Saxon AJ, Ling W, Hillhouse M, et al: Buprenorphine/naloxone and methadone effects on laboratory indices of liver health: a randomized trial. Drug Alcohol Depend 128(1–2):71–76, 2013 22921476

Schottenfeld RS, Chawarski MC, Mazlan M: Maintenance treatment with buprenorphine and naltrexone for heroin dependence in Malaysia: a randomised, double-blind, placebo-controlled trial. Lancet 371(9631):2192–2200, 2008 18586174

Seifert J, Metzner C, Paetzold W, et al: Detoxification of opiate addicts with multiple drug abuse: a comparison of buprenorphine vs. methadone. Pharmacopsychiatry 35(5):159–164, 2002 12237786

Soyka M, Horak M, Dittert S, et al: Less driving impairment on buprenorphine than methadone in drug-dependent patients? J Neuropsychiatry Clin Neurosci 13(4):527–528, 2001 11748323

Soyka M, Lieb M, Kagerer S, et al: Cognitive functioning during methadone and buprenorphine treatment: results of a randomized clinical trial. J Clin Psychopharmacol 28(6):699–703, 2008 19011441

Stoller KB, Bigelow GE, Walsh SL, et al: Effects of buprenorphine/naloxone in opioid-dependent humans. Psychopharmacology (Berl) 154(3):230–242, 2001 11351930

Strain EC, Walsh SL, Preston KL, et al: The effects of buprenorphine in buprenorphine-maintained volunteers. Psychopharmacology (Berl) 129(4):329–338, 1997 9085402

Strain EC, Walsh SL, Bigelow GE: Blockade of hydromorphone effects by buprenorphine/naloxone and buprenorphine. Psychopharmacology (Berl) 159(2):161–166, 2002 11862344

Strain EC, Moody DE, Stoller KB, et al: Relative bioavailability of different buprenorphine formulations under chronic dosing conditions. Drug Alcohol Depend 74(1):37–43, 2004 15072805

Tracqui A, Kintz P, Ludes B: Buprenorphine-related deaths among drug addicts in France: a report on 20 fatalities. J Anal Toxicol 22(6):430–434, 1998 9788517

Walsh SL, Comer SD, Lofwall MR, et al: Effect of buprenorphine weekly depot (CAM2038) and hydromorphone blockade in individuals with opioid use disorder: a randomized clinical trial. JAMA Psychiatry June 22, 2017 [Epub ahead of print] 28655025

Wedam EF, Bigelow GE, Johnson RE, et al: QT-interval effects of methadone, levo-methadyl, and buprenorphine in a randomized trial. Arch Intern Med 167(22):2469–2475, 2007 18071169

Weiss RD, Potter JS, Fiellin DA, et al: Adjunctive counseling during brief and extended buprenorphine-naloxone treatment for prescription opioid dependence: a 2-phase randomized controlled trial. Arch Gen Psychiatry 68(12):1238–1246, 2011 22065255

Ziaaddini H, Nasirian M, Nakhaee N: Comparison of the efficacy of buprenorphine and clonidine in detoxification of opioid-dependents. Addict Health 4(3–4):79–86, 2012 24494140

Ziedonis DM, Amass L, Steinberg M, et al: Predictors of outcome for short-term medically supervised opioid withdrawal during a randomized, multicenter trial of buprenorphine-naloxone and clonidine in the NIDA clinical trials network drug and alcohol dependence. Drug Alcohol Depend 99(1–3):28–36, 2009 18805656

4

Patient Assessment

Petros Levounis, M.D., M.A.
Jonathan Avery, M.D.

THE ASSESSMENT of a patient for buprenorphine treatment is essentially the same as the assessment of any patient with a substance use disorder. In this chapter, we describe the complete evaluation of a patient and cover a broad range of issues that may impact addiction treatment. Everyday clinical practice often dictates a symptom-focused evaluation, and treating patients with buprenorphine is not an exception. For example, we include a brief discussion of physical examination as part of a complete patient assessment. However, the majority of psychiatrists do not routinely conduct physical examinations; typically, they collaborate with internists and other primary care physicians who cover this aspect of the patient's medical care. Treating patients with buprenorphine should not change your way of evaluating your patients and managing your practice.

Establishing a Relationship

When the clinician is interviewing a patient who has an opioid use disorder (OUD), a matter-of-fact, nonjudgmental, and respectful approach works best. Many patients have been discriminated against or mistreated because of their substance use disorder. Understandably, they may be mistrustful of clinicians and may not be eager to talk about events and activities that are embarrassing and often illegal. Open the interview by asking about the patient's level of comfort. For example, you may want to say, "How are you feeling?" "Are you feeling any withdrawal symptoms?" "When was the last time you used any opioids?" This approach helps to establish you as considerate and compassionate and may influence how likely the patient will be to retain information you give—as well as how likely he or she will be to open up about sensitive problems and to return to your office. Establishing a trusting and secure relationship is one of the most powerful elements of successful addiction treatment and is critical in the management of any chronic relapsing disorder (Najavits and Weiss 1994).

Recognize that some information is difficult to talk about and acknowledge the patient's discomfort. For example, at some point you may say, "You seemed to get quiet when I asked that." Assure confidentiality and tell the patient that you are asking because you are concerned for his or her health. We have found that being genuinely interested and curious about your patient's life provides the most powerful means of smoothing out awkward feelings and allowing your patient to open up about his or her drug history. Using curiosity as your primary approach to the patient also helps you persist in getting full answers to difficult questions and following up on qualified answers. For example, if the answer to the question "Have you ever injected heroin?" is "Not really," you may then ask the patient to tell you all about the last time he or she injected. In some cases, it may be easier to lead with assumptive questions, such as "When was the last time you injected heroin?"

Taking a History of Drug Use

THE BASICS

Patients who use heroin and/or prescription opioids often use other substances as well. When taking a drug history, inquire about both legal and illegal substances. Asking specifically about each class of drugs, as well as about each possible source such as dealers, friends and family, prescriptions, the Internet, herbal stores, and over-the-counter medications can give surprising and valuable results. For each drug, you should gather information about 1) frequency of use, 2) amount used, 3) route of administration, 4) acute response to the effects of the drug, and 5) changes in use over time. Typically, start with questions about legal drugs (nicotine, alcohol, prescription pills) and then progress to illegal drugs (e.g., cannabis, heroin, hallucinogens, cocaine, and crystal methamphetamine). Patients are less likely to be defensive when describing their use of legal drugs, and the discussion may then progress more easily into areas associated with illegal drugs and illegal activities. Another way of obtaining the drug history is to start with the first psychoactive agent used and work chronologically through the patient's experience with substances of abuse. Either way, information about the most recent use, including use in the weeks and days just before the assessment, is likely to be the most helpful in evaluating the patient for buprenorphine treatment. In general, assumptive, open-ended questions generate more detailed and productive information. For example, you may ask, "How are things at home since you started drinking regularly?" or "What has been going on in your life since you lost your job?"

Opioids are abused by all routes of administration, including intravenous, oral, inhalation (snorting), smoking, subcutaneous (skin "popping"), and intramuscular routes. Heroin is often used intravenously, but in recent years more and more people inhale heroin. This shift in the pattern of use may be due to the AIDS epidemic and the associated danger of infection from contaminated needles. It also may be due to the increase in the purity of heroin, which is now potent enough to give the user an adequate "high" even if it is inhaled and not injected. Prescription opioids are typically taken orally but may also be snorted, chewed, or crushed and injected. Pills are crushed to circumvent the mechanism that delays the release of the active ingredients in long-acting formulations such as OxyContin (an acrylic-coated formulation of oxycodone). See Table 4–1 for a list of the most commonly abused opioids and Table 4–2 for other commonly abused substances.

Family participation in the evaluation is ideal but often not an option. Patients often have been cut off from contact with their loved ones because of their substance use disorders. However, when family members come to the office, they tend to offer very useful information and insights into the patient's illness. They also can become great allies in carrying out the patient's treatment plan, helping him or her both logistically and emotionally, and can act as your liaison in the patient's home.

CONSEQUENCES

Almost all patients who misuse opioids have experienced opioid withdrawal at some point in their lives. Although they are very familiar with the actual symptoms and consequences of intoxication and withdrawal, they may not be familiar with the medical terms, and these should be explained. It also may be necessary to explain to the patient what is meant by tolerance—that is, that with time, greater amounts of the drug are needed to achieve the same effect, or there is a diminished effect from the same amount of the drug.

Asking the patient about the different consequences of his or her use is useful in two ways. First, it helps paint a multidimensional picture of the patient's life and thus establish past and current levels of psychosocial functioning. Second, and perhaps more important, it helps the patient identify losses in his or her life, which may increase motivation for change. We often review five areas of consequences of drug use with patients:

TABLE 4–1.   **Commonly abused opioids**

Diacetylmorphine (heroin)

Codeine

Oxycodone (OxyContin, Percodan, Percocet, Tylox)

Hydrocodone (Vicodin, Lortab)

Morphine (MS Contin, Oramorph)

Hydromorphone (Dilaudid)

Meperidine (Demerol)

Fentanyl (Sublimaze, Actiq)

Propoxyphene (Darvon)

Methadone (Dolophine)

Opium

Kratom (leaves of *Mitragyna speciosa*)

TABLE 4–2.   **Other commonly abused substances**

Nicotine

Alcohol

Benzodiazepines

Cocaine

Methamphetamine (crystal meth)

Cannabis

Phencyclidine (PCP)

"Club drugs" (ecstasy, ketamine, γ-hydroxy-butyrate)

Emerging drugs of abuse (e.g., synthetic cathinones, synthetic cannabinoids, *Salvia divinorum*)

Noncontrolled substances (e.g., clonidine, dextromethorphan)

1. *Medical consequences* may include hepatitis C, HIV infection, and other infections (e.g., endocarditis, abscesses), as well as injuries from falls and burns secondary to intoxication. Medical comorbidities are discussed further in Chapter 11, "Medical Comorbidity."
2. *Psychiatric consequences* may include opioid-induced depression, sexual dysfunction, and sleep disorders. Although opioids are less likely to result in symptoms of mental illness than are most other drugs of abuse, differentiating between substance-induced and independent psychiatric disorders can be challenging. This topic is discussed further in Chapter 10, "Psychiatric Comorbidity."
3. *Interpersonal and family consequences* may include separation or divorce and estrangement from parents, siblings, and children.
4. *Financial and employment consequences* may include bankruptcy, loss of job, and loss of a professional license.
5. *Legal consequences* may include arrests for driving under the influence (DUI) or driving while intoxicated (DWI), incarceration, parole or probation, and loss of custody of children.

PREVIOUS TREATMENTS AND RECOVERY EFFORTS

Before getting into the patient's previous medical treatments, the clinician needs to know whether the patient has tried to stop using by himself or herself. Frequently, people with OUDs have tried to quit on their own, often with the help of home products and over-the-counter medications such as antidiarrheal agents and sleeping aids, with buprenorphine or methadone bought off the street, or with no pharmacological help at all, that is, going "cold turkey." (The expression "cold turkey" comes from the piloerection and characteristic clammy appearance of the skin during opioid withdrawal.) If this is the case, ask what happened. Ask about the severity and duration of any withdrawal symptoms and how the patient expects to feel differently with medical treatment.

Some patients also may have a history of involvement with mutual help groups, which are sometimes called self-help groups or 12-step groups, such as Alcoholics Anonymous and Narcotics Anonymous. Finding out how long the patient has been attending meetings and how many meetings he or she attends each week can give you an indication of the patient's motivation for treatment. If the patient has been attending mutual help meetings consistently, has formally joined a group, and has a sponsor, then he or she is more likely to be committed to the recovery process.

Reviewing with the patient previous medical treatments typically involves the following four areas:

1. *Management of the withdrawal syndrome,* which includes inpatient hospital admissions and outpatient community-based programs

2. *Rehabilitation* in 28-day or other residential treatment facilities
3. *Outpatient counseling* or psychotherapy
4. *Long-term pharmacotherapy*, which includes maintenance with methadone (a μ opioid receptor agonist), maintenance with buprenorphine (a μ opioid receptor partial agonist), or treatment with oral or extended-release injectable naltrexone (a μ opioid receptor antagonist).

You also may ask the patient about his or her longest period of abstinence, how it was attained, and what worked to sustain it. Inquiring about drug cravings and triggers to relapse (including emotions, people, places, and things) helps the patient remember the major obstacles to sobriety. The review of triggers signals to the patient that serious effort will be required to identify, avoid, and cope with these powerful culprits of drug relapse. It also alerts the clinician to the patient's specific vulnerabilities that will need to be addressed in a comprehensive treatment plan (see Chapter 5, "Clinical Use of Buprenorphine").

MNEMONIC FOR TAKING HISTORY OF DRUG USE

One way to keep in mind the different elements of taking a history of drug use is by remembering the acronym TRAPPED (Welsh 2003), which stands for the following:

- Treatment history (inpatient, outpatient; methadone, buprenorphine, naltrexone)
- Route of administration (intravenous, intranasal, intramuscular)
- Amount (in dollars, "bags," or milligrams)
- Pattern of use (changes over time)
- Prior abstinence (with or without medical help)
- Effects (medical, psychiatric, psychosocial)
- Duration of use (including most recent use)

MEDICAL, PSYCHIATRIC, FAMILY, AND PSYCHOSOCIAL HISTORY

Apart from the direct medical consequences of drug use discussed earlier in this chapter, the medical history also includes significant acute and chronic medical illnesses as well as operations, allergies, and current medications. The inventory of current medications should list not only medications prescribed to the patient but also medications prescribed to others (often family members or friends) that the patient may be taking from others' medicine cabinets and prescription medications that the patient may be buying on the street. This list also should include over-the-counter preparations, dietary supplements, and herbal pills.

TABLE 4–3. **The stages of change**

1. Pre-contemplation—"I don't have a problem. Why should I quit?"

2. Contemplation—"Someday, I may want to think about quitting."

3. Preparation (Determination)—"I'm seriously planning to quit in the next few weeks."

4. Action—"I have just stopped using and work hard to stay clean."

5. Maintenance—"I have been sober for several months."

The psychiatric history consists of the review of psychiatric hospitalizations, outpatient treatments, and psychiatric medications. Be sure to inquire about treatment delivered by nonpsychiatrists, such as a primary care physician who prescribes an antidepressant or a psychologist who provides psychotherapy. Chapter 10 discusses psychiatric assessment in detail.

It is well established that both substance use disorders and other psychiatric conditions such as depression, schizophrenia, and bipolar disorder have significant genetic components. A detailed family history therefore contributes valuable information to aid in our understanding of the patient's vulnerabilities and helps us distinguish between a primary psychiatric disorder and a substance-induced psychiatric disorder (Pickens and Svikis 1988).

The psychosocial history, sometimes also referred to as personal history, completes the comprehensive history portion of the patient assessment. It consists of gathering information about the patient's childhood development, education, employment, military service, physical or sexual abuse, run-ins with the law, spouse or partner, children, housing and living situation, and religion and spirituality. Several elements of the psychosocial history have already been covered in this chapter, given that addiction tends to interfere with—and often destroy—many aspects of a person's life.

MOTIVATION FOR CHANGE

According to the Transtheoretical Model of Change developed by Prochaska and DiClemente (1982), patients have different levels of motivation for changing their substance use. The five stages of change are listed in Table 4–3. Although many patients seem to progress sequentially through the stages of change from pre-contemplation to maintenance, clinicians often treat patients who skip stages or sometimes go back to an earlier stage despite considerable early gains toward motivation for sobriety. For example, a patient may be working hard on the action stage of change, during which he or she may be attending meetings and taking medication; however, a slip with heroin use may severely disappoint and discourage the patient, who may then experience a setback and return to the contemplation stage: "Do I really want to stop using? Maybe I'm meant to be a heroin addict and I should just accept it." Most patients—and, in fact, most people—are ambivalent about change. Ambivalence is a normal part of the human experience, not a defect of will as people once thought. We also now know that exploring people's ambivalence is a critical element in enhancing their motivation.

Individuals progress through the stages of change in numerous ways and use many strategies, and Miller and Rollnick's (2013) work on motivational interviewing throughout the years has provided clinicians with an evidence-based way to aid patients in this process. The motivational interviewing approach is an empathic and supportive interviewing style that helps individuals resolve ambivalence toward making change by increasing intrinsic motivation for change. Every interaction—including the assessment phase—aims to actively engage individuals in their treatment.

It is important to remember, however, that an additional stage of change may be relapse. With addiction being a chronic relapsing illness, it is reasonable to expect that some patients will relapse. Relapse is part of the natural history of the illness and of the recovery process, and as such it plays a significant role in the progression of a person through the change cycle. Patients who relapse typically reenter the stages of change at the contemplation level and may progress more rapidly during subsequent treatment (Levounis et al. 2017).

Physical Examination

The physical examination is particularly helpful in identifying and caring for the intravenous drug user. Needle marks and sclerosed veins (track marks) on the upper extremities, secondary to chronic heroin injecting, can be concealed easily by long-sleeved shirts but become apparent on physical examination. Skin infections can lead to cellulitis and abscesses that, unless they are discovered and treated in a timely fashion, may progress to even more serious conditions. Furthermore, the physical examination is essential in the medical treatment of the patient who also has hepatitis C and/or HIV infection.

Physical examination is also helpful in identifying the presence and severity of opioid intoxication (e.g., constricted pupils) and opioid withdrawal (e.g., dilated pupils). Sinusitis and chronic cough are also consistent with chronic opioid use. Basic assessment and management of the patient with OUD and co-occurring medical illnesses are discussed in Chapter 11.

Laboratory Examination

Certain laboratory test results can raise the clinician's level of suspicion of alcohol and drug misuse. Abnormal liver function test results (especially an elevated aspartate transaminase to alanine transaminase ratio and an elevated γ-glutamyl-transferase level), elevated red blood cell mean corpuscular volume, and carbohydrate-deficient transferrin are all associated with alcohol use disorder. Antibodies to HIV, hepatitis B virus, and hepatitis C virus may indicate intravenous drug use.

Urine toxicology examinations (UTs) are helpful in the evaluation and treatment of the substance-abusing patient. Heroin and codeine metabolize into morphine, which is the substance detected in urine. Codeine metabolizes into morphine slowly, so it can be present as either codeine or morphine (or both) in urine. However, heroin (diacetylmorphine) is never found in urine because it hydrolyzes very quickly to morphine. Occasionally, the intermediate product in this hydrolysis, 6-monoacetylmorphine (6-MAM), is transiently detected in urine, and the test for this is sometimes used in forensic settings. If urine is positive for 6-MAM, the patient certainly used heroin; however, if 6-MAM detection is negative, then the test gives no information about heroin use. Routine UTs for opioids typically test only for morphine and codeine, so tests for semisynthetic or synthetic opioids such as oxycodone, hydrocodone, hydromorphone, and fentanyl often have to be ordered separately. UTs also test for cocaine, benzodiazepines, and cannabis, but if the patient uses such substances sporadically, he or she may not have used near the time of sample collection and the result may be negative (see Chapter 5).

Detecting drugs in hair, saliva, and sweat samples has attracted great attention as alternatives to UTs. However, the current clinical usefulness of these methods is limited, and they are used primarily in experimental settings.

Diagnosis

The *Diagnostic and Statistical Manual of Mental Disorders*, 5th Edition (DSM-5; American Psychiatric Association 2013) provides detailed criteria for establishing the diagnosis of a substance use disorder. All of the DSM-5 substance use disorders require clinically significant impairment or distress and the presence of at least two physical, psychological, or social consequences of the drug use. DSM-5 includes several specifiers to further characterize the substance use disorders; these specifiers relate mostly to *course* (e.g., early remission, sustained remission) and *severity* (based on the number of criteria endorsed). For OUD, there is also a specifier to indicate whether or not the individual is on maintenance therapy. (Please see Box 4–1 for the criteria for OUD.) DSM-5 also provides diagnostic criteria for clinical presentations that are directly related to substance use, such as intoxication and withdrawal, along with descriptive specifiers. Although this is the formal language, it is important to note that other terms, including *substance dependence* and *substance abuse* (from older editions of DSM) and *substance addiction*, are commonly used.

Box 4–1.   DSM-5 Diagnostic Criteria for Opioid Use Disorder

A. A problematic pattern of opioid use leading to clinically significant impairment or distress, as manifested by at least two of the following, occurring within a 12-month period:

1. Opioids are often taken in larger amounts or over a longer period than was intended.
2. There is a persistent desire or unsuccessful efforts to cut down or control opioid use.
3. A great deal of time is spent in activities necessary to obtain the opioid, use the opioid, or recover from its effects.
4. Craving, or a strong desire or urge to use opioids.
5. Recurrent opioid use resulting in a failure to fulfill major role obligations at work, school, or home.
6. Continued opioid use despite having persistent or recurrent social or interpersonal problems caused or exacerbated by the effects of opioids.
7. Important social, occupational, or recreational activities are given up or reduced because of opioid use.
8. Recurrent opioid use in situations in which it is physically hazardous.
9. Continued opioid use despite knowledge of having a persistent or recurrent physical or psychological problem that is likely to have been caused or exacerbated by the substance.
10. Tolerance, as defined by either of the following:
    a. A need for markedly increased amounts of opioids to achieve intoxication or desired effect.
    b. A markedly diminished effect with continued use of the same amount of an opioid.
    Note: This criterion is not considered to be met for those taking opioids solely under appropriate medical supervision.
11. Withdrawal, as manifested by either of the following:
    a. The characteristic opioid withdrawal syndrome (refer to Criteria A and B of the criteria set for opioid withdrawal, [DSM-5] pp. 547–548).
    b. Opioids (or a closely related substance) are taken to relieve or avoid withdrawal symptoms.
    Note: This criterion is not considered to be met for those individuals taking opioids solely under appropriate medical supervision.
    Specify if:
    In early remission: After full criteria for opioid use disorder were previously met, none of the criteria for opioid use disorder have been met

for at least 3 months but for less than 12 months (with the exception that Criterion A4, "Craving, or a strong desire or urge to use opioids," may be met).

In sustained remission: After full criteria for opioid use disorder were previously met, none of the criteria for opioid use disorder have been met at any time during a period of 12 months or longer (with the exception that Criterion A4, "Craving, or a strong desire or urge to use opioids," may be met).

Specify if:

On maintenance therapy: This additional specifier is used if the individual is taking a prescribed agonist medication such as methadone or buprenorphine and none of the criteria for opioid use disorder have been met for that class of medication (except tolerance to, or withdrawal from, the agonist). This category also applies to those individuals being maintained on a partial agonist, an agonist/antagonist, or a full antagonist such as oral naltrexone or depot naltrexone.

In a controlled environment: This additional specifier is used if the individual is in an environment where access to opioids is restricted.

Coding based on current severity: Note for ICD-10-CM codes: If an opioid intoxication, opioid withdrawal, or another opioid-induced mental disorder is also present, do not use the codes below for opioid use disorder. Instead, the comorbid opioid use disorder is indicated in the 4th character of the opioid-induced disorder code (see the coding note for opioid intoxication, opioid withdrawal, or a specific opioid-induced mental disorder). For example, if there is comorbid opioid-induced depressive disorder and opioid use disorder, only the opioid-induced depressive disorder code is given, with the 4th character indicating whether the comorbid opioid use disorder is mild, moderate, or severe: F11.14 for mild opioid use disorder with opioid-induced depressive disorder or F11.24 for a moderate or severe opioid use disorder with opioid-induced depressive disorder.

Specify current severity:

305.50 (F11.10) **Mild:** Presence of 2–3 symptoms.

304.00 (F11.20) **Moderate:** Presence of 4–5 symptoms.

304.00 (F11.20) **Severe:** Presence of 6 or more symptoms.

Source. Reprinted from American Psychiatric Association: *Diagnostic and Statistical Manual of Mental Disorders*, 5th Edition, Arlington, VA, American Psychiatric Association, 2013. Copyright © 2013 American Psychiatric Association. Used with permission.

Buprenorphine Versus Methadone: Regulatory Criteria and Limitations

The regulatory criteria for the use of buprenorphine differ from the criteria for methadone use in the treatment of OUD. Although buprenorphine can be prescribed to anyone age 16 years and older who currently meets criteria for OUD, methadone treatment requires that patients be at least 18 years old, currently meet criteria for OUD, and have been addicted for at least 1 year before admission to treatment.

Buprenorphine for the treatment of OUD can be prescribed at the office or clinic of any physician who has a valid waiver from the U.S. Drug Enforcement Administration. In comparison, methadone for the treatment of OUD can be administered only at a federally approved and regulated clinic, an opioid treatment program (OTP) facility. (OTPs are increasingly offering buprenorphine as a treatment options as well.) This difference gives buprenorphine a tremendous practical and social advantage. Clinicians can now provide mainstream treatment for opioid addiction as part of their everyday practice, and patients can address their substance use problems within the privacy and comfort of the patient-clinician relationship.

On the other hand, methadone treatment in an OTP facility, which requires daily attendance for at least the first several months of treatment, may be best for patients who require a highly structured environment. For example, patients who have multiple substance use disorders and/or other psychiatric conditions that require more comprehensive care usually benefit from the daily encounters, monitoring, services, and routines of an OTP (Schottenfeld et al. 2005). In general, methadone treatment in an OTP may be more appropriate than buprenorphine in an office-based treatment practice for patients who are less stable and less motivated, with a lower level of functioning and a higher need for psychosocial supports. Table 4–4 summarizes the selection considerations for selecting office-based buprenorphine treatment versus OTP-based methadone treatment.

Another option that has recently become more widely available is buprenorphine treatment provided in an OTP. This may be the best choice for a patient who prefers buprenorphine to methadone but may not have the stability required for office-based buprenorphine treatment. Some patients are most successful when they begin buprenorphine treatment in the highly structured environment of an OTP and then move to an office-based clinic or private office when they are psychiatrically, socially, and medically ready for the transition.

Going forward, other formulations of buprenorphine, including the recently approved buprenorphine implant Probuphine, may be an option for individuals with OUD. Such formulations may provide long-term, consistent treatment for individuals (Sigmon and Bigelow 2017).

TABLE 4–4.   Selection considerations: buprenorphine vs. methadone

	Buprenorphine in office-based treatment	Methadone in an opioid treatment program
Criteria	Current diagnosis of OUD	Current diagnosis and 1 year history of OUD
Age	16 years and older	18 years and older
Reliability	Higher	Lower
Motivation	Higher	Lower
Social needs	Lower	Higher
Level of function	Higher	Lower

Note.   OUD = opioid use disorder.

Certain individuals may not be appropriate for or want treatment with buprenorphine or methadone. This may be because of issues ranging from medical comorbidities to patient preference to issues with noncompliance to inability to use opioid replacement treatment because of work regulations. Naltrexone, especially extended-release injectable naltrexone, may be appropriate for these individuals (see Chapter 9, "Methadone, Naltrexone, and Naloxone") (Gastfriend 2011). Other individuals will attempt to use various psychosocial treatments (e.g., 12-step groups, cognitive-behavioral therapy) without medications, although the evidence for nonpharmacological approaches to OUD is poor, and these approaches may not have a significant impact on outcome (Levounis 2015).

Appropriateness of Office-Based Buprenorphine Treatment

The majority of patients who have an OUD should be considered for treatment with buprenorphine. Specifically, the risks and benefits of buprenorphine therapy should be balanced against the alternatives of nontreatment or other forms of treatment (Fishman et al. 2010). Although several pharmacological and nonpharmacological interventions (methadone and naltrexone, cognitive-behavioral therapy, and 12-step facilitation; see Chapter 5) have been shown to be useful, buprenorphine is recommended as a first-line treatment of OUD because of its efficacy, safety, and tolerability profile (see Chapter 3, "Efficacy and Safety of Buprenorphine"). A patient should be considered an appropriate candidate for treatment with buprenorphine under the following conditions (Gordon et al. 2007; Kraus et al. 2011):

- The patient meets criteria for the diagnosis of OUD
- The patient is interested in office-based treatment of his or her illness
- The patient understands the risks and benefits (as well as the induction requirements) of the medication
- The patient demonstrates motivation for change

Multiple studies have shown that buprenorphine treatment is successful in a wide variety of office practices and clinics (Barry et al. 2009; Fiellin et al. 2008; Kraus et al. 2011; Schuckit 2016). The decision to initiate buprenorphine treatment for a patient at your setting also depends on how well your resources match the patient's needs. For example, a patient who has multiple and significant medical problems may be better served in a medical office that offers buprenorphine treatment than in a private psychiatric office. Conversely, a patient who has borderline personality disorder may not be treated as successfully by a clinician who is not trained in psychiatry. If the patient has a significant chronic pain syndrome as well as an OUD, then medication management may be best addressed in a pain management specialist's office. If the patient has a significant benzodiazepine use disorder and is taking high-dose benzodiazepines, buprenorphine may not be the best option given the risk of respiratory suppression, and the patient may be served better by initially completing medically assisted withdrawal for benzodiazepines. And if the patient's severity of addiction requires a higher level of care, such as an intensive outpatient program or partial hospitalization, then referral to an addiction treatment center or an OTP (as discussed in the previous section, "Buprenorphine Versus Methadone: Regulatory Criteria and Limitations") may be indicated.

Conclusion

Several factors improve the chances for successful office-based treatment. The ideal buprenorphine candidate adheres to the treatment plans, is medically and psychiatrically healthy, lives in a stable and supportive psychosocial environment, attends mutual help meetings regularly, does not use alcohol or other drugs, and does not have a history of multiple previous treatments and relapses. Very few patients will meet these criteria, however, and the question the clinician should be asking is not whether one patient is a better buprenorphine candidate than another patient but whether a particular individual will be better off with or without buprenorphine treatment. If your practice is suitable for the patient and you have access to additional resources (e.g., a medical specialist or an intensive outpatient program), then office-based buprenorphine treatment is one of the very best options you can offer to your patient with OUD.

Clinical Pearls

* Assess your patients for buprenorphine therapy the same way you assess all your patients.

* Explore the patient's motivation and identify his or her stage of change.

* Establish the diagnosis of OUD using the DSM-5 criteria.

* Regard buprenorphine as your first-line treatment of OUD but also consider other pharmacological and nonpharmacological options.

References

American Psychiatric Association: Diagnostic and Statistical Manual of Mental Disorders, 5th Edition. Arlington, VA, American Psychiatric Association, 2013

Barry DT, Irwin KS, Jones ES, et al: Integrating buprenorphine treatment into office-based practice: a qualitative study. J Gen Intern Med 24(2):218–225, 2009 19089500

Fiellin DA, Moore BA, Sullivan LE, et al: Long-term treatment with buprenorphine/naloxone in primary care: results at 2–5 years. Am J Addict 17(2):116–120, 2008 18393054

Fishman MJ, Shulman GR, Mee-Lee D, et al: ASAM Patient Placement Criteria: Supplement on Pharmacotherapies for Alcohol Use Disorders. Baltimore, MD, Lippincott Williams and Wilkins, 2010

Gastfriend DR: Intramuscular extended-release naltrexone: current evidence. Ann NY Acad Sci 1216:144–166, 2011 21272018

Gordon AJ, Trafton JA, Saxon AJ, et al: Implementation of buprenorphine in the Veterans Health Administration: results of the first 3 years. Drug Alcohol Depend 90(2–3):292–296, 2007 17493771

Kraus ML, Alford DP, Kotz MM, et al: Statement of the American Society Of Addiction Medicine Consensus Panel on the use of buprenorphine in office-based treatment of opioid addiction. J Addict Med 5(4):254–263, 2011 22042215

Levounis P: Is pharmacotherapy ever "all you need" to stay sober? Psychiatry News, July 17, 2015. Available at: http://psychnews.psychiatryonline.org/doi/full/10.1176/appi.pn.2015.PP7b7. Accessed August 7, 2017.

Levounis P, Arnaout B, Marienfeld C (eds): Motivational Interviewing for Clinical Practice. Arlington, VA, American Psychiatric Association Publishing, 2017

Miller WR, Rollnick S: Motivational Interviewing: Helping People Change, 3rd Edition. New York, Guilford, 2013

Najavits LM, Weiss RD: Variations in therapist effectiveness in the treatment of patients with substance use disorders: an empirical review. Addiction 89(6):679–688, 1994 8069169

Pickens RW, Svikis DS (eds): Biological Vulnerability to Drug Abuse. National Institute on Drug Abuse Research Monograph 89 (DHHS Publ No ADM 90-1590). Rockville, MD, National Institute on Drug Abuse, 1988. Available at http://archives.drugabuse.gov/pdf/monographs/89.pdf. Accessed July 1, 2010.

Prochaska JO, DiClemente CC: Transtheoretical therapy: towards a more integrative model of change. Psychotherapy 19(3):276–288, 1982

Schottenfeld RS, Chawarski MC, Pakes JR, et al: Methadone versus buprenorphine with contingency management or performance feedback for cocaine and opioid dependence. Am J Psychiatry 162(2):340–349, 2005 15677600

Schuckit MA: Treatment of opioid-use disorders. N Engl J Med 375(4):357–368, 2016 27464203

Sigmon SC, Bigelow GE: Food and Drug Administration approval of sustained-release buprenorphine for treatment of opioid dependence: realizing its potential. 112(3):386–387, 2017 27561982

Welsh CJ: "Trapped": a mnemonic for taking a substance use history (letter). Acad Psychiatry 27(4):289, 2003 14989212

5

Clinical Use of Buprenorphine

Ricardo Restrepo, M.D., M.P.H.
Petros Levounis, M.D., M.A.

IN THIS CHAPTER, we review the clinical use of buprenorphine in the treatment of opioid use disorder (OUD). This is a "how to" chapter. We first present a brief overview of the pharmacology of buprenorphine and some general considerations in setting up the treatment, then describe in detail the practical aspects of buprenorphine induction, stabilization, and maintenance therapy. We also briefly describe the option of using buprenorphine for opioid medically supervised withdrawal (MSW), although this approach has considerable limitations and drawbacks, as discussed in Chapter 3 ("Efficacy and Safety of Buprenorphine"). We hope that this chapter will be used as a quick reference to the nuts and bolts of using buprenorphine to treat patients with OUD.

The *Diagnostic and Statistical Manual of Mental Disorders*, 5th Edition (DSM-5; American Psychiatric Association 2013) no longer uses the terms *substance abuse* and *substance dependence*; rather, it refers to *substance use disorders*. The criteria for an OUD are generally the same as in DSM-IV (American Psychiatric Association 1994). The diagnostic criteria for DSM-IV abuse and dependence were combined in DSM-5 except for two changes: 1) the criterion for recurrent legal problems has been removed, and 2) a new criterion for craving, or a strong desire or urge, to use opioids has been added. A patient must meet at least 2 diagnostic criteria out of 11 to qualify as having an OUD. Severity is characterized as *mild* if 2 or 3 criteria are met, *moderate* if 4 or 5 criteria are met, and *severe* if 6 or more criteria are met.

Three case examples and related questions are presented at the end of this chapter for additional consideration. For discussion of this case, please see Chapter 15, "Comments on the Case Vignettes."

Buprenorphine Formulations

New formulations approved for the treatment of OUD by the U.S. Food and Drug Administration (FDA) have entered the market in various doses since the orphan drug exclusive marketing protection rights expired on Subutex and Suboxone in October 2009 (Table 5–1). These formulations are 1) buprenorphine (three generic versions), often referred to as the *mono* product, and 2) a buprenorphine-naloxone (BUP/NX) combination (Suboxone, Zubsolv, Bunavail, and three generic versions), the *combo* product. The mono product is available in sublingual tablet doses of 2 mg (Figure 5–1) and 8 mg (Figure 5–2) of buprenorphine; the combo product is available in sublingual tablet and film as well as buccal film with different doses depending on the formulations. Suboxone and generic forms are available in doses of 2 mg buprenorphine/0.5 mg naloxone (Figure 5–3) or 8 mg buprenorphine/2 mg naloxone (Figure 5–4). Zubsolv sublingual tablets are available in doses of 0.7 mg buprenorphine/0.18 mg naloxone (Figure 5–5), 1.4 mg buprenorphine/0.36 mg naloxone (Figure 5–6), 2.9 mg buprenorphine/0.71 mg naloxone (Figure 5–7), 5.7 mg buprenorphine/1.4 mg naloxone (Figure 5–8), 8.6 mg buprenorphine/2.1 mg naloxone (Figure 5–9), and 11.4 mg buprenorphine/2.9 mg naloxone (Figure 5–10). Bunavail buccal film is available in doses of 2.1 mg buprenorphine/0.3 mg naloxone, 4.2 mg buprenorphine/0.7 mg naloxone, and 6.3 mg buprenorphine/1 mg naloxone (Figures 5–11, 5–12, and 5–13). These two new formulations provide higher bioavailability than other formulations, meaning more buprenorphine enters the bloodstream, requiring lower doses (Table 5–2). For practical purposes, when clinicians refer to the combo product as "8 mg of bup" or "2 mg of bup," it is understood that what they mean is 8 mg of buprenorphine with 2 mg of naloxone or 2 mg of buprenorphine with 0.5 mg of naloxone, respectively.

In 2016, the FDA approved Probuphine, a 6-month buprenorphine implant (Figures 5–14 and 5–15), as the first implant for the maintenance treatment of OUD. Approval of a depot buprenorphine monthly injection is pending.

Other buprenorphine formulations available for pain management—but not approved for the treatment of OUD in the United States—are injectable buprenorphine (Buprenex), buccal film (Belbuca), and extended-release trans-

TABLE 5–1. **Buprenorphine products for treatment of opioid use disorder**

Brand name	Formulation	Available doses
Subutex (brand name discontinued in 2011 in the United States)	Buprenorphine sublingual tablets, including generic equivalents	2 mg buprenorphine 8 mg buprenorphine
Suboxone tablets (brand name discontinued in 2012 in the United States)	Buprenorphine and naloxone sublingual tablets, including generic equivalents	2 mg buprenorphine/ 0.5 mg naloxone 8 mg buprenorphine/ 2 mg naloxone
Suboxone film	Buprenorphine and naloxone sublingual film (may also be administered by buccal route)	2 mg buprenorphine/ 0.5 mg naloxone 4 mg buprenorphine/ 1 mg naloxone 8 mg buprenorphine/ 2 mg naloxone 12 mg buprenorphine/ 3 mg naloxone
Zubsolv	Buprenorphine and naloxone sublingual tablets	0.7 mg buprenorphine/ 0.18 mg naloxone 1.4 mg buprenorphine/ 0.36 mg naloxone 2.9 mg buprenorphine/ 0.71 mg naloxone 5.7 mg buprenorphine/ 1.4 mg naloxone 8.6 mg buprenorphine/ 2.1 mg naloxone 11.4 mg buprenorphine/ 2.9 mg naloxone
Bunavail	Buprenorphine hydrochloride and naloxone hydrochloride buccal film	2.1 mg buprenorphine/ 0.3 mg naloxone 4.2 mg buprenorphine/ 0.7 mg naloxone 6.3 mg buprenorphine/ 1 mg naloxone
Probuphine	Buprenorphine hydrochloride implant	Four implant rods, each containing 80 mg of buprenorphine HCl, for a total of 320 mg

TABLE 5–2.   Equivalent doses of buprenorphine/naloxone combination products

Buprenorphine/naloxone combination products	Equivalent doses					
Suboxone sublingual tablets, including generic equivalents		2 mg buprenorphine/0.5 mg naloxone		8 mg buprenorphine/2 mg naloxone		
Suboxone sublingual film		2 mg buprenorphine/0.5 mg naloxone	4 mg buprenorphine/1 mg naloxone	8 mg buprenorphine/2 mg naloxone	12 mg buprenorphine/3 mg naloxone	
Zubsolv sublingual tablets	0.7 mg buprenorphine/0.18 mg naloxone	1.4 mg buprenorphine/0.36 mg naloxone	2.9 mg buprenorphine/0.71 mg naloxone	5.7 mg buprenorphine/1.4 mg naloxone	8.6 mg buprenorphine/2.1 mg naloxone	11.4 mg buprenorphine/2.9 mg naloxone
Bunavail buccal film		2.1 mg buprenorphine/0.3 mg naloxone	4.2 mg buprenorphine/0.7 mg naloxone	6.3 mg buprenorphine/1 mg naloxone		
Probuphine implant				4 implant rods, each containing 80 mg of buprenorphine HCl, for a total of 320 mg		

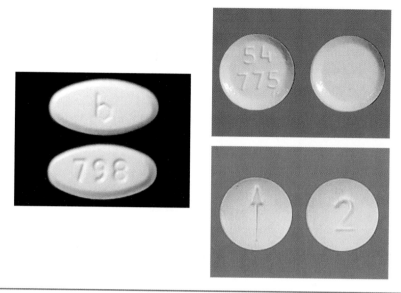

FIGURE 5–1.   Three generic presentations of the 2-mg buprenorphine tablet (2-mg mono product).

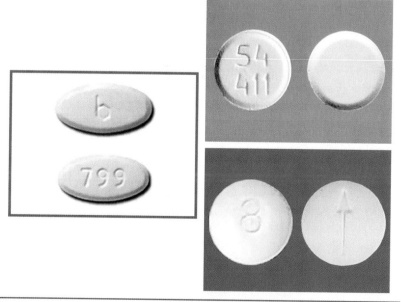

FIGURE 5–2.   Three generic presentations of the 8-mg buprenorphine tablet (8-mg mono product).

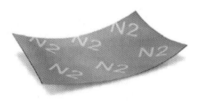

FIGURE 5–3.   **Suboxone 2-mg buprenorphine/0.5-mg naloxone sublingual film (2-mg combo product). © Indivior UK Limited. All rights reserved.**

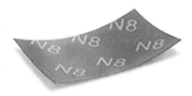

FIGURE 5–4.   **Suboxone 8-mg buprenorphine/2-mg naloxone sublingual film (8-mg combo product). © Indivior UK Limited. All rights reserved.**

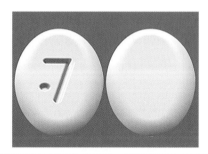

FIGURE 5–5.   **Zubsolv 0.7-mg buprenorphine/0.18-mg naloxone sublingual tablet. © Orexo US Inc. Used with permission.**

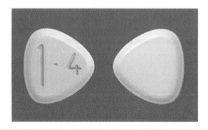

FIGURE 5–6.   **Zubsolv 1.4-mg buprenorphine/0.36-mg naloxone sublingual tablet. © Orexo US Inc. Used with permission.**

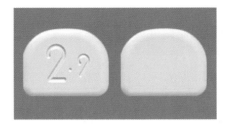

FIGURE 5–7.   **Zubsolv 2.9-mg buprenorphine/0.71-mg naloxone sublingual tablet.** © Orexo US Inc. Used with permission.

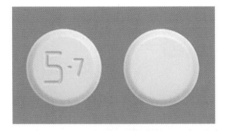

FIGURE 5–8.   **Zubsolv 5.7-mg buprenorphine/1.4-mg naloxone sublingual tablet.** © Orexo US Inc. Used with permission.

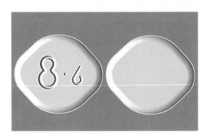

FIGURE 5–9.   **Zubsolv 8.6-mg buprenorphine/2.1-mg naloxone sublingual tablet.** © Orexo US Inc. Used with permission.

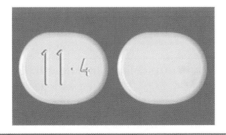

FIGURE 5–10.   **Zubsolv 11.4-mg buprenorphine/2.9-mg naloxone sublingual tablet.** © Orexo US Inc. Used with permission.

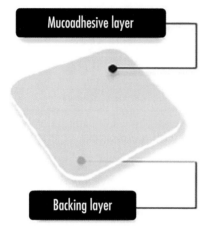

BEMA technology breakdown

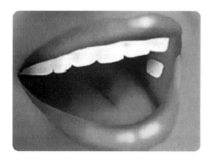

BEMA drug delivery

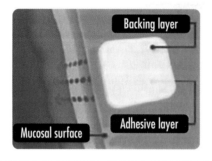

BEMA film placement

FIGURE 5–11.   **Bunavail drug delivery overview: BioErodible MucoAdhesive (BEMA) technology.** © BDSI 207. Used with permission.

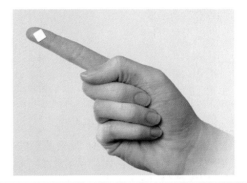

FIGURE 5–12.   **Bunavail buccal film size.** © BDSI 207. Used with permission.

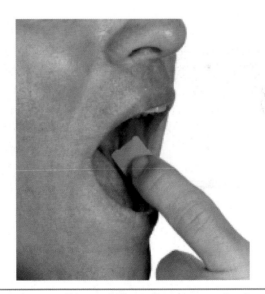

FIGURE 5–13.   **Bunavail buccal film adherence to cheek mucous membrane.** © BDSI 207. Used with permission.

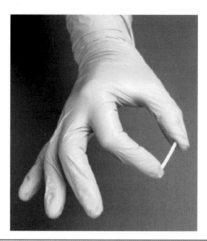

FIGURE 5–14.   **Probuphine implant. © Braeburn Pharmaceuticals, Inc. All rights reserved.**

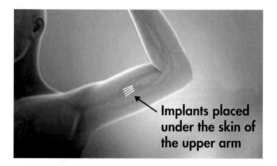

FIGURE 5–15.   **Placement of Probuphine. © Braeburn Pharmaceuticals, Inc. All rights reserved.**
The implants are inserted by a health care professional under the skin of the inside of the patient's upper arm. The implants are small, flexible, and about the size of a matchstick.

dermal film (Butrans). These formulations are approved for the management of moderate to severe chronic pain.

Pharmacology Overview

Buprenorphine is a long-acting partial agonist at the μ opioid receptor. The medication has high affinity, slow dissociation, and low intrinsic activity at the μ receptor. The partial agonist effects of buprenorphine on the μ receptor increase linearly with increasing doses of the drug, until moderate doses result in a plateau of pharmacological effects and further increases in doses result in no additional effect. The advantage of this ceiling effect is that buprenorphine carries a lower risk of abuse, addiction, and serious side effects (e.g., respiratory depression) compared with full opioid agonists. On the other hand, buprenorphine can precipitate opioid withdrawal in a person who is physiologically dependent on a full opioid agonist (see Chapter 2, "General Opioid Pharmacology"), so patients need to be monitored during induction therapy in order to avoid such precipitated withdrawal. Buprenorphine is also an antagonist at κ opioid receptors, an agonist at δ opioid receptors, and a partial agonist at opiate receptor–like 1 (ORL-1; nociceptin) receptors. The contributions of these actions to the OUD profile of buprenorphine are unclear.

Buprenorphine has poor oral bioavailability, which is the main reason the sublingual tablet and film and, most recently, the buccal film were developed. In addition, the BUP/NX combination formulation was developed to discourage diversion for intravenous use. The BUP/NX sublingual formulation or buccal film, taken as indicated, has an almost exclusively buprenorphine effect—naloxone absorbed by the sublingual or mucous membrane route does not precipitate withdrawal because it has minimal sublingual bioavailability. However, if a patient attempts to get "high" by dissolving the film or crushing the combination tablet and injecting the resulting product, naloxone will precipitate opioid withdrawal because it has excellent intravenous bioavailability (see Chapter 2). An expert panel convened by the Center for Substance Abuse Treatment (part of the federal Substance Abuse and Mental Health Services Administration) recommended that the BUP/NX combination sublingual tablets and films be used for all treatment purposes—including induction, stabilization, and maintenance. The buccal film was approved only for maintenance—with the exception of use in pregnant patients. For pregnant women, the mono product is preferred over the BUP/NX combination. The very limited data on sublingual naloxone exposure in pregnancy are not sufficient to evaluate a drug-associated risk (see Chapter 14, "Women's Health and Pregnancy").

For the rest of this chapter, we use the term *buprenorphine* to refer to the BUP/NX combination products unless otherwise specified.

Buprenorphine Induction

The goal of buprenorphine induction and stabilization is to find the lowest dosage of buprenorphine at which the patient 1) discontinues or markedly reduces use of other opioids, 2) experiences a decrease in cravings for opioid use, 3) has no opioid withdrawal symptoms, 4) has minimal or no side effects from the medication, and 5) starts feeling that his or her life is no longer out of control.

Buprenorphine induction must be managed carefully because withdrawal symptoms can arise from either too little or too much medication, resulting in spontaneous or precipitated withdrawal, respectively. Undermedication will not treat the patient's opioid withdrawal symptoms adequately, and overmedication may bring on the very symptoms from which the patient is seeking relief (Center for Substance Abuse Treatment 2004). Furthermore, underdosing buprenorphine may lead the patient to try to self-medicate withdrawal symptoms with other opioids, alcohol, or benzodiazepines. Overdosing buprenorphine during the induction phase may result in potentially significant respiratory depression when it is co-administered with other central nervous system (CNS) depressants such as benzodiazepines or alcohol.

After buprenorphine induction, when the patient has been stabilized with an appropriate dosage of the medication, buprenorphine maintenance is usually the preferred treatment, but some patients may elect to undergo MSW. One of the most significant advantages of buprenorphine is that the patient does not have to make this decision at the start of therapy, a time when, typically, he or she is in the midst of a crisis. Instead, the decision can be made several weeks later, when the patient's condition has stabilized. Whether the patient ultimately decides to continue taking the medication or discontinue taking it, the initial steps are the same: induction and stabilization (Kraus et al. 2011).

Clinician Choices

OBTAINING THE BUPRENORPHINE

Clinicians have the option of either 1) keeping a supply of medication in the office for the induction or 2) instructing the patient to fill a prescription for the first doses in a pharmacy and then bring the medication to the office, where it will be administered. Either way, secure access to the medication by establishing a list of pharmacies in your area that are familiar with the medication. If the first option is followed and a supply of buprenorphine tablets or soluble films is kept in the office, the physician and the institution must keep detailed records as required by federal and state laws. These laws mandate specific conditions for maintaining supplies of controlled substances for administration or dispensing (see Chapter 8, "Referral, Logistics, and Diversion"). Unless you work in a hospital or other institution with adequate on-site pharmacy resources, the option whereby the clinician gives the patient a prescription for the first day's dosage may be preferable. However, asking the patient to fill the prescription and bring the medication back to the office implies a delay in the first day's dosing and a risk that the patient might not return with the filled prescription. Another option is to fax or e-mail an encrypted order of the prescription to the pharmacy and have the medication delivered to your office.

DECIDING BETWEEN MONO AND COMBO TABLETS

In most circumstances, induction can begin with the BUP/NX combination tablet. As previously mentioned in the section "Pharmacology Overview," there is essentially no naloxone bioavailability by the sublingual route, so the patient will not experience precipitated withdrawal from the naloxone contained in the first dose of BUP/NX. Induction with buprenorphine mono tablets should generally be avoided; it can be done in very limited circumstances, such as patients with demonstrated allergy to naloxone or in pregnant patients who are not candidates for methadone use. If the buprenorphine mono formulation is used for induction in patients who are not pregnant, we recommend switching to BUP/NX as soon as possible to reduce the risk of diversion of the medication.

CHOOSING THE DAY OF THE WEEK

Monday through Wednesday in the morning is the ideal time to start the induction. An early morning appointment decreases the risk of opioid use before the office visit, and starting early in the week allows more opportunities for follow-up assessment visits. Avoid induction during the weekend unless your work setting has the personnel and infrastructure needed to treat patients at that time.

SELECTING THE SETTING

An American Society of Addiction Medicine (2015) guideline recommends observing the initial buprenorphine induction directly in the clinician's office and monitoring the patient's progress by regular office visits during the stabilization and maintenance phases of the patient's treatment. However, as more experience has been gained with this medication, a new treatment setting for the induction has been suggested. It is defined as a home buprenorphine induction, in which the patient initiates the medication off-site after a clinician completes the initial assessment and provides instructions (Cunningham et al. 2011; Lee et al. 2009). However, more clinical data are needed before recommending this alternative as a routine procedure. Whichever approach you choose, it is helpful to partner with a colleague who is also certified to prescribe buprenorphine and can cover your practice when necessary. For more details, see the section "Buprenorphine Induction Not Directly Observed by the Clinician: Home Induction."

PATIENT INSTRUCTIONS

Preparing for the Induction

Following assessment of the patient and the decision to initiate buprenorphine treatment (see Chapter 4, "Patient Assessment"), you need to give your patient instructions in preparation for induction to buprenorphine treatment. The most important direction is that the patient needs to arrive at the office in the state of withdrawal. Explain that withdrawal depends on many factors, such as level of tolerance, amount of use, and the type of opioid(s) abused. Ask your patient not to take any opioids for symptomatic relief while preparing for the induction. Be clear with your language and list opioids for the patient, using trademarked names, generic names, and street name of the drugs to avoid confusion.

Taking the Pills

Explain to the patient that buprenorphine is a sublingual tablet or soluble film, which takes about 2–10 minutes to dissolve depending on the formulation. The tablet or soluble film is dissolved under the tongue. The patient should not chew or swallow the medication and should not talk or drink until the entire tablet or film has dissolved. Absorption improves with a moist mouth. Taking more than one tablet or film at the same time can be uncomfortable and may result in a bad taste with poor absorption. Advise the patient to take one tablet or film at a time until he or she completes the full dosage for the day.

Level of Withdrawal

The patient should experience mild to moderate withdrawal before taking the first buprenorphine sublingual dose. As a general rule, the longer the physician can delay the first dose of buprenorphine, the easier and less complicated the induction will be (Casadonte 2009).

In order to reliably assess withdrawal symptoms, we recommend that the clinician use the Clinical Opiate Withdrawal Scale (COWS; Figure 5–16) to evaluate the patient's withdrawal symptoms prior to induction because patients may exaggerate their symptoms to avoid discomfort. COWS items include both signs (objective items such as resting pulse, pupil size, tremor, runny nose or tearing, yawning, sweating, and gooseflesh skin) and symptoms (subjective items such as anxiety or irritability, restlessness, bone or joint aches, and gastrointestinal upset). Each item is scored from 0–4 or 0–5, and the total score is interpreted as follows (Wesson and Ling 2003):

5–12	Mild withdrawal
13–24	Moderate withdrawal
25–36	Moderately severe withdrawal
>36	Severe withdrawal

In addition to using COWS, the clinician can provide the patient with a subjective scale, the Subjective Opiate Withdrawal Scale (SOWS; Figure 5–17). The symptoms are rated by the patient on a scale of 0 (not at all present) to 4 (an extreme feeling) (Handelsman et al. 1987). The patient may complete this

	Times:	___	___	___	___
Resting pulse rate: (record beats per minute) Measured after patient has been sitting or lying for 1 minute. 0 pulse rate 80 or below 1 pulse rate 81–100 2 pulse rate 101–120 4 pulse rate > 120					
Sweating: over past half-hour not accounted for by room temperature or patient activity. 0 no report of chills or flushing 1 subjective report of chills or flushing 2 flushed or observable moistness on face 3 beads of sweat on brow or face 4 sweat streaming off face					
Restlessness: observation during assessment. 0 able to sit still 1 reports difficulty sitting still, but is able to do so 3 frequent shifting or extraneous movements of legs/arms 5 unable to sit still for more than a few seconds					
Pupil size: 0 pupils pinned or normal size for room light 1 pupils possibly larger than normal for room light 2 pupils moderately dilated 5 pupils so dilated that only the rim of the iris is visible					
Bone or joint aches: if patient was having pain previously, only the additional component attributed to opiate withdrawal is scored. 0 not present 1 mild diffuse discomfort 2 patient reports severe diffuse aching of joints/ muscles 4 patient is rubbing joints or muscles and is unable to sit still because of discomfort					
Runny nose or tearing: not accounted for by cold symptoms or allergies. 0 not present 1 nasal stuffiness or unusually moist eyes 2 nose running or tearing 4 nose constantly running or tears streaming down cheeks					

Patient's name:_____ Date: _____
Buprenorphine induction:
Enter scores at time zero, 30 minutes after first dose, 2 hours after first dose, etc.

FIGURE 5–16. **Clinical Opiate Withdrawal Scale (COWS).**

Gastrointestinal (GI) upset: over last half-hour. 0 no GI symptoms 1 stomach cramps 2 nausea or loose stool 3 vomiting or diarrhea 5 multiple episodes of diarrhea or vomiting				
Tremor: observation of outstretched hands. 0 no tremor 1 tremor can be felt, but not observed 2 slight tremor observable 4 gross tremor or muscle twitching				
Yawning: observation during assessment. 0 no yawning 1 yawning once or twice during assessment 2 yawning three or more times during assessment 4 yawning several times/minute				
Anxiety or irritability: 0 none 1 patient reports increasing irritability or anxiousness 2 patient obviously irritable or anxious 4 patient so irritable or anxious that participation in the assessment is difficult				
Gooseflesh skin: 0 skin is smooth 3 piloerection of skin can be felt or hairs standing up on arms 5 prominent piloerection				
Total scores with observer's initials:				
Score: 5–12 = mild 13–24 = moderate 25–36 = moderately severe > 36 = severe withdrawal				

FIGURE 5–16.   **Clinical Opiate Withdrawal Scale (COWS).** *(continued)*
Flow sheet for measuring symptoms over a period of time during buprenorphine induction. For each item, write in the number that best describes the patient's sign or symptom. Rate it on just its apparent relationship to opiate withdrawal. For example, if heart rate is increased because the patient was jogging just before assessment, the increased pulse rate would not be added to the score.
Source.   Template from the American Society of Addiction Medicine.

Please score each of the 16 items below according to how you feel now (circle one number).

Scale: 0=not at all 1=a little 2=moderately 3=quite a bit 4=extremely

| Date: |
| Time: |

	Symptom	Score				
1	I feel anxious	0	1	2	3	4
2	I feel like yawning	0	1	2	3	4
3	I am perspiring	0	1	2	3	4
4	My eyes are teary	0	1	2	3	4
5	My nose is running	0	1	2	3	4
6	I have goose bumps	0	1	2	3	4
7	I am shaking	0	1	2	3	4
8	I have hot flushes	0	1	2	3	4
9	I have cold flushes	0	1	2	3	4
10	My bones and muscles ache	0	1	2	3	4
11	I feel restless	0	1	2	3	4
12	I feel nauseous	0	1	2	3	4
13	I feel like vomiting	0	1	2	3	4
14	My muscles twitch	0	1	2	3	4
15	I have stomach cramps	0	1	2	3	4
16	I feel like using now	0	1	2	3	4
	TOTAL (range 0–64):					

FIGURE 5–17. Subjective Opiate Withdrawal Scale (SOWS).

Source. Handelsman et al. 1987.

form in the waiting room and thus easily provide the clinician with a quick first estimate of the level of opioid withdrawal.

Induction With Patients Dependent on Short-Acting Opioids

In general, the patient can begin buprenorphine therapy 12–16 hours after the last use of a short-acting opioid (e.g., heroin, hydrocodone, immediate-release oxycodone). Before receiving the first dose of buprenorphine, the patient needs to exhibit objective opioid withdrawal symptoms (a COWS score of >12). If there is no or little clinical evidence of mild to moderate opioid withdrawal, reassess the last use of opioids and consider asking the patient to either 1) return another day or 2) wait in the office until evidence of withdrawal is clear. A third option, allowing the patient to leave the office and return later that day, with clear instructions to not take any opioids while he or she is away from the office, is not recommended because there is the possibility that the patient will use more opioids and/or not return.

The clinician needs to know the new formulations approved for induction and be ready to start the medication at the corresponding dose (See Table 5–2). Once mild to moderate withdrawal is established, the patient is given 2–4 mg of buprenorphine. After the initial dose, it is recommended that the clinician monitor the patient in the office for 2 hours to confirm that opioid withdrawal symptoms subside and do not reemerge. The length of time the patient is monitored in the office varies depending on the clinician's familiarity with the patient and experience with the medication. Relief of opioid withdrawal symptoms should begin within 30–45 minutes after the first dose. If symptoms start to subside, a second dose of 2–4 mg is typically administered, and frequently, the patient is instructed to take additional buprenorphine at home as needed for symptom relief. The maximum amount of buprenorphine at the end of the first day of induction ranges from 8 mg to 12 mg (Sullivan and Fiellin 2008). If symptoms of opioid withdrawal worsen or reemerge after the first dose of buprenorphine, precipitated withdrawal is a likely explanation (see subsection "Managing Precipitated Withdrawal" below). Advise your patient to avoid driving or operating other machinery until he or she is familiar with the effects of the medication.

Induction With Patients Dependent on Intermediate- and Long-Acting Opioids

In general, patients who are using intermediate-acting opioids (e.g., sustained-release oxycodone, fentanyl) should first be given buprenorphine 18–24 hours after their last use of the intermediate-acting opioid; for patients using long-acting opioids (e.g., methadone), we recommend waiting 36–48 hours after last use of the full agonist.

If the patient attends a methadone program, confirm his or her dosage, management, and the rationale for switching from methadone to buprenorphine with both the patient and the patient's counselor. Methadone has a very long duration of action and accumulates in tissue stores, resulting in an increased risk of precipitated withdrawal during buprenorphine induction. Current clinical practice recommends that patients first taper—slowly—their methadone use to no more than 30 mg/day (or its equivalent if the patient is taking another long-acting opioid or an intermediate-acting opioid). We then recommend holding the dosage of methadone to 30 mg/day for a minimum of 1 week in order to establish a steady state. Next, discontinue methadone use and evaluate the patient frequently, possibly daily for 2–3 days, until mild to moderate signs and symptoms of opioid withdrawal develop (a COWS score of >12). At that point, you can safely administer the first buprenorphine dose of 2–4 mg and proceed with the induction as described in the previous subsection.

If the patient does not tolerate a methadone taper to 30 mg/day, it is still possible to start buprenorphine use; however, in this case the judgment of the clinician will guide the induction process. As described above, the first dose of buprenorphine should not be given until there is clear evidence of opioid withdrawal, and the patient may require very close monitoring to avoid or manage any precipitated withdrawal (see the next subsection). The scientific literature on this topic is limited, with few guidelines on how to safely switch patients from methadone dosages higher than 30 mg/day to buprenorphine treatment (Glasper et al. 2005; Salsitz et al. 2010).

Managing Precipitated Withdrawal

If opioid withdrawal worsens or reemerges shortly after the first dose of buprenorphine, the medication has most likely precipitated a withdrawal syndrome due to its high affinity for the μ opioid receptor and resultant displacement of the full opioid agonist from the receptor. Precipitated withdrawal is not a medical emergency but can be very uncomfortable. It rarely occurs if the clinician is careful to withhold the first buprenorphine dose until the patient shows clear signs of moderate opioid withdrawal. The preferred strategy in the management of precipitated withdrawal is to administer additional doses of buprenorphine, 2 mg every 1–2 hours, in an attempt to provide enough agonist effect to suppress the withdrawal. Increasing the dosage of the medication responsible for the adverse effect may seem counterintuitive, especially to the affected patient, but it makes both pharmacological and clinical sense. Once buprenorphine has precipitated withdrawal, the medication cannot be taken back; therefore, pushing the dosage to achieve an agonist response is the best alternative.

In rare circumstances when the induction needs to be stopped, as in the case of a patient who refuses to take any more buprenorphine, supportive treatments for the patient's withdrawal symptoms are necessary. The following medications can be used: clonidine, 0.1 mg every 8 hours (or lofexidine outside the United States) to reduce autonomic withdrawal symptoms while monitoring the patient's blood pressure; antiemetics for nausea; dicyclomine for abdominal cramps; hydroxyzine for agitation; loperamide for diarrhea; trazodone for insomnia; and nonsteroidal anti-inflammatory agents such as ibuprofen for myalgias and arthralgias. Ask the patient to return to the office the next day for a follow-up visit and possibly a new buprenorphine induction attempt.

Subsequent Days of Induction

After the first day of buprenorphine induction, the procedures for patients dependent on short-, intermediate-, or long-acting opioids are the same. A review of the patient's subjective experience on the first day of buprenorphine induction, a COWS score check, and a clinical evaluation may be used to determine the need for dosage adjustment, depending on the withdrawal or overmedication symptoms experienced by the patient. If the patient continues to experience withdrawal symptoms, he or she should receive the total dose used on the first day and additional 2- to 4-mg increments of buprenorphine until a total dose of 12–16 mg is achieved on the second day of induction. If the patient feels sedated and overmedicated at the end of the first day, lower the daily dose by 2–4 mg. If neither withdrawal nor overmedication symptoms are observed on the second day, repeat the total dose from the first day. A good night's sleep is a good measure of adequate coverage.

Sometimes the induction takes more than 2 days. You may ask the patient to come back to the office for further dose adjustments, or you may review the clinical status over the telephone or by e-mail and adjust as needed. Dose adjustments follow the same principles as above: raise the dosage if withdrawal symptoms continue and/or cravings for opioids occur and lower the dosage if adverse effects occur. If the patient experiences withdrawal symptoms or cravings after taking a total of 16 mg on the second day, first assess whether the patient is taking the medication correctly (letting it dissolve under the tongue, locating it with a moist mouth, not talking until it is dissolved). If so, then the dose should be increased slowly. Wait at least 5 days before any increase after 16 mg/day. Dosages higher than 24 mg/day have not been demonstrated to provide clinical advantages for the purpose of OUD treatment (Substance Abuse and Mental Health Services Administration 2016). The maximum daily dose is 32 mg of buprenorphine by the end of the first week, but the majority of patients stabilize with 8–16 mg/day.

Do not assume that the patient has not used any other opioids since the first day of induction—ask your patient if he or she has used any opioids since leaving the office. Suspect active opioid use if the patient continues experiencing opioid withdrawal symptoms and/or difficulties with medication adherence. A urine toxicology examination for drugs of abuse may be indicated to guide clinical interventions.

Buprenorphine Induction Not Directly Observed by the Clinician: Home Induction

The current U.S. national prescribing guidelines published by the Center for Substance Abuse Treatment of the Substance Abuse and Mental Health Services Administration describe observed buprenorphine induction as the standard of practice. The unobserved or home induction is an approach that began occurring when increasing numbers of patients were treated with buprenorphine and clinicians became more comfortable using the medication. If you are just starting to prescribe the medication and/or your patient is unstable, do not start induction outside of your office. If a patient has expressed significant fear of withdrawal, he or she may not be a good candidate for home induction because of the possibility of starting buprenorphine too early and causing a precipitated withdrawal.

A few studies of unobserved buprenorphine induction with positive outcomes have been reported in the scientific literature (Lee et al. 2014). Note that before you move in this direction, you need to provide significant patient education, including a detailed handout that covers how and when to start buprenorphine. The ideal candidate to start buprenorphine induction without direct clinician observation is one who has been treated by the clinician previously, has had a previous observed induction without complications, is known to be reliable, demonstrates clear documented knowledge of the risks of unobserved induction, and is willing to come to the office in the event of problems.

If you face problematic office logistics after seeing a patient in your office, you can prescribe buprenorphine for home induction. In this case, it is expected that you will provide explicit written instructions on how and when to start buprenorphine, with clear agreement that the patient will maintain telephone contact with your office and/or your group. Always document these interactions and make a clear agreement with your patient that he or she will visit your office the day after or a maximum of 2 days after starting buprenorphine. All telephone calls and contacts should be documented in the clinician's medical record.

Although home induction may be growing, we must emphasize that there are limited safety data on not maintaining the patient under direct observation. In the few studies that have reported on this practice, unobserved induction does not seem to be associated with disproportionate adverse events or lower treatment retention rates when compared with observed induction.

Special Cases

PREGNANT WOMEN AND NEONATES

Decades of clinical experience have shown that methadone is a safe treatment of OUD for pregnant women. Buprenorphine has also been found to be both safe and effective in pregnancy. Use of the mono product is preferred over the BUP/NX combination because of the theoretical concern for teratogenic effects from naloxone. Mono buprenorphine does not contain naloxone, which can cause fetal and maternal hormonal changes (Soyka 2013). It also reduces the potential that the medication could result in maternal and fetal withdrawal symptoms if the patient tries to use the drug intravenously (see also Chapter 14). There are case studies showing that buprenorphine is safe and effective for the treatment of neonatal abstinence syndrome (Kraft et al. 2016). In more recent studies (Jones et al. 2010, 2014; Thomas et al. 2014;), buprenorphine maintenance during pregnancy was associated with improved maternal and fetal outcomes compared with no medication-assisted treatment. Rates of neonatal abstinence syndrome are similar among infants born to methadone- versus buprenorphine-maintained mothers, but symptoms were less severe for infants whose mothers were treated with buprenorphine maintenance (see Chapter 14).

ADOLESCENTS

When treating adolescents, clinicians should always try to engage the adolescent and his or her parents or guardians and prepare the treatment with them. The goal is to maximize treatment adherence and prevent relapses. However, most states have laws that allow adolescents to seek treatment for substance use disorders without parental consent; in these cases, the adolescents' confidentiality should be respected. The first line of treatment for adolescents with OUD is psychosocial intervention. Buprenorphine is an effective treatment approved by the FDA for patients 16 years and older with severe OUD (Marsch et al. 2016; Subramaniam et al. 2011) (see Chapter 13, "Opioid Use by Adolescents").

OPIOID USE DISORDER WITHOUT PHYSIOLOGICAL DEPENDENCE

People who have OUD but are not currently physically dependent can also benefit from treatment with buprenorphine. For example, someone who has been addicted to heroin for many years but has not used for the past 6 months while incarcerated is at high risk for relapse on release from prison. Also, patients who binge on opioids but do not meet criteria for physiological dependence (tolerance or withdrawal) may still meet criteria for OUD according to DSM-5 because of severe psychosocial deterioration. Re-induction with buprenorphine may also be appropriate for a patient who recently completed an MSW and has begun to use opioids occasionally. In this case, there would be no reason to delay treatment until the patient has resumed daily use and is again physically dependent. Buprenorphine treatment can address such patients' cravings and keep them safe.

Buprenorphine induction for patients who are not physiologically dependent on opioids starts with 2 mg of buprenorphine. The dose is then raised by 2-mg increments during the following days until the patient is comfortable and cravings abate. You may repeat a target dose of buprenorphine that was successful during previous stabilization and maintenance phases.

Buprenorphine Stabilization

The stabilization phase lasts 1–2 months. During this period, patients are seen regularly, every 1–3 weeks, in order to find a homeostatic state in the opioid system. Adjust the dosage of buprenorphine, if needed, to determine the minimum dosage necessary to eliminate withdrawal symptoms, markedly decrease cravings, and minimize side effects. Once you achieve initial control of withdrawal symptoms and craving, further dose increases should be approached in a very conservative manner. Because of the drug's long half-life (24–60 hours, mean elimination half-life of 37 hours), it may take 10–14 days to achieve the full benefit of an increased dosage. More frequent increases may therefore result in unnecessary and excessive doses.

The average daily dose is 8–16 mg of buprenorphine, but some patients require as much as 24–32 mg/day. If a patient continues to have significant cravings and/or withdrawal symptoms at 32 mg/day, consider discontinuing buprenorphine and treating the patient with methadone.

During the stabilization phase, discuss with the patient the importance of engaging in psychosocial treatments and 12-step programs (see Chapter 7, "Psychosocial and Supportive Treatment"). This is an appropriate point at which to reinforce the message that the patient should not expect buprenorphine to eliminate all of his or her problems and that the most successful outcomes are seen in patients who combine medication with psychosocial treatment and other recovery efforts.

Buprenorphine Maintenance

Buprenorphine maintenance lasts several months or years depending on the patient's individual needs. Many opioid-dependent patients require treatment with buprenorphine indefinitely, not unlike patients with diabetes requiring in-sulin treatment or bipolar patients needing lithium maintenance. During this time, continue to review the benefits and adverse effects of buprenorphine; pe-riodically run liver function tests and urine toxicology screens to check for bu-prenorphine metabolite (norbuprenorphine); conduct pregnancy tests; continue with pill counts; and counsel the patient on relapse prevention, phys-ical well-being, and mental health (see also Chapter 7).

After completion of the stabilization phase, most patients continue with the same dosage, typically 8–16 mg/day. However, several medical and psycho-social factors may dictate a change in dosage. Medical factors include signifi-cant weight increase or decrease, progression of liver disease, changes in other prescription medications, and pregnancy or menopause. As patients stabilize further and feel healthy, their life circumstances get better, finances recover, re-lationships blossom, and coping skills improve. As a result, patients may have fewer opioid cravings, have a lower risk of relapse, and need less medication. Even if complete MSW is not the goal of treatment, discuss with your patient the possibility of working toward a lower dosage of buprenorphine as long as he or she still feels comfortable and safe from relapse. Reassure the patient that he or she can always return to the maintenance dosage if needed (see also Chapter 6, "Buprenorphine Treatment in Office-Based Settings").

Dosing Strategies

Once the patient is stable and the buprenorphine maintenance daily dose is es-tablished, he or she may switch to a less-than-daily dosing schedule (Johnson et al. 2003). Buprenorphine can be taken sublingually safely and effectively on an alternate-day dosing schedule (every 48 hours) by doubling the maintenance dose (e.g., if the patient is taking 8 mg/day, switch to 16 mg on Mondays and Wednesdays and 24 mg on Fridays) (Amass et al. 1994). Alternative schedules include dosing every 72 hours by tripling the maintenance dose (Bickel et al. 1999) or dosing every 96 hours by quadrupling the maintenance dose (Petry et al. 2000, 2001). The efficacy of thrice-weekly dosing has been well docu-mented; however, more data are needed before these other dosing schedules can be recommended (Amass et al. 2001; Pérez de los Cobos et al. 2000).

Although daily dosing is generally recommended to improve medication adherence, less-than-daily dosing regimens are also clinically useful for several reasons:

1. Alternate-day dosing schedules have been shown to be preferred by some patients to daily dosing.
2. Thrice-weekly dosing has been shown to be safe and effective.

3. In an opioid treatment program (OTP), these dosing schedules decrease the risk of diversion because they reduce the need for take-home medication. In addition, monitoring and ensuring compliance with medication can be done at the clinic if diversion is suspected.

4. Less-than-daily dosing schedules may be an incentive to patients, such as working parents with demanding schedules, contingent on abstinence from illicit drugs and compliance with treatment, as with methadone.

It is likely that the benefits of less-than-daily dosing schedules with buprenorphine will be more advantageous when buprenorphine is dispensed in an OTP facility, but these schedules may also be considered for buprenorphine treatment in an office-based setting (Marsch et al. 2005).

On the other hand, although once-daily dosing is an effective treatment to block opioid craving and relapse, in some cases more frequent dosing may be advised. Some patients report that buprenorphine works well through the morning, but they experience a recurrence of thoughts and urges to use late in the afternoon or early in the evening. One effective strategy is to keep the same daily dose but to have the patient divide the tablet and the dosing—that is, change from one 8-mg tablet every morning to a half-tablet (4 mg) every morning and another half-tablet (4 mg) in the mid- or late afternoon. It has been suggested that the recurrence of thoughts and urges to use is a psychological effect in individuals who have been using short-acting opioids with multiple doses every day for many years. In other words, twice-daily dosing is a way for patients to feel better psychologically about buprenorphine's effectiveness by mirroring their long-term drug use pattern. However, it is possible that there is also a pharmacological explanation for this complaint—as in the case of pain management, when it is usually necessary to recommend divided daily doses.

Drug-Drug Interactions

Buprenorphine has such high affinity for the μ opioid receptor that it will displace most full opioid agonists and may thus precipitate withdrawal. Although this concept has been reviewed multiple times in buprenorphine training curricula (including this book), the likelihood of buprenorphine-precipitated withdrawal is low, and even when it does occur, it is mild in intensity and short in duration. For a detailed discussion of the interaction of buprenorphine with full opioid agonists, see Chapter 2 and Chapter 12 ("Acute and Chronic Pain").

The opioid antagonist naltrexone is approved by the FDA for the treatment of opioid and alcohol use disorder but should not be combined with buprenorphine. Naltrexone has adequate oral bioavailability and could potentially precipitate withdrawal in a patient who is taking buprenorphine.

There is a potential synergistic effect in combining CNS depressants with buprenorphine, especially when taken intravenously. In a study conducted with rats (Nielsen and Taylor 2005), the ceiling effect of buprenorphine disappeared when buprenorphine was combined with high doses of benzodiazepines. The combination of buprenorphine and diazepam resulted in respiratory depression similar to the effect of full agonists. Although the combination of buprenorphine and benzodiazepines or other CNS depressants is not contraindicated, patients taking buprenorphine who also take sedatives (either prescribed by a clinician or purchased illegally) are at increased risk of respiratory depression (Lintzeris et al. 2007; McCance-Katz et al. 2010; Nielsen et al. 2007). A medical advisory published by Reckitt Benckiser (2012), the manufacturer of Suboxone and Subutex, advises the following:

- Consider reducing the dosage of either buprenorphine or the benzodiazepine or both
- Educate the patient about the potential danger
- Treat co-occurring psychiatric disorders, such as depression and/or anxiety
- Avoid prescribing benzodiazepines whenever possible

For a detailed discussion of the interaction of buprenorphine with benzodiazepines and other sedating agents, please see also the subsection "Overdose and Buprenorphine" in Chapter 3.

Medically Supervised Withdrawal (Detoxification) With Buprenorphine

The treatment of opioid withdrawal by administering a medication taper and eventually discontinuing it is sometimes called *medically supervised withdrawal* (MSW) and sometimes *detoxification*. Strictly speaking, the term detoxification is a misnomer because opioids are not in themselves neurotoxic (as compared, for example, with alcohol, which is directly toxic to the nervous system), but the term detoxification has prevailed both in the medical literature and the community. The use of buprenorphine for MSW is increasing (Dunn et al. 2011; Gowing et al. 2017; Helm et al. 2008; Horspool et al. 2008; Ridge et al. 2008; Sigmon et al. 2013; Weiss et al. 2011), yet there is little standardization of buprenorphine MSW designs and limited evidence of its long-term efficacy.

Buprenorphine can be used for MSW from opioids safely and effectively in both inpatient and outpatient settings. Studies support that buprenorphine is more effective and is better tolerated than clonidine for the treatment of opioid withdrawal (Ziedonis et al. 2009). Before the FDA approval of sublingual buprenorphine, the analgesic formulation was administered by injection and used for opioid withdrawal. At the present time, the injectable formulation is not recommended because of the clinical advantages of the sublingual preparation (American Psychiatric Association 2007). Since the approval of sublingual buprenorphine for the treatment of OUD, the FDA has specifically stated that the parenteral formulation should no longer be used for this purpose.

Both buprenorphine and methadone have long action and proven effectiveness in MSW. Buprenorphine has the additional advantage of being very safe because of its ceiling effect. However, well-designed studies comparing buprenorphine and methadone for opioid withdrawal are limited (Polydorou and Kleber 2008).

The management of opioid withdrawal can be divided into three scenarios: 1) rapid MSW in 3 or fewer days, 2) MSW in 4–30 days, and 3) MSW in more than 30 days. All approaches require that patients experience mild to moderate opioid withdrawal (a COWS score of >12) before the first dose of 2–4 mg of buprenorphine is administered. Equally important is that all approaches recommend that patients engage in some form of psychosocial treatment and support after completion of MSW.

The average daily dose of buprenorphine on the first and second days of MSW ranges between 8 mg and 12 mg; on the third day the patient is given 6 mg of buprenorphine; then the medication is discontinued (Cheskin et al. 1994). Alternatively, the buprenorphine dosage can be decreased in decrements of 2 mg/day over the following days if necessary (Horspool et al. 2008). Two 5-day protocols have been shown to be safe and efficacious in treating acute withdrawal, with the higher-dosage buprenorphine schedule (8, 8, 8, 4, and 2 mg/day on days 1–5) demonstrating moderate superiority over the lower-dosage protocol (2, 4, 8, 4, and 2 mg/day on days 1–5) (Oreskovich et al. 2005). Information on the long-term efficacy of these interventions is limited.

The moderate-length MSW approach allows patients to undergo induction and stabilization before medication tapering begins. Patients first stabilize with an adequate buprenorphine dosage according to their withdrawal severity, cravings, adverse effects, and other drug use. On the basis of one of the few randomized double-blind studies (Sigmon et al. 2013) of patients undergoing MSW from prescription OUD, buprenorphine doses should be gradually reduced over a period of 4 or more weeks instead of more quickly over a shorter period of time. In this study, participants reduced their doses of buprenorphine over a period of 1, 2, or 4 weeks. Patients who gradually reduced their dose of buprenorphine over a 4-week period had higher rates of remaining abstinent from opioids after MSW than did patients with a shorter "taper" time of 1 or 2 weeks. Patients who successfully completed MSW were maintained on daily oral naltrexone to prevent relapse.

The average daily dose of buprenorphine on a moderate MSW schedule is 8 mg. The Clinical Trials Network (CTN), a project sponsored by the National Institute on Drug Abuse, has used a 13-day MSW schedule that is suitable for

TABLE 5–3.   **National Institute on Drug Abuse Clinical Trials Network buprenorphine withdrawal protocol**

Study day	1	2	3	4	5	6	7	8	9	10	11	12	13
Combination[a] daily dose (mg)	4[b]	8	16	14	12	10	8	6	6	4	4	2	2

[a]Buprenorphine-naloxone.
[b]Plus additional 4 mg, as needed.
Source.   Ling et al. 2005.

inpatient and outpatient settings (Table 5–3). On the first day, 4 mg of bu-prenorphine and an additional 4 mg, if needed, are administered; on the second day, 8 mg is given; and on the third day, 16 mg is given. For the next 4 days (days 4 through 7), buprenorphine dosages are decreased in decrements of 2 mg/day, reaching 8 mg on the seventh day of MSW. Then the daily dose is decreased gradually by 2 mg every 2 days. During the last 2 days (days 12 and 13) of the CTN protocol, the patient takes 2 mg of the medication per day (Ling et al. 2005). This CTN protocol is only one of the MSW schedules using buprenor-phine sublingual tablets that are suggested in the literature (Dunn et al. 2011), and the comparative effectiveness of the approaches is largely unknown. A study of 364 patients with opioid dependence (Katz et al. 2009) compared a brief 5-day buprenorphine detoxification protocol with an extended 30-day protocol. The results suggested that longer MSW schedules improve treatment engagement, increase the chances for successful completion of MSW, and fa-cilitate transition to long-term addiction treatment.

Withdrawal symptoms associated with a more gradual reduction in bu-prenorphine dosage, over a period longer than 30 days, are less severe than they are with shorter MSW protocols. The medical literature reports less illicit opi-oid use and greater treatment retention with longer MSW schedules (Horspool et al. 2008; Sigmon et al. 2013; Sullivan and Fiellin 2008).

As previously mentioned (see subsection "Managing Precipitated With-drawal"), the clinician can also use additional non-opioid medications for symptomatic relief of opioid withdrawal during the MSW with buprenor-phine, if clinically indicated. Clinical evidence of insomnia, anxiety, restless-ness, nausea, vomiting, diarrhea, and muscle cramps has justified the use of ancillary medications.

Buprenorphine Taper and Discontinuation

Sometimes, gradual reduction or tapering from the patient's buprenorphine maintenance doses is planned by both patients and clinicians. It is unclear whether tapering a stable buprenorphine dosage is best accomplished with a short- or a long-term discontinuation schedule. A study of 516 patients taking buprenorphine found a modest advantage of a 7-day taper versus a 28-day taper, with 44% versus 30% of patients having opioid-free urine specimens, respectively, at the end of the taper (Ling et al. 2009). It is important to underscore that discontinuation of buprenorphine is frequently an ineffective treatment of OUD; in a study by Ling et al. (2009), only 12% (with a 7-day taper) to 13% (with a 28-day taper) of the subjects remained opioid free at the 3-month follow-up.

The Prescription Opioid Addiction Treatment Study (POATS) is the first randomized controlled study of medication treatment for patients dependent on prescription opioids. The study looked at more than 650 individuals who were dependent on prescription opioids and sought outpatient treatment. In Phase I of the study, all participants received a 2-week buprenorphine stabilization followed by a 2-week taper. Participants who had an unfavorable outcome in Phase I were given an additional 12 weeks of buprenorphine maintenance followed by a 4-week taper. In both phases, the study assessed opioid drug use during the first 8 weeks after discontinuation of buprenorphine via self-report assessments and urinary drug screens. The study showed that patients are most likely to reduce opioid use during buprenorphine treatment. However, if patients are tapered off buprenorphine, even after 12 weeks of treatment, the likelihood of an unsuccessful outcome is high, even in patients receiving counseling in addition to standard medical management. Sigmon et al. (2013) reported between 29% and 63% improvement after a 2- to 4-week buprenorphine taper in prescription opioid abusers, whereas only 7% of POATS participants were abstinent at the end of Phase I. Consistent with prior literature, nearly half of POATS participants were abstinent or reduced their use at the end of the period covered, but most (>90%) relapsed within 8 weeks after buprenorphine was tapered off (Weiss et al. 2011).

Some patients can taper down to 2 mg or 4 mg (sublingual tablets or equivalent of other formulations) but cannot completely discontinue buprenorphine without uncomfortable withdrawal symptoms. Patients who discontinue buprenorphine should be monitored and assessed for cravings and adherence to psychosocial therapies. The clinician can offer alternative forms of pharmacotherapy to help the patient remain abstinent in the long term and should always explain to the patient the possibility of restarting buprenorphine if clinically indicated (Fiellin et al. 2014).

Conclusion

Treating OUD with buprenorphine is technically simple and straightforward. The treatment has three phases: induction, stabilization, and maintenance. During induction, the patient works closely with the clinician to avoid withdrawal symptoms (spontaneous or precipitated) and to ensure a smooth transition. Maximizing symptom relief and minimizing adverse effects is the balancing act of the stabilization phase. During the maintenance phase, the focus shifts from dose adjustments to promotion of a healthy lifestyle, investment in various psychosocial treatments, and fulfillment of the patient's personal goals. The majority of patients feel mild to moderate discomfort for a few hours during the first day of induction, but this is quickly followed by profound relief and gratitude once they experience the beneficial effects of the medication. For clinicians, effecting this dramatic transformation can be one of the most rewarding and gratifying aspects of medical practice.

Clinical Pearls

- Always use the buprenorphine-naloxone formulation except in pregnant patients (who may receive the mono buprenorphine formulation if necessary).

- If the patient is physiologically dependent on opioids, make sure that he or she is in mild to moderate withdrawal before starting the induction. The longer you can delay the first dose of buprenorphine, the easier and less complicated the induction will be.

- Start the induction with 2–4 mg of buprenorphine and raise the dosage over the first couple of days of induction to a target daily dosage of 8–16 mg; the maximum dosage is 24–32 mg/day.

- Stabilize the patient over 1–3 weeks. If further dose adjustments are needed, 1) increase the dosage to manage cravings or withdrawal symptoms or 2) lower the dosage, as tolerated, to reduce side effects or for patient preference. Because of buprenorphine's long half-life, dose increases should occur no more frequently than once a week.

- Avoid using other opioid agonists or opioid antagonists while the patient is taking buprenorphine. Drug-drug interactions with most other classes of drugs can be managed with dose adjustments.

- If you decide to use buprenorphine for medically supervised withdrawal, keep in mind that the longer the taper, the greater the chance of success.

Case 1

Sally is a 21-year-old sophomore at a local college. She makes an appointment after seeing your name on a buprenorphine provider locator list on the Internet. In the office, she is taciturn and makes little eye contact. You learn that she started occasional use of prescription pain pills in high school when "everyone was doing it on the weekends." Three months ago, a friend gave her "Oxys." She is worried now because she uses them almost daily. She says, "I feel lousy if I don't get them." She recently failed two exams and has stopped her daily jogging routine. She admits to occasional marijuana use and has a few drinks on weekends but denies use of other drugs:. "I tried to stop, but I can't. My parents are going to kill me...."

1. Does Sally demonstrate DSM-5 criteria for opioid use disorder (OUD)?

2. How would you rate the severity of her opioid use problem?

3. Does she meet legal criteria for opioid agonist therapy?

4. Is her age an issue?

Case 2

Mark is a married 45-year-old postal worker who comes to your office saying, "Someone told me you write for BUP." He has been receiving methadone treatment for the last 5 years but has a new postal route and tells you, "I can't make it to the clinic and keep my job. I've been on 120 mg of methadone and have been clean for the last 3 years." He says you can call the clinic to verify that he has been compliant. "I have to be on time for work!" he adds. He does not attend Alcoholics Anonymous, Narcotics Anonymous, or any other supportive group meetings.

1. What steps are recommended to convert someone from methadone treatment to buprenorphine treatment?

Case 3

Thom is a 28-year-old married firefighter with OUD. He developed OUD 2 years ago after receiving opioids for a back injury. He found that opioids helped his pain and his mood. He needed higher and higher amounts each day, and finds he is unable to control his use any longer. His work and friendships have suffered from his use. You meet with him for the first time and find out that he recently converted to buprenorphine treatment under the care of a different physician but complains of the other prescriber's "requirements."

1. Would you feel comfortable prescribing buprenorphine?

2. What are your requirements (ancillary therapy or support in and out of your office), if any, of someone for whom you are prescribing buprenorphine?

CASE 3 (CONTINUED)

Thom has been coming to your "BUP group" fairly consistently for the past 3 months. Two weeks ago, he had a positive test result for cocaine on his urine toxicology screen. He also missed his group meeting last week.

1. Did you ask Thom to sign a treatment agreement when you took over his case?

2. Did you delineate your limits for exclusion from your practice?

3. Is this a rule violation?

4. Is this a clinical problem?

5. What will be your next step?

References

Amass L, Bickel WK, Higgins ST, et al: Alternate-day dosing during buprenorphine treatment of opioid dependence. Life Sci 54(17):1215–1228, 1994 8164503

Amass L, Kamien JB, Mikulich SK: Thrice-weekly supervised dosing with the combination buprenorphine-naloxone tablet is preferred to daily supervised dosing by opioid-dependent humans. Drug Alcohol Depend 61(2):173–181, 2001 11137282

American Psychiatric Association: Diagnostic and Statistical Manual of Mental Disorders, 4th Edition. Washington, DC, American Psychiatric Association, 1994

American Psychiatric Association: Practice guideline for the treatment of patients with substance use disorders, 2nd edition. Am J Psychiatry 164 (4 suppl):5–123, 2007. Available at: http://www.psychiatryonline.com/pracGuide/pracGuideTopic_5.aspx. Accessed April 23, 2016.

American Psychiatric Association: Diagnostic and Statistical Manual of Mental Disorders, 5th Edition. Arlington, VA, American Psychiatric Association, 2013

American Society of Addiction Medicine: ASAM National Practice Guideline For the Use of Medications in the Treatment of Addiction Involving Opioid Use. Rockville, MD, American Society of Addiction Medicine, June 1, 2015. Available at: www.asam.org/docs/default-source/practice-support/guidelines-and-consensus-docs/asam-national-practice-guideline-supplement1b630f9472bc604-ca5b7ff000030b21a.pdf?sfvrsn=0. Accessed August 8, 2017.

Bickel WK, Amass L, Crean JP, et al: Buprenorphine dosing every 1, 2, or 3 days in opioid-dependent patients. Psychopharmacology (Berl) 146(2):111–118, 1999 10525745

Casadonte PP: Buprenorphine induction, in Physicians Clinical Support System–Buprenorphine (PCSS-B), Clinical Guidance. October 27, 2009. Available at: http://pcssmat.org/wp-content/uploads/2014/02/PCSS-MATGuidanceBuprenorphineInduction.Casadonte.pdf. Accessed August 6, 2017.

Center for Substance Abuse Treatment: Clinical Guidelines for the Use of Buprenorphine in the Treatment of Opioid Addiction. Treatment Improvement Protocol (TIP) Series 40. DHHS Publ No (SMA) 04-3939. Rockville, MD, Substance Abuse and Mental Health Services Administration, 2004. Available at: www.naabt.org/documents/TIP40.pdf. Accessed August 6, 2017.

Cheskin LJ, Fudala PJ, Johnson RE: A controlled comparison of buprenorphine and clonidine for acute detoxification from opioids. Drug Alcohol Depend 36(2):115–121, 1994 7851278

Cunningham CO, Giovanniello A, Li X, et al: A comparison of buprenorphine induction strategies: patient-centered home-based inductions versus standard-of-care office-based inductions. J Subst Abuse Treat 40(4):349–356, 2011 21310583

Dunn KE, Sigmon SC, Strain EC, et al: The association between outpatient buprenorphine detoxification duration and clinical treatment outcomes: a review. Drug Alcohol Depend 119(1–2):1–9, 2011 21741781

Fiellin DA, Schottenfeld RS, Cutter CJ, et al: Primary care-based buprenorphine taper vs maintenance therapy for prescription opioid dependence: a randomized clinical trial. JAMA Intern Med 174(12):1947–1954, 2014 25330017

Glasper A, Reed LJ, de Wet CJ, et al: Induction of patients with moderately severe methadone dependence onto buprenorphine. Addict Biol 10(2):149–155, 2005 16191667

Gowing L, Ali R, White JM: Buprenorphine for managing opioid withdrawal. Cochrane Database of Systematic Reviews 2017, Issue 2. Art. No. CD002025, DOI: 10.1002/14651858.CD002025.pub5

Handelsman L, Cochrane KJ, Aronson MJ, et al: Two new rating scales for opiate withdrawal. Am J Drug Alcohol Abuse 13(3):293–308, 1987 3687892

Helm S, Trescot AM, Colson J, et al: Opioid antagonists, partial agonists, and agonists/antagonists: the role of office-based detoxification. Pain Physician 11(2):225–235, 2008 18354714

Horspool MJ, Seivewright N, Armitage CJ, et al: Post-treatment outcomes of buprenorphine detoxification in community settings: a systematic review. Eur Addict Res 14(4):179–185, 2008 18583914

Johnson RE, Strain EC, Amass L: Buprenorphine: how to use it right. Drug Alcohol Depend 70(2 suppl):S59–S77, 2003 12738351

Jones HE, Kaltenbach K, Heil SH, et al: Neonatal abstinence syndrome after methadone or buprenorphine exposure. N Engl J Med 363(24):2320–2331, 2010 21142534

Jones HE, Dengler E, Garrison A, et al: Neonatal outcomes and their relationship to maternal buprenorphine dose during pregnancy. Drug Alcohol Depend 134:414–417, 2014 24290979

Katz EC, Schwartz RP, King S, et al: Brief vs. extended buprenorphine detoxification in a community treatment program: engagement and short-term outcomes. Am J Drug Alcohol Abuse 35(2):63–67, 2009 19199166

Kraft WK, Stover MW, Davis JM: Neonatal abstinence syndrome: pharmacologic strategies for the mother and infant. Semin Perinatol 40(3):203–212, 2016 26791055

Kraus ML, Alford DP, Kotz MM, et al: Statement of the American Society of Addiction Medicine Consensus Panel on the use of buprenorphine in office-based treatment of opioid addiction. J Addict Med 5(4):254–263, 2011 22042215

Lee JD, Grossman E, DiRocco D, et al: Home buprenorphine/naloxone induction in primary care. J Gen Intern Med 24(2):226–232, 2009 19089508

Lee JD, Vocci F, Fiellin DA: Unobserved "home" induction onto buprenorphine. J Addict Med 8(5):299–308, 2014 25254667

Ling W, Amass L, Shoptaw S, et al: A multi-center randomized trial of buprenorphine-naloxone versus clonidine for opioid detoxification: findings from the National Institute on Drug Abuse Clinical Trials Network. Addiction 100(8):1090–1100, 2005 16042639

Ling W, Hillhouse M, Domier C, et al: Buprenorphine tapering schedule and illicit opioid use. Addiction 104(2):256–265, 2009 19149822

Lintzeris N, Mitchell TB, Bond AJ, et al: Pharmacodynamics of diazepam co-administered with methadone or buprenorphine under high dose conditions in opioid dependent patients. Drug Alcohol Depend 91(2–3):187–194, 2007 17624687

McCance-Katz EF, Sullivan LE, Nallani S: Drug interactions of clinical importance among the opioids, methadone and buprenorphine, and other frequently prescribed medications: a review. Am J Addict 19(1):4–16, 2010 20132117

Marsch LA, Bickel WK, Badger GJ, et al: Buprenorphine treatment for opioid dependence: the relative efficacy of daily, twice and thrice weekly dosing. Drug Alcohol Depend 77(2):195–204, 2005 15664721

Marsch LA, Moore SK, Borodovsky JT, et al: A randomized controlled trial of buprenorphine taper duration among opioid-dependent adolescents and young adults. Addiction 111(8):1406–1415, 2016 26918564

Nielsen S, Taylor DA: The effect of buprenorphine and benzodiazepines on respiration in the rat. Drug Alcohol Depend 79(1):95–101, 2005 15943948

Nielsen S, Dietze P, Lee N, et al: Concurrent buprenorphine and benzodiazepines use and self-reported opioid toxicity in opioid substitution treatment. Addiction 102(4):616–622, 2007 17286641

Oreskovich MR, Saxon AJ, Ellis ML, et al: A double-blind, double-dummy, randomized, prospective pilot study of the partial mu opiate agonist, buprenorphine, for acute detoxification from heroin. Drug Alcohol Depend 77(1):71–79, 2005 15607843

Pérez de los Cobos J, Martin S, Etcheberrigaray A, et al: A controlled trial of daily versus thrice-weekly buprenorphine administration for the treatment of opioid dependence. Drug Alcohol Depend 59, 223–233, 2000 10812283

Petry NM, Bickel WK, Badger GJ: A comparison of four buprenorphine dosing regimens using open-dosing procedures: is twice-weekly dosing possible? Addiction 95(7):1069–1077, 2000 10962771

Petry NM, Bickel WK, Badger GJ: Examining the limits of the buprenorphine interdosing interval: daily, every-third-day and every-fifth-day dosing regimens. Addiction 96(6): 823–834, 2001 11399214

Polydorou S, Kleber HD: Detoxification of opioids, in The American Psychiatric Publishing Textbook of Substance Abuse Treatment, 4th Edition. Edited by Galanter M, Kleber HD. Washington, DC, American Psychiatric Publishing, 2008, pp 265–287

Reckitt Benckiser: Medical Advisory and Best-Practices Update. Richmond, VA, Reckitt Benckiser Pharmaceuticals, August 2012. Available at: www.accessdata.fda.gov/drugsatfda_docs/nda/2012/022410Orig1s006.pdf. Accessed August 8, 2017.

Ridge G, Gossop M, Lintzeris N, et al: Factors associated with the prescribing of buprenorphine or methadone for treatment of opiate dependence. J Subst Abuse Treat 37(1):95–100, 2008 19004598

Salsitz EA, Holden CC, Tross S, et al: Transitioning stable methadone maintenance patients to buprenorphine maintenance. J Addict Med 4(2):88–92, 2010 21769026

Sigmon SC, Dunn KE, Saulsgiver K, et al: A randomized, double-blind evaluation of buprenorphine taper duration in primary prescription opioid abusers. JAMA Psychiatry 70(12):1347–1354, 2013 24153411

Soyka M: Buprenorphine use in pregnant opioid users: a critical review. CNS Drugs 27(8):653–662, 2013 23775478

Subramaniam GA, Warden D, Minhajuddin A, et al: Predictors of abstinence: National Institute of Drug Abuse multisite buprenorphine/naloxone treatment trial in opioid-dependent youth. J Am Acad Child Adolesc Psychiatry 50(11):1120–1128, 2011 22024000

Substance Abuse and Mental Health Services Administration: Sublingual and transmucosal buprenorphine for opioid use disorder: review and update. SAMHSA Advisory 15(1):1–12, 2016

Sullivan LE, Fiellin DA: Narrative review: buprenorphine for opioid-dependent patients in office practice. Ann Intern Med 148(9):662–670, 2008 18458279

Thomas CP, Fullerton CA, Kim M, et al: Medication-assisted treatment with buprenorphine: assessing the evidence. Psychiatr Serv 65(2):158–170, 2014 24247147

Weiss RD, Potter JS, Fiellin DA, et al: Adjunctive counseling during brief and extended buprenorphine-naloxone treatment for prescription opioid dependence: a 2-phase randomized controlled trial. Arch Gen Psychiatry 68(12):1238–1246, 2011 22065255

Wesson DR, Ling W: The Clinical Opiate Withdrawal Scale (COWS). J Psychoactive Drugs 35(2):253–259, 2003 12924748

Ziedonis DM, Amass L, Steinberg M, et al: Predictors of outcome for short-term medically supervised opioid withdrawal during a randomized, multicenter trial of buprenorphine-naloxone and clonidine in the NIDA clinical trials network drug and alcohol dependence. Drug Alcohol Depend 99(1–3):28–36, 2009 18805656

6

Buprenorphine Treatment in Office-Based Settings

Jeffrey D. Baxter, M.D.
Dong Chan Park, M.D.

TO DATE, thousands of medical providers from a variety of specialties have taken steps to integrate buprenorphine treatment into their office practices (Dick et al. 2015). However, many barriers to the further expansion of treatment remain. Surveys have shown that concerns about lack of time and support prevent providers from adopting this treatment modality. Other providers cite as a further barrier a lack of knowledge about how to provide effective treatment to patients struggling with opioid use disorder (OUD). Even providers who have completed the mandatory training to receive a waiver to prescribe buprenorphine often feel underprepared to support patients with OUD (Barry et al. 2009; Hutchinson et al. 2014; Netherland et al. 2009; Walley et al. 2008). But research also has shown that once providers gain some positive experience with the treatment and its impact on patients, interest in providing the treatment expands (Green et al. 2014).

The purpose of this chapter is to provide some practical guidance on how to approach treatment of OUD with buprenorphine in office-based settings. A provider does not have to be a certified addiction specialist to provide effective treatment with buprenorphine. With some modest additions and adaptations, most of the techniques providers use to manage other conditions also will work well in managing OUD.

Topics presented in this chapter include the following:

1. Managing OUD as a chronic illness
2. Strategies for office-based buprenorphine treatment
3. Recovery monitoring through history and with toxicology testing
4. Managing problem behaviors and responding to relapse
5. Transitioning patients off of buprenorphine and into different levels of care

Managing OUD as a Chronic Illness

One practical strategy for organizing buprenorphine treatment is to utilize clinical approaches helpful for managing chronic medical conditions. McLellan et al. (2000) outlined the many ways in which substance use disorders (SUDs) share features with chronic illnesses such as asthma, diabetes, and hypertension. Each can be a lifelong condition, with periods of good control interspersed with periods of poor control. Genetics, family systems, culture, and social environments all play roles in the development of these conditions, putting some individuals at higher risk than others. Individual behaviors contribute as well, with daily choices about diet, exercise, cigarette smoking, and drug misuse affecting disease progression and severity. For all of these conditions, effective treatments are available, but more than half of patients do not adhere to treatment recommendations. Many patients stop taking medications, lose motivation for exercise, and make unhealthy choices regarding food, smoking, and drug use.

Providers with experience helping patients manage chronic illness know that progress is achieved most often in small, incremental steps and that it is often interspersed with setbacks. Sustaining good health and recovery requires behavioral changes that develop over time with effort on the part of both the patient and the provider.

The Limitations of Traditional Addiction Treatment

McLellan et al. (2000) pointed out that the manner in which addiction treatment has been structured and the ways in which it is portrayed in popular culture work against the understanding of SUDs as chronic illnesses. Patients with SUDs are frequently directed to short-term detoxification treatment lasting less than 1 week. When patients complete these programs, both the patients and their families expect them to be free of SUDs and to not return to drug use. Similarly, many patients enroll in short-term inpatient programs, often 30 days in duration, but when they return to their home environment, many relapse to drug use, to the frustration of themselves and those around them. If the progression of SUDs were more like that of pneumonia or any other acute, time-limited condition, such dramatic results might be seen from short-term treatments. For example, even patients with more severe forms of pneumonia who require hospitalization and intravenous antibiotics are cleared of the infection within a few weeks.

The same is not true for chronic conditions such as diabetes and hypertension. Patients may require short-term hospitalization when these illnesses are poorly controlled or are causing health complications. But no one would expect diabetes or hypertension to resolve completely after a 7- or 30-day inpatient treatment. When patients with these conditions are stable enough to be released from the hospital, all require ongoing treatment and monitoring to help keep their conditions under control and prevent future complications. They need support to help take medications correctly. They need assistance to monitor blood sugar, blood pressure, and peak flow measurements. They need education on how to prevent exposures that put them at risk and how to adjust treatment when their conditions worsen. And they need guidance on how to sustain healthier lifestyles. Experienced providers recognize that this work will need to continue for prolonged periods and will require investment over time by the patients, their families, and all members of the clinical team.

APPLYING THE PRINCIPLES OF CHRONIC DISEASE MANAGEMENT

In managing moderate to severe OUD, these same principles that apply to chronic diseases also apply to OUD. In the words of Dr. McLellan, for treatment to be effective, "it is essential that practitioners adapt the care and medical monitoring strategies currently used in the treatment of other chronic illnesses to the treatment of drug dependence" (McLellan et al. 2000, p. 1,694).

The following list highlights a number of general principles for the management of chronic conditions that can be applied to the treatment of OUD:

- Patients with chronic conditions need ongoing care; shorter-term, higher-intensity treatments will not be sufficient to maintain control of the condition
- Regular monitoring is needed to maintain control, prevent complications, and detect relapse

- The intensity of monitoring should vary with the severity of the condition
- Clinicians should collaborate with patients to identify goals of treatment and strategies for recovery
- Relapse should be anticipated, and a plan should be developed to respond quickly to get the condition back under control
- Family and social networks should be included in treatment whenever possible
- All patients should be screened and monitored for mental health issues
- All members of the care team, from across many disciplines and professional backgrounds, should be involved
- Linkages to specialty medical and behavioral services should be provided when needed
- Clinicians should help patients access recovery resources available in the community
- Clinicians should use motivational enhancement techniques to improve adherence and outcomes
- Clinicians should support treatment goals beyond complete abstinence from drug use, such as decreases in drug use, improvements in health and productivity, and investment in family and other responsibilities

REDUCING HARM FROM DRUG USE

Another helpful strategy is to work with patients to reduce harm to themselves and others resulting from SUDs. Abstinence from drug use is the most common goal set by patients and providers. The complete cessation of drug use is the ideal outcome of treatment and is the only certain way to prevent the complications and consequences of drug misuse. But it is also helpful to pursue a broader range of harm reduction goals, many of which can be accomplished while the patient is working toward complete and sustained abstinence. For example, decreasing the frequency of opioid use, other drug use, alcohol use, and tobacco use may decrease the risk of medical complications, overdose, and exposure to infectious diseases. Patients may be able to return to work, care for their families, and continue with school or fulfill other responsibilities that had been neglected. Medical and mental health conditions may be identified and treatment initiated. Patients may decrease conflict with family and avoid illegal activities and their consequences. And patients may be better able to engage in behavioral treatment, 12-step peer support, and other programs that will help them work toward achieving and sustaining abstinence. All of these are valuable goals that can reduce the risks to individuals, families, and communities prior to complete abstinence from opioids and other drugs.

Similarly, treatment for other chronic conditions is initiated for the express purpose of reducing risks and complications. For patients with asthma, inhaled corticosteroids reduce the frequency of life-threatening exacerbations, even before patients are ready to quit smoking. For patients with diabetes, insulin reduces the risks of hyperglycemia and end-organ damage even before patients have successfully improved their diets or lost weight. Antihypertensive medications reduce the risk of heart and kidney disease while patients with high blood pressure work on establishing regular exercise routines. None of these treatments eliminates the chronic medical condition, but all of them are considered valid, valuable methods to help patients live longer, healthier lives. Specifically, some patients on methadone maintenance benefit from ongoing treatment despite occasional lapses with illicit opioid use because methadone decreases complications and improves functioning. Some patients on buprenorphine treatment can be expected to have similar results, presenting significant functional improvement despite occasional substance misuse. In these cases, providers need to continuously assess whether ongoing office-based treatment is both safe and appropriate.

Strategies for Office-Based Buprenorphine Treatment

SCHEDULE FOLLOW-UP APPOINTMENTS AT REGULAR INTERVALS

Follow-up visits may take place with a number of different members of the care team. In medical offices, collaborative care delivered through a nurse care coordinator has been shown to be efficient and effective (Alford et al. 2011; LaBelle et al. 2016). In psychiatric or other behavioral offices, care may be shared with behavioral treatment specialists. Many providers also use treatment groups or other structured treatment programs, such as relapse prevention curricula or intensive outpatient programs. The frequency of the visits should increase when patients are unstable or otherwise need more support.

SET TREATMENT GOALS AND MONITOR PROGRESS

At each visit, set treatment goals that are incremental, reasonable, and specific, as well as achievable between visits. Goals also should be tailored to the treatment phase. For example, in the early induction and stabilization phases, using the medication safely, achieving abstinence, and eliminating the risky behaviors associated with drug abuse will be a priority. Once the patient has achieved some stability, work with him or her to set longer-term goals in a variety of areas that reflect the broader definition of recovery. Explore each patient's goals for improving his or her mental and physical health, relationships, employment, education, and ability to meet other roles and responsibilities. With each visit, assist the patients in breaking down these larger goals into incremental, achievable steps and monitor for progress. Finally, remember that patients may make progress on many of these goals before achieving complete abstinence.

HELP PATIENTS ACHIEVE BEHAVIOR CHANGE

Motivational interviewing (MI) is an effective technique for helping patients achieve sustained behavior change. A discussion of the full range of MI skills is beyond the scope of this chapter. Providers interested in developing their skills should review *Motivational Interviewing: Helping People Change*, third edition (Miller and Rollnick 2012) and *Motivational Interviewing for Clinical Practice* (Levounis et al. 2017). These books will provide insight for providers supporting patients trying to change behaviors related to substance use or other health issues.

Following the principles of MI, the clinician should guide patients through the process of setting goals and developing plans to achieve those goals. Avoid dictating the treatment goals as much as possible to minimize defensive reactions from patients. Open-ended questions that may help guide these sessions could include the following:

- What are your goals in entering treatment?
- What steps will you take to achieve those goals?
- What would be a good first step toward achieving those goals?
- What do you want to accomplish between now and our next visit?
- What has worked for you in the past to help you make progress?

Recognize improvements and success rather than always focusing on slips and failures. Keep patients talking about what has worked and how it worked, because strategies that worked before are likely to work again. Acknowledge that change is gradual and that sustained change takes time and effort.

ADDRESS COMORBIDITIES

Address physical and mental health comorbidities as part of treatment for the OUD. Coordinate care with medical and psychiatric providers outside of the buprenorphine office setting.

Developing a Recovery Monitoring System

RECOVERY MONITORING THROUGH HISTORY

McLellan et al. (2005) recommended structuring visits using a *recovery monitoring* approach. They argued that these objectives are different from those of inpatient SUD treatment, which takes place in controlled settings, and defined the objectives of outpatient SUD treatment as falling into four general categories:

1. Patients should be engaged and should participate in treatment
2. Patients should reduce and/or eliminate drug use
3. Patients should see improvements in health and physical and social functioning
4. Patients should reduce the negative impacts of their substance use on family, community, and the broader society

These categories provide a framework for treatment planning in outpatient buprenorphine treatment. Providers experienced with treating chronic medical problems such as asthma or diabetes will notice that these objectives are broader than is typical for standard medical care, in which improvements in measurements of disease severity, such as hemoglobin A1c or peak flow measurements, are often the primary goal.

To operationalize this approach, providers could develop a set of standardized questions from each of these four domains, to be answered at every follow-up visit:

1. How many treatment sessions have you attended in the last week/month?
2. How many days in the last week/month have you used opioids? Other drugs/alcohol?
3. How many appointments for medical or mental health care have you attended in the last week/month?
4. How many days in the last week/month have you been able to work, care for family, or meet other responsibilities?
5. How many days in the last month have you had conflicts with family, neighbors, or law enforcement?

Questions like these can form the core of every follow-up appointment and should be supplemented by monitoring of specific goals established by patients.

Standardized tools exist for monitoring SUD symptom severity (e.g., the Addiction Severity Index [ASI], Behavior and Symptom Identification Scale [BASIS-24]), but these can be impractical for office settings that do not specialize in SUD or mental health treatment. Still, the use of a tool such as the Patient Health Questionnaire (PHQ-9) to monitor depressive symptoms may be a valuable addition to recovery monitoring for patients for whom depression is an ongoing issue.

RECOVERY MONITORING WITH TOXICOLOGY SCREENING

There are two general goals for the use of toxicology screening in buprenorphine treatment: 1) to confirm the presence of the buprenorphine being prescribed and 2) to confirm the absence of other opioids and illicit drugs.

Although some patients may complain that drug screening feels like an invasion of privacy, others express appreciation for the monitoring and request that it be performed regularly. The manner in which drug screening is presented may impact how well it is accepted by patients. Therefore, the provider should include a discussion of expectations for drug testing in the initial treatment agreement and use language that normalizes this testing as a standard part of monitoring for the safety and effectiveness of buprenorphine treatment. If concerns arise, comparisons to the management of other medical conditions may help. No patient would have confidence in a provider's care if he or she prescribed insulin without regularly checking blood glucose measurements and hemoglobin A1c levels or prescribed lithium without measuring serum lithium levels. Similarly, it would be irresponsible and unsafe to provide SUD treatment without monitoring for adherence and ongoing drug misuse.

The following subsection provides a short introduction to techniques for toxicology testing. Providers interested in more information should review the monograph *Urine Drug Testing in Clinical Practice: The Art and Science of Patient Care* by Gourlay et al. (2015). A recent version of this monograph is available for free online, with CME available, at www.udtmonograph6.com/cme.html.

Basic Drug Screening Techniques

The two most commonly used methods for drug screening are immunoassays and gas (or liquid) chromatography–mass spectrometry (GC-MS/LC-MS) (Moeller et al. 2008). Drug screening in office-based buprenorphine treatment is most often performed using urine samples, although oral swabs for saliva testing are available. Immunoassays work in the same way that over-the-counter pregnancy tests and rapid "strep" screens do: An antibody to the drug metabolite is linked to a color indicator and then bonded to elution paper. When the paper absorbs a liquid that contains drug metabolites, these metabolites bind to the antibodies and cause the indicator to change color. There are many benefits to this type of testing. Immunoassays are inexpensive and easy to perform and can be used in many clinical settings, including providers' offices and other outpatient treatment program settings. Specific tests have been developed for a number of opioids, including oxycodone, fentanyl, methadone, and buprenorphine.

However, there are a number of limitations to immunoassay drug testing. First, immunoassays are qualitative tests, providing only a positive or negative result. They provide no information about the level of drug metabolite in a sample, and they read positive only when the amount of drug metabolite in the fluid tested reaches a certain threshold level, or cutoff. The cutoff for opioid metabolites is set quite high in many standard screens, meaning that a patient may demonstrate a false-negative result when levels of metabolite are lower

TABLE 6–1.   **Federal workplace drug testing cutoff values[a] and detection time in urine**

	Initial cutoff level by immunoassay (ng/mL)	Confirmatory level by GC-MS (ng/mL)	Typical detection time in urine (days)
Opioid metabolites (morphine, heroin)	2,000	2,000	2–3
Cocaine metabolite (benzoylecgonine)	300	150	2–4
Marijuana metabolite (Δ-9-THC)	50	15	3–30
Amphetamines	1,000	500	2
Phencyclidine	25	25	8

Note.   GC-MS=gas chromatography–mass spectrometry; Δ-9-THC=Δ-9-tetrahydrocannabinol.
[a]Values used in U.S. Department of Transportation testing.
Source.   Adapted from Moeller et al. 2008.

than the cutoff. Table 6–1 shows the threshold levels for drug metabolites used in U.S. Department of Transportation testing and the average time it takes after drug use for the metabolites to be detected in urine. Cutoffs vary for commercial drug testing kits that are not used for testing under federal guidelines. Note that the cutoff levels for opiate metabolites are set quite high to prevent false-positive screening results from opiates found in low levels in some foods (e.g., poppy seeds)

It is also possible to have false-positive results due to the presence of other substances and medications that cross-react with the components of the immunoassay. Table 6–2 lists some common substances that may cause false-positive immunoassay screening results. This list is not exhaustive; please see Manchikanti et al. (2008) and Moeller et al. (2008) for more detailed information. Providers should note that although many agents cross-react with the amphetamine screen, the metabolite for cocaine, benzoylecgonine, is unique. Only cocaine and medications that contain cocaine, and not other topical anesthetics, should cause a positive result. Most buprenorphine providers have mechanisms in place to follow up any questionable positive results by confirming or clearing them with GC-MS testing.

Finally, it is important to recognize that standard opiate immunoassay screens detect only morphine and drugs that are metabolized to morphine: heroin, codeine, and all morphine products. Semisynthetic opioids such as the commonly misused pharmaceutical opioids oxycodone and hydrocodone occasionally, but

TABLE 6–2.   **Common substances and medications that may cause false-positive immunoassay results**

Opiates	Benzodiazepines	Marijuana	Amphetamines	Phencyclidine
Dextromethorphan	Oxaprozin	Dronabinol	Bupropion	Dextromethorphan
Diphenhydramine[a]	Sertraline	Efavirenz	Chlorpromazine	Diphenhydramine
Quinine		Hemp-containing foods	Ephedrine	Doxylamine
Quinolones		NSAIDs	Phenylephrine	Ibuprofen
Rifampin		Proton pump inhibitors	Phenylpropanolamine	Imipramine
Verapamil[a]		Riboflavin	Pseudoephedrine	Ketamine
			Promethazine	Meperidine
			Ranitidine	Tramadol
			Selegiline	Venlafaxine
			Trazodone	

Note.   NSAIDs=nonsteroidal anti-inflammatory drugs.
[a]False-positive result on methadone screen only.
Source.   Adapted from Moeller et al. 2008.

TABLE 6–3.   **Common opioids and their most prevalent metabolites**

Drug	Metabolites
Morphine	Morphine, morphine glucuronides
Heroin (diacetylmorphine)	6-Monoacetylmorphine, morphine
Codeine	Norcodeine, morphine
Oxycodone	Noroxycodone, oxymorphone, oxycodol
Hydrocodone	Norhydrocodone, hydromorphone, hydrocodol
Hydromorphone	Hydromorphone glucuronides
Buprenorphine	Norbuprenorphine, buprenorphine glucuronides
Methadone	EDDP
Meperidine	Normeperidine
Propoxyphene	Norpropoxyphene
Fentanyl	Norfentanyl

Note.   EDDP=2-ethylidene-1,5-dimethyl-3,3-diphenylpyrrolidine.
Source.   Adapted from Manchikanti et al. 2008; Nagar and Raffa 2008.

not reliably, cross-react and give a positive opiate screening result. Specific testing should be done to detect semisynthetic opioids. Fully synthetic opioids, such as methadone and fentanyl, are not detected by standard opiate screens and also require testing specifically for these agents. Table 6–3 lists the most prevalent metabolites of the most common opioid agents. These metabolites are reported specifically only with GC-MS testing, not with immunoassays.

Testing for Buprenorphine

Buprenorphine taken sublingually is metabolized primarily to norbuprenorphine. Metabolites are active at the μ opioid receptor and therefore may enhance the effect of the medication (Brown et al. 2011). Neither buprenorphine nor its metabolites are detected by standard opiate immunoassays. Providers should test for the buprenorphine metabolite, norbuprenorphine, to provide some objective evidence that patients are taking the medication. When immunoassays are used, providers should be careful to note whether the test detects buprenorphine, norbuprenorphine, or both agents. As with all immunoassays, false-positive results are possible because of cross-reactivity with other substances, and false-negative results are possible if the levels in the patient's urine fall below cutoff.

Many providers are measuring buprenorphine and norbuprenorphine levels and then looking at the ratio of the metabolite to the parent compound. Patients initiating buprenorphine treatment show higher levels of the parent compound, buprenorphine. When buprenorphine is taken regularly, the levels of norbuprenorphine surpass the levels of buprenorphine, often by a factor of 4 or more (Hull et al. 2008). Some studies have demonstrated that with chronic dosing, levels of the parent compound fall to very low levels that may be below the detectable thresholds of certain immunoassays (Hull et al. 2008). Therefore, patients taking buprenorphine regularly may show a false-negative result for buprenorphine if the test measures only the parent compound.

On the other hand, samples that show very high levels of the unchanged parent compound with very low or absent levels of the metabolite may indicate that a patient has dissolved a tablet into the urine sample (Hull et al. 2008). It should be noted that for individual patients, urine buprenorphine levels vary widely with timing of administration, levels of hydration, and individual rates of urine production and drug metabolism. There is no reliable way to use drug levels to determine precisely how much buprenorphine a person is taking. This testing may be most helpful to identify patients who have no buprenorphine metabolites in their system or to provide additional information in the evaluation of patients who are not meeting treatment goals or who complain of inadequate dosing.

Finally, urine drug testing also presents a number of logistical issues that buprenorphine providers must consider:

- Will testing be done on site or at a referral laboratory?
- If testing is done on site, will patients be observed while providing the samples to prevent substitution?
- Will other quality control measures such as urine temperature, specific gravity, and creatinine levels be available?
- By what mechanism, and in what circumstances, will screening immunoassays be sent for GC-MS or LC-MS confirmation?
- Will testing be done randomly or only at the time of office visits?
- What will happen if the patient is found to have substituted a urine sample?
- How will patients pay for this monitoring if they are uninsured or if their insurance does not pay for this service?

Where available, it is helpful to develop relationships with a referral laboratory, preferably one with some experience in drug testing. Providers with links to hospital laboratories may be able to call on the hospital laboratory staff with questions. In many areas, there are private drug testing companies with professional toxicologists that will manage the entire testing process. Providers should monitor testing procedures, however, because many laboratories offer large, multicomponent panels and then charge per item tested. As the number of items tested and the use of GC-MS and LC-MS increase, the cost of each screening can get quite high.

Managing Problem Behaviors and Responding to Relapse

Time invested in reviewing treatment agreements, establishing strong therapeutic relationships, and developing clear treatment plans will prevent many problem behaviors. That being said, it is helpful to plan ahead and prepare providers and support staff to provide clear, consistent responses when problems do occur. In all situations, safety is the most important priority. Providers must respond immediately to any behavior that seriously compromises the safety of patients or those around them. For example, threatening behavior against other patients or staff or criminal behavior such as selling drugs or forging prescriptions would usually result in discharge from the treatment after investigation of the incidents.

Short of serious safety concerns, however, it is important to remember that change is a process that happens gradually and often involves both steps forward and steps backward in order to make progress. Prompt, graded responses to less serious behaviors, coupled with motivation enhancement, will maintain safety and retain patients in treatment. Minimal problems, such as a missed counseling visit, may be managed easily by a focused discussion with the treating provider. A brief lapse may require a temporary increase in the frequency of monitoring visits and urine screens and/or a dosage adjustment. A more serious relapse may indicate the need for a major review of the treatment plan, with the addition of more counseling services and/or a significant increase in participation in mutual support groups, as described below.

Problem behaviors fall into five general categories:

1. *Violations of office policies*, including inappropriate interactions with office staff, noncompliance with financial responsibilities associated with treatment, calling in to report lost or stolen medications, calls for early refills, and nonemergency calls after office hours
2. *Noncompliance with treatment plans*, including unapproved increases in buprenorphine dosing, missed office appointments or missed visits with consultants, declining to allow communication with other treatment providers, failing to provide urine samples for drug screening, and failing to participate in behavioral treatment as requested
3. *Continued misuse of opioids*, including unapproved use of opioid pain medications
4. *Misuse of non-opioid illegal drugs* such as methamphetamine or cocaine, problem alcohol use, and unapproved use of other medications with the potential for misuse
5. *Criminal behavior*, such as alteration of prescriptions, diversion of prescribed buprenorphine, selling or sharing other medications or illegal drugs, or theft

When problem behaviors arise that do not cause immediate safety concerns, it is important to verify and document the behavior and review this information with the patient. Many providers begin by reviewing the details of the problem behavior along with the treatment agreement and the most recent treatment plan to make sure that all parties have the same expectations and goals. Patients also should have the opportunity to tell their side of the story. In specialty behavioral and substance abuse treatment settings, it is common to implement a written *behavior contract* (which is discussed in further detail in Chapter 8, "Referral, Logistics, and Diversion"), which identifies the problem behavior, the expected remedy, the time period in which it is expected that the situation will be remedied, and the consequences if insufficient action is taken. In other settings, this formal process may be too time-consuming, and in these settings or in the case of less serious problems, a verbal review of similar information documented in the progress note may be more practical.

As with chronic illnesses such as diabetes or depression, when patients are nonadherent or not meeting treatment goals, the most common responses are to increase monitoring and increase the intensity of treatment. Patients might be seen once or twice a week for a time, with more frequent drug screens and limited medication supplies. Providers can mandate participation in 12-step programs or other formal behavioral or psychiatric treatment. For patients struggling to stabilize substance misuse or mental health symptoms, participation in structured intensive outpatient programs or inpatient hospitalization may be required. It is important to explain that any increase in the intensity and requirements of treatment is not punitive and is primarily to ensure the patient's ultimate success in treatment.

Occasional opioid misuse during the first week or two of treatment is not unusual and may require a dosage adjustment, but it rarely implies a serious treatment problem. However, ongoing misuse of opioids should prompt a careful review of adherence to buprenorphine dosing, the adequacy of that dose, medication dosing technique, and the adequacy of counseling or other recovery efforts. Relapses to opioid misuse after a period of stability typically occur in response to unexpected psychosocial stressors. A review of the circumstances and the patient's response to them may reveal some previously unidentified risk factors and/or a patient's psychopathology, which may call for modification of the treatment plan. A temporary intensification of treatment services—in frequency, in intensity, or both—may be adequate to help the patient restore his or her previous level of functioning.

Behavior associated with buprenorphine diversion should result in increased frequency of visits and screening tests to monitor drug use, short-interval prescriptions, and random callbacks to count the number of pills or films left in the patient's bottle. Additional strategies are discussed further in Chapter 8.

It is not uncommon for some patients to stop all use of opioids (other than buprenorphine) but then present with evidence of a new or intensified problem with alcohol or other drugs. These problems are best managed by counseling, pharmacology, and/or participation in a 12-step program. Patients should be told that sobriety from all illicit drugs is the goal of treatment and that the ongoing use or misuse of alcohol or other drugs is likely to undermine the success of their buprenorphine treatment program. That being said, occasional social drinking or marijuana use should not be grounds for the termination of buprenorphine treatment. Some patients may take months or even years to establish complete sobriety. The clinician should look for signs of progress toward full recovery and sobriety but recognize that progress may be slow and may occur at different rates with different substances. In particular, cigarette smoking accounts for the majority of mortality in patients in treatment for SUDs, and it is not uncommon for nonsmokers to initiate smoking when quitting opioid use (Baca and Yahne 2009). Providers should pay attention and provide appropriate counseling and resources for any smoking-related issue.

Ongoing problem use of alcohol and sedatives poses the additional risk of respiratory suppression and overdose. Patients with problem alcohol and/or benzodiazepine use require clinical attention for those problems in the form of medications and/or MI and, for severe cases, will need a referral to an inpatient facility for withdrawal treatment. Continued struggle with problem alcohol use or sedative abuse should prompt a review of the patient's suitability for office-based buprenorphine treatment.

Transitioning Patients off Buprenorphine and on to Different Levels of Care

Ultimately, providers will need to weigh the risks and benefits of office-based treatment with buprenorphine for each patient and discuss with their patients whether it is both safe and appropriate to continue. Except in the most unusual or extreme circumstances, termination of office-based buprenorphine treatment should be the last response to problem behaviors. At the same time, however, providers must be realistic about the complexity of problems that they can manage in their office setting and be ready to offer a referral to a higher level of care such as inpatient withdrawal treatment facility, methadone maintenance treatment, or a residential program. For example, patients who cannot administer or store buprenorphine safely despite added levels of supervision and services such as visiting nurse may not be suitable for office-based buprenorphine treatment. Patients who, after a series of interventions to intensify treatment and monitoring, are unable to meet minimum treatment goals such as reducing very dangerous levels of polysubstance misuse or who are unable to adhere to other important treatment expectations may require a higher level of care. For patients who continue to misuse sedatives or alcohol, clinicians should explore alternative treatments for their OUD, such as opioid antagonist therapy, which is discussed in further detail in Chapter 9 ("Methadone, Naltrexone, and Naloxone"). Continued buprenorphine treatment within the structure of a methadone program or a residential therapeutic community also may be a better option for some patients.

Once the provider and the patient make the determination that buprenorphine will be discontinued in an office-based setting, questions often arise about how to transition patients to higher levels of care. Treatment programs for substance use may have long waiting periods, and patients may be reluctant to change treatment modalities. Except in cases where there are serious safety concerns or criminal activities, it is important to avoid abruptly stopping buprenorphine treatment and causing withdrawal, and also to avoid allegations of abandonment. Transitioning patients to higher levels of care should be done safely and ethically. Ideally, patients will have been set up with the next program before their buprenorphine is discontinued. The current principles of medical ethics by the American Medical Association mandate that providers 1) notify the patient of discontinuation in advance to allow the patient to secure another provider and 2) facilitate transfer of care (Council on Ethical and Judicial Affairs 2016). Many interpret this guideline as providing for the following protocol:

1. Provide patients, in writing, with the reasons why their treatment is recommended to change, a warning about the potential for withdrawal symptoms and the risks associated with relapse to drug misuse, and contact information for local substance abuse treatment centers
2. Provide a transitional supply of buprenorphine to cover the patient for a reasonable period of time (e.g., 30 days, but can be extended depending on the typical waiting time to secure treatment in higher levels of care)
3. Offer to transfer records to a new treatment center after receiving legal documentation from the patient for release of information
4. Mail the notification via certified mail with a receipt request and retain a copy of the notification and the receipt in the patient's file

Buprenorphine can be tapered off over the course of a few weeks and then substituted with the opioid antagonist naltrexone after waiting 10 days after the last dose of buprenorphine. If the patient becomes unstable, admission to inpatient withdrawal treatment or other inpatient treatment may be needed to ensure the patient's safety and to facilitate beginning another form of treatment. On the other hand, buprenorphine can be continued at the current dose if a patient is being referred to a methadone maintenance program. Patients should always be reminded to seek emergency care in case of crises. Even if a patient declines any and all referrals to alternative treatments, he or she should be provided with a naloxone rescue kit and be informed of the risks of an overdose death.

Clinical Pearls

- Substance use disorders are best conceptualized as being analogous to other chronic medical conditions such as diabetes: they are best managed by setting reasonable goals, agreeing on a long-term treatment plan, and employing other psychosocial treatments and supports.

- Monitoring recovery by careful history and urine testing at each visit is recommended. Providers should understand the limit of immunoassays and be equipped to follow up aberrant results with GC-MS testing.

- Relapses are not uncommon, especially early in the treatment, and should be managed by increasing intensity and/or frequency of treatment and/or a dosage adjustment.

- There are a number of problem behaviors that threaten the success of office-based buprenorphine treatment. Some of them can be resolved by reviewing the treatment contract and goals, implementing more psychosocial treatments, and/or referring to a higher level of care.

- Termination of office-based buprenorphine treatment should be a last resort and should be done safely and ethically with appropriate referrals.

CASE 4

Eddie is a 25-year-old cab driver who initiated buprenorphine 6 months ago. He began using intravenous heroin in his teens and has a history of truancy but denies any history of criminal behavior. He has been driving his cab for 3 years. Nonetheless, you never feel quite comfortable when he is on your appointment schedule. He "lost" one of his prescriptions 2 months ago, and you agreed to replace it but warned him that you would not do it again. As he walks into your office, you see that his last urine test was positive for morphine. He becomes defensive and angry when you ask him about his urine test results. "No way, doc! It's a mistake in your test...."

1. What are your strengths and weaknesses in understanding and interpreting toxicology?

2. What do you do now?

3. What interview style do you use if you perceive your patient as resistant?

4. What action will you take?

5. Is transfer to a more structured program (possibly a methadone clinic) the next step?

CASE 5

Henrietta is a 43-year-old automobile mechanic with OUD who has been in treatment with buprenorphine/naloxone in your clinic for a year. She comes to your Thursday evening buprenorphine group and says that she is "back on track"—by which she means that she is back to work, paying her bills, and rebuilding her repair shop business. She admits that she drinks to relax at the end of the day. Exploration of her alcohol intake reveals that she drinks four or five beers every evening. She adds, "I finish off a case on weekends, but drinking has never been a problem, doc." She does not attend Alcoholics Anonymous (AA) or Narcotics Anonymous. "All they talk about is problems—I'm all set." She has a husband and three children, ages 5–9. She is happy with her work, but her husband has told her that she should cut back on her drinking or he might have to leave "again."

1. Is Henrietta's drinking a problem?

2. Should she undergo withdrawal treatment from alcohol?

3. If you continue buprenorphine therapy, would you change her treatment plan?

4. How would you address attendance at AA meetings?

5. Would 12-step facilitation be effective in this case?

References

Alford DP, LaBelle CT, Kretsch N, et al: Collaborative care of opioid-addicted patients in primary care using buprenorphine: five-year experience. Arch Intern Med 171(5):425–431, 2011 21403039

Baca CT, Yahne CE: Smoking cessation during substance abuse treatment: what you need to know. J Subst Abuse Treat 36(2):205–219, 2009 18715746

Barry DT, Irwin KS, Jones ES, et al: Integrating buprenorphine treatment into office-based practice: a qualitative study. J Gen Intern Med 24(2):218–225, 2009 19089500

Brown SM, Holtzman M, Kim T, et al: Buprenorphine metabolites, buprenorphine-3-glucuronide and norbuprenorphine-3-glucuronide, are biologically active. Anesthesiology 115(6):1251–1260, 2011 22037640

Council on Ethical and Judicial Affairs: AMA Principles of Medical Ethics: I. Chicago, IL, American Medical Association, 2016

Dick AW, Pacula RL, Gordon AJ, et al: Growth in buprenorphine waivers for physicians increased potential access to opioid agonist treatment, 2002–11. Health Aff (Millwood) 34(6):1028–1034, 2015 26056209

Gourlay DL, Heit HA, Caplan YH: Urine Drug Testing in Clinical Practice: The Art and Science of Patient Care. Bridgewater, NJ, The Center for Independent Healthcare Education, 2015. Available at http://www.udtmonograph6.com/cme.html. Accessed November 2, 2016.

Green CA, McCarty D, Mertens J, et al: A qualitative study of the adoption of buprenorphine for opioid addiction treatment. J Subst Abuse Treat 46(3):390–401, 2014 24268947

Hull MJ, Bierer MF, Griggs DA, et al: Urinary buprenorphine concentrations in patients treated with suboxone as determined by liquid chromatography-mass spectrometry and CEDIA immunoassay. J Anal Toxicol 32(7):516–521, 2008 18713521

Hutchinson E, Catlin M, Andrilla CH, et al: Barriers to primary care physicians prescribing buprenorphine. Ann Fam Med 12(2):128–133, 2014 24615308

LaBelle CT, Han SC, Bergeron A, et al: Office-based opioid treatment with buprenorphine (OBOT-B): statewide implementation of the Massachusetts Collaborative Care Model in community health centers. J Subst Abuse Treat 60:6–13, 2016 26233698

Levounis P, Arnaout B, Marienfeld C: Motivational Interviewing for Clinical Practice. Arlington, VA, American Psychiatric Association Publishing, 2017

Manchikanti L, Atluri S, Trescot AM, et al: Monitoring opioid adherence in chronic pain patients: tools, techniques, and utility. Pain Physician 11 (2 suppl):S155–S180, 2008 18443638

McLellan AT, Lewis DC, O'Brien CP, et al: Drug dependence, a chronic medical illness: implications for treatment, insurance, and outcomes evaluation. JAMA 284(13):1689–1695, 2000 11015800

McLellan AT, McKay JR, Forman R, et al: Reconsidering the evaluation of addiction treatment from retrospective follow-up to concurrent recovery monitoring. Addiction 100:447–458, 2005 15784059

Miller WR, Rollnick S: Motivational Interviewing: Helping People Change, 3rd Edition. New York, Guilford, 2012

Moeller KE, Lee KC, Kissack JC: Urine drug screening: practical guide for clinicians. Mayo Clin Proc 83(1):66–76, 2008 18174009

Nagar S, Raffa RB: Looking beyond the administered drug: metabolites of opioid analgesics. J Fam Pract 57 (6 suppl):S25–S32, 2008 18655760

Netherland J, Botsko M, Egan JE, et al: Factors affecting willingness to provide buprenorphine treatment. J Subst Abuse Treat 36(3):244–251, 2009 18715741

Walley AY, Alperen JK, Cheng DM, et al: Office-based management of opioid dependence with buprenorphine: clinical practices and barriers. J Gen Intern Med 23(9):1393–1398, 2008 18592319

7

Psychosocial and Supportive Treatment

Peter D. Friedmann, M.D., M.P.H., DFASAM, FACP
Tae Woo Park, M.D., M.Sc.

OPIOID USE DISORDER can be a complex behavioral disorder that affects multiple dimensions of a person's life, so it is no surprise that its treatment is often a complex, multidimensional intervention. Long-term recovery requires a level of commitment and effort that can go beyond simple adherence with buprenorphine treatment, and experienced buprenorphine providers have learned that psychosocial counseling can be an essential part of office-based treatment. Furthermore, although buprenorphine providers are not required to provide adjunctive psychosocial treatments, the Drug Addiction Treatment Act of 2000 (DATA 2000) does require that they "have the capacity to refer addiction treatment patients for appropriate counseling" (p. 114), and several state Medicaid programs require counseling for buprenorphine coverage.

In this chapter, we give an overview of treatment options for ambulatory patients who receive office-based buprenorphine therapy. Counseling can take several forms—not all of which have been thoroughly tested—and some subgroups of patients may benefit more than others from psychosocial treatment. Trial and error and multiple "doses" of treatment over a long period of time are often necessary to facilitate lasting behavioral change. A basic understanding of treatment options for clinicians can assist patients in achieving favorable outcomes. A case example and related questions are presented at the end of this chapter for additional consideration. For discussion of the case, please see Chapter 15, "Comments on the Case Vignettes."

Does Professional Counseling Improve Outcome?

Research on the efficacy of psychosocial treatment for patients receiving methadone maintenance therapy first identified the relationship between treatment improvement and professional counseling (McLellan et al. 1993). Patients who received professional counseling had better outcomes then those who did not. However, a subsequent meta-analysis found that adjunctive psychosocial treatment was not effective in reducing opioid use or improving treatment retention (Amato et al. 2011). Among tested psychosocial treatment modalities, general supportive counseling and contingency management have the best evidence of efficacy in methadone maintenance treatment (Dugosh et al. 2016). In the broader substance use disorder population, psychosocial treatment involving confrontational counseling, nonspecific drug counseling, and nonspecific psychotherapy are ineffective, whereas cognitive-behavioral therapy (CBT), contingency management, and other manual-guided behavioral therapies such as motivation enhancement therapy (MET), 12-step facilitation (TSF), and behavioral marital therapy are associated with significant improvements in treatment (Miller and Wilbourne 2002; O'Farrell and Fals-Stewart 2002).

The largest and most scientifically rigorous random assignment trial comparing the effect of different types of psychosocial treatments in substance use disorders was Project MATCH (Matching Alcoholism Treatments to Client Heterogeneity), funded by the National Institute on Alcohol Abuse and Alcoholism (NIAAA). Although this study focused on individuals with alcohol dependence and not opioid dependence, its findings are commonly accepted as relevant across the addictive disorders. Individuals in Project MATCH were randomly assigned to manual-guided individual CBT, MET, or TSF therapy. All of the subjects showed significant improvement, and the three counseling approaches were thought to be equally effective (Allen et al. 1997).

The evidence for the efficacy of adjunctive psychosocial interventions is less robust in buprenorphine treatment. Several studies of buprenorphine maintenance found no benefit from CBT, contingency management, or additional drug counseling compared with manualized standard medical management (Fiellin et al. 2006, 2013; Ling et al. 2013; Weiss et al. 2011). A subgroup analysis suggested that prescription opioid users receiving CBT might have more weeks abstinent from all drugs compared with those receiving medical management, an effect not found in heroin users (Cutter et al. 2015). In two trials that tested a computer-based psychosocial treatment based on the community reinforcement approach (CRA) in buprenorphine maintenance patients, CRA improved outcomes compared with standard drug counseling (Bickel et al. 2008), and CRA plus contingency management improved outcomes compared with contingency management alone (Christensen et al. 2014).

The control condition used in most of these null trials was manualized standard medical management (Fiellin et al. 2006, 2013; Weiss et al. 2011). Medical management consisted of regular visits of approximately 20 minutes with the buprenorphine prescriber and involved assessing treatment response and recommending abstinence and self-help participation. Thus, medical management was not an inert control condition. It is unknown whether additional counseling or CBT are effective compared with minimal or no counseling. Additionally, the duration of trials was 24 weeks or less. Treatments of longer duration may have greater efficacy (Zhang et al. 2003).

Although counseling must be available to buprenorphine patients, 40% or more of patients do not attend formal counseling (Finch et al. 2007), and many choose self-help groups only. With the possible exception of CBT for prescription opioid users, no particular counseling approach can be recommended as superior to standard medical management for different phases of treatment or patient subgroups. In the following sections, we describe a variety of manual-guided individual and group therapies that have been found to be effective in other substance use disorder populations.

Assessment for Professional Treatment

Many treatment programs use the American Society of Addiction Medicine patient placement criteria to determine the appropriate intensity of treatment services. These criteria assess patients' severity of illness in six dimensions:

1. Acute intoxication or withdrawal potential
2. A medical condition that may distract from or complicate recovery
3. Comorbid emotional or behavioral problems
4. Treatment acceptance and resistance (insight and compliance)
5. Relapse potential (craving or history of relapses)
6. Recovery environment (structured and supportive)

Arguably, the most important dimensions for deciding on the setting and intensity of rehabilitative services are the comorbid emotional and/or behavioral problems and recovery environment. Comorbid emotional and/or behavioral problems, whether or not they fulfill the criteria for a psychiatric disorder in the *Diagnostic and Statistical Manual of Mental Disorders*, 5th edition (DSM-5; American Psychiatric Association 2013), are endemic among substance-using patients. Recovery environment refers to whether the individual has a supportive place to live (i.e., a drug-free environment) and a structured daily routine (e.g., a job, school, or even attending daily Alcoholics Anonymous [AA] meetings). Often, patients with co-occurring disorders or unstable recovery environments require more intensive treatment settings such as intensive outpatient treatment, partial hospitalization (9–25 hours/week), or residential treatment. Patients with limited emotional and/or behavioral comorbidity, a structured daily routine, and a supportive environment can usually receive outpatient treatment (<9 hours/week). Assessment by a qualified addiction treatment professional is usually necessary to determine the appropriate level of care. Patients who apply for outpatient buprenorphine treatment should be assessed from this perspective to determine whether they are stable enough for outpatient care and whether they require a higher level of intensity of care (see Chapter 4, "Patient Assessment").

Professional Treatment Versus Recovery Groups

The addiction treatment system includes both professional treatment programs that are full-fledged health care entities and informal recovery groups, most of which are based on the 12 steps. Recovery groups are the most cost-effective and widely available secular source of social support available to recovering persons. Clinicians are urged to encourage involvement in these groups as an essential source of social support and practical advice about living with the disease and controlling its symptoms. In some communities, care from a buprenorphine clinician along with recovery group involvement may be the only available treatment options. That said, some recovery groups have philosophies that buprenorphine patients sometimes find difficult to accept (e.g., buprenorphine treatment is not abstinence). It is a common misconception that recovery groups such as AA and Narcotics Anonymous (NA) alone are a form of addiction treatment. Although referral to recovery groups is an important component of the overall treatment plan, involvement in these groups alone does not constitute optimal treatment.

Residential and Intensive Outpatient Programs

Selecting an appropriate setting for addiction treatment depends on the recovery environment. For example, patients who are homeless will likely benefit most from a residential program. Short-term (e.g., 28-day) inpatient programs are often modeled after the Minnesota Model, which focuses on initiation of recovery using a 12-step orientation. Long-term residential programs (lasting longer than 3 months) commonly use elements from the well-known *therapeutic community* model developed by such programs as Phoenix House (www.phoenixhouse.org) and Samaritan Daytop Village (www.samaritanvillage.org). Modified therapeutic communities are also prevalent in prisons and correctional transitional programs. Therapeutic communities create a highly structured therapeutic milieu in which group and individual therapy are delivered along with behavioral modification through progressive responsibilities and privileges and comprehensive rehabilitative services. These programs reduce crime and drug use and increase employment among individuals who complete them (National Institute on Drug Abuse 2002), but attrition is high—only 15%–25% of patients complete the full course of treatment (Keen et al. 2001).

All addiction treatment programs offer some combination of group, individual, and/or family therapy. Many programs offer groups that focus on insight building and education, although little evidence supports their effectiveness. In general, quality programs offer group treatment and individual treatment that have one or more of the following components:

1. Recovery orientation focused on initiation of the 12 steps
2. Cognitive-behavioral orientation with a focus on understanding, avoiding, and coping with triggers for relapse
3. Motivation enhancement orientation with a focus on resolving ambivalence and increasing readiness for behavioral change

Some programs offer family or marital therapy to reduce negative family dynamics and codependence that could lead to relapse. These evidence-based counseling methods are preferable to supportive care or solely psychoeducational approaches.

Concerns about cost have led to a decline in the availability of inpatient and residential treatment. Nonetheless, patients with neither a structured daily routine (e.g., patients who are unemployed) nor a supportive environment (e.g., patients who are homeless, live in a drug-encouraging neighborhood, or have an addicted significant other) require a treatment plan that provides the needed structure and support. The result is that many patients who formerly received inpatient services are now housed in either sober houses or shelters and receive outpatient treatment. Intensive outpatient or daytime hospital programs can provide a fully structured plan of activities and a supportive therapeutic milieu. For patients without access to formal treatment, attending an AA or NA meeting every day for 90 days ("making the 90-in-90") can provide some measure of structure and support.

Toxicological monitoring is an important aspect of the structure in formal treatment programs. In some modalities, such as therapeutic communities or methadone treatment programs, verified progress in treatment leads to increased privileges, such as unsupervised visitation or methadone take-home doses. Objective testing for substance use is essential for verifying self-reports and for facilitating and monitoring progress. Case management with access to psychological, medical, and psychiatric consultation and employment assistance is another evidence-based practice to look for in quality programs.

Choosing a Professional Treatment Program

The Substance Abuse and Mental Health Services Administration's Substance Abuse Treatment Facility Locator (which can be found online at https://findtreatment.samhsa.gov/locator/home) and local directories maintained by state departments of health or state substance abuse agencies are helpful tools for selecting qualified programs. However, just like with choosing any specialist for your patient, selecting quality substance abuse treatment providers is neither trivial nor easy. As with selecting other specialists, asking knowledgeable colleagues, patients, and their families for recommendations is advisable. Ideally, you should search for programs with a multidisciplinary approach and treatment providers who are comfortable with addiction pharmacotherapy that combines the following:

- Evidence-based counseling
- A longitudinal approach across the entire continuum of care
- Case management
- A comprehensive array of psychosocial services either on site or via referral
- A patient-centered approach that recognizes the importance of evening hours, transportation, and child care to facilitate access

High-quality programs routinely include screening for co-occurring psychiatric conditions and, if needed, provide referral or treatment on site. Once the patient accesses the program, it is essential that the patient sign a release of information statement so that the clinician can proactively establish communication with the primary treatment provider. This communication allows clarification of roles in the formulation and implementation of a treatment plan, care coordination, and ongoing sharing of information relevant to treatment progress (e.g., toxicology results and treatment participation). If documented in the chart, time spent in these coordination activities can be used to justify current procedural terminology evaluation and management coding (see Chapter 8, "Referral, Logistics, and Diversion").

Facilitating Outpatient Treatment and/or Recovery Group Involvement

HANDLING RESISTANCE TO TREATMENT: MOTIVATION ENHANCEMENT THERAPY

Often, patients resist recommendations for counseling or 12-step involvement. MET approaches offer a very powerful method for dealing with resistant or ambivalent patients. On the basis of the stages of change paradigm, this approach to counseling recognizes that ambivalence is a normal part of the change and recovery process and that the clinician's behavior can either facilitate or impede progress toward recovery. A supportive, nonjudgmental patient-clinician relationship is especially important in these cases. Because of the negative interactions many such patients have had with the health care system, they are often guarded and quick to sense disrespect from health care providers. Interview style may be as important as content. With a resistant patient, the clinician should convey concern, empathy, and respect through the use of open-ended questions, active listening, and repeating back the patient's words and ideas so that he or she knows the clinician has listened (reflective listening) (Miller and Rollnick 2012). Affirmation of the patient's positive statements and modest successes (arriving at the appointment, duration of abstinence, challenges overcome, improvements in health, and positive lifestyle changes) will build both the therapeutic relationship and the patient's self-efficacy (Barnes and Samet 1997).

Resistance should be viewed as a natural response whenever someone is being asked to change behaviors. When patients resist going to counseling or meetings, the clinician needs to explore motivation and attitudes toward recovery and negotiate for acceptable alternatives in a motivational style (Barnes and Samet 1997; Miller and Rollnick 2012). The clinician should accept that he or she cannot impose his or her personal views on the patient but must invite the patient to consider new perspectives. Resistance should be a clue for the clinician to change strategy: to ask more open-ended questions, listen more, emphasize respect for the patient, ask for the patient's perspective on the problem, ask the patient to suggest solutions, and discuss the pros and cons of change. Finally, it is important to emphasize the personal responsibility of the patient, because in the final analysis, the patient must accept and carry out the recovery plan. To use an analogy: the clinician serves as a coach on the sideline, helping to instill motivation and offering strategy, but the patient is the one on the field. For patients who lack self-efficacy, especially those with prior failed attempts at change, the clinician is an important source of hope, support, encouragement, and alternative strategies. The MET approach was incorporated as one of the manual-guided behavioral therapies employed in Project MATCH; copies of the manual (Miller et al. 1995) are available from NIAAA at http://pubs.niaaa.nih.gov/publications/match.htm. The Miller and Rollnick (2012) text is also a valuable and highly accessible resource for the buprenorphine practitioner.

The clinician should assess and consider the patient's agenda. However, a patient-centered approach does not mean the absence of disagreement; on the contrary, it can make confrontation more effective. For example, if the clinician believes that lack of counseling places the recovering patient at risk for relapse, that belief should be stated directly and the patient should be asked to respond. Recommendations should be framed as specific responses to needs. Feedback should reinforce the areas in which the patient is doing well, express direct concern about overconfidence and the relationship between the concerning behavior and possible consequences, and seek the patient's reaction. If the patient disagrees, management of the patient's opioid use disorder should be negotiated with the same concern used in addressing patients with coronary artery disease who resist changing a sedentary lifestyle. In both cases, judgmental, hardline approaches often produce no clinical benefit and may alienate the patient. A menu of possible options should be presented, and the clinician should negotiate to reach a solution that is acceptable to both clinician and patient. In the final analysis, behavior change is hard work, and the patient should be applauded and supported for any positive change. In a supportive, ongoing relationship, future meetings hold the possibility of helping the resistant patient recognize and address his or her risky behaviors.

WORKING WITH 12-STEP RECOVERY GROUPS

Twelve-step fellowships such as AA and NA are the most widely available form of long-term support for recovery. The 12 steps outline a process of personal change. These steps move the recovering person from initial acceptance of the diagnosis through self-exploration and on to action. Because one of the most difficult tasks of recovery is breaking loose from perceived "friends" who use alcohol or other drugs, 12-step groups, in addition to focusing on the personal changes necessary for recovery, help establish substance-free social networks. Some therapists offer specific treatment designed to assist patients in the process of connecting to mutual support programs. The TSF manual that was used in Project MATCH is available from NIAAA (Nowinski et al. 1995) and provides more details on some of the recommendations described in the next subsection.

FACILITATING INVOLVEMENT IN 12-STEP GROUPS

By encouraging involvement in 12-step groups, the clinician can have an effective role in facilitating recovery (Friedmann et al. 1998). The clinician should encourage the patient to look for a home group in which he or she feels comfortable. The patient should be reminded that every group is different and to try different meetings until one feels right. The patient should be encouraged to regularly participate in the home group and to search for a sponsor and gather a list of telephone numbers from group members. NA focuses on heroin and other opioids, but some buprenorphine patients are more comfortable at AA meetings. This circumstance is understandable because of concerns about encountering the "wrong people" at NA meetings and because some NA groups do not recognize buprenorphine patients as being in recovery. In general, contemporary AA groups are accustomed to polysubstance use and welcome anyone who seeks recovery. Occasionally, buprenorphine patients encounter other AA/NA members who challenge their buprenorphine treatment and insist that the patient is not legitimately sober.

The Sponsor: An Important Ongoing Source of Support

The clinician should strongly support a recovering patient's search for a sponsor (Nowinski et al. 1995). The sponsor, an AA/NA member who has been abstinent for a year or more, is a role model and informal guide to the program. It is important to explain to the patient that the use of sponsors is one of the oldest and most important and effective traditions in 12-step programs. The sponsor will support recovery and confront behavior indicative of imminent relapse. The sponsor should be of the same gender as the patient (or the opposite gender for a patient who identifies as gay or lesbian) and the same age or older. If the patient is having trouble finding a sponsor, he or she should continue to attend meetings, and when announcements are requested, state simply that he or she needs a sponsor. A patient who has difficulty speaking in front of a group should be encouraged to arrive early and stay late and casually let people know that he or she is looking for a sponsor.

The Telephone List: An Essential Tool for Managing High-Risk Situations and Slips

The telephone list is especially important for new members and for those without a sponsor. The clinician should urge the patient to gather a list of telephone numbers from other members who are prepared to give their contact information to new members. Using the telephone is one of the cornerstones of 12-step therapy. Reassure the patient that members expect to give out their telephone numbers and expect to get calls. The clinician should remind patients to call their sponsor or other members whenever they have an urge to drink or use drugs; whenever they feel lonely, angry, tired, or have other negative feelings; whenever they feel overly good (and perhaps complacent) about their sobriety;

and as soon as possible after a relapse. Often, there is no need to explain the reason for calling. The telephone list can also include supportive sober friends or family.

At each visit, the clinician should ask in a nonjudgmental manner about the number of meetings per week the patient is attending, the level of participation in the meetings, and any contact with a sponsor. Clinician concern about a sudden drop-off in meeting attendance, a lack of participation, loss of contact with the sponsor, or possible signs of relapse should be expressed in a direct and empathic manner.

ADDRESSING RESISTANCE TO AA/NA

Resistance to AA/NA is common. Some patients genuinely take issue with 12-step groups, typically complaining that they do not like the religiosity of traditional groups, that they cannot tolerate the cigarette smoke, or that their substance problem is not severe enough to need AA/NA. The clinician should have a repertoire of appropriate responses for reluctant patients. Patients who object to smoking should be directed to nonsmoking meetings, which are growing in number. The clinician needs to urge patients who object to spirituality to seek out meetings with a less overtly spiritual tone; atheist meetings; or, where available, Rational Recovery (https://rational.org), SMART Recovery (www.smartrecovery.org), Meditation and Recovery meetings, or similar secular recovery groups. The clinician should explain that belief in the 12 steps or in a higher power is less important than simply going to meetings and seeking supportive, nonusing friends. For patients who are uncomfortable with the spiritual aspects of a 12-step program, clinicians need to emphasize the practical wisdom reflected in its many slogans, a few of which are discussed below (Nowinski et al. 1995):

- *One day at a time.* This slogan is useful for patients who get caught up in lamenting the past or planning the future. It emphasizes that the key to sobriety is to focus on the present situation and to avoid drug use today. Although anniversaries of sobriety are important, what is most important is whether you drink or use drugs today, not whether you drank or used drugs yesterday or will drink or use drugs tomorrow.
- *First things first.* This slogan says that if the patient does not stay sober, nothing else will matter. This is useful for patients who get distracted from their recovery work by other life problems and responsibilities. It is important to emphasize that everyone has multiple obligations, but sobriety must be the first commitment.
- *Fake it 'til you make it.* Twelve-step groups acknowledge that many of their suggestions may not appeal or make sense to the newly recovering person. This slogan asks the member to accept on faith that the advice will make

sense eventually. This slogan is useful with patients who resist going to meetings, working the steps, and following the sponsor's advice. A related slogan, *Take what you need and leave the rest*, encourages patients to derive from these groups the ideas and support that they think will aid their recovery and to ignore unhelpful aspects of the program.

However, 12-step groups are not for everyone, and the clinician should reassure patients that meeting attendance is neither essential to continuing the patient-clinician relationship nor the only path to recovery.

Cognitive-Behavioral Therapy and Relapse Prevention Counseling

Relapse is a process in which the return to alcohol or drug use results from a series of maladaptive responses to stressors or stimuli (Marlatt and Gordon 1985). The initial return to use (a *lapse* or *slip*) results when the recovering person inadequately copes with emotions, situations, or cues that create craving—an inner need or desire for the substance. The predominant triggers for relapse are negative affective states (e.g., frustration, anger, fatigue, boredom, stress), family conflict (e.g., marital fights), social pressure such as that at parties or in bars, and social isolation (Connors et al. 1996; Miller 1996). Twelve-step groups use the expressions *people, places, and things* and *HALT: don't get Hungry, Angry, Lonely, or Tired* to represent the idea of relapse triggers.

After the first instance of drug use, the individual may experience guilt, shame, and/or anxiety. These negative feelings can lead to an attitude that there is nothing more to lose, resulting in relapse to heavy use to assuage the negative feelings. Although the term *slipping* used by 12-step groups does not differentiate between an initial lapse and full-blown relapse, the recovering patient should be urged to see past the negative feelings brought on by initial use and understand their potential for harm. The clinician is in a position to educate the patient to recognize high-risk situations, craving, and slips and to help develop a coping plan.

Plan to Cope With Emergencies: High-Risk Situations, Craving, and Slips

CBT approaches have proved particularly effective in helping patients avoid relapse and build successful and healthy coping skills. Recovering patients commonly experience high-risk situations, such as life crises, drug offers, craving, and slips, as they struggle to maintain sobriety (Kadden et al. 1995). Craving can be triggered by negative or positive emotions; physical distress; or people, places, and things that remind the patient of drugs. The clinician should emphasize that craving is an uncomfortable but normal part of recovery and is nothing to be ashamed of. The clinician should counsel patients that cravings last only a few minutes to hours and eventually weaken and disappear if the patient does not give in. While advocating avoidance of high-risk situations and people, the clinician must acknowledge that avoidance is not always possible. For example, major life changes and crises are inevitable. Thus, coping skills and planning are essential for stable recovery.

Relapse prevention counseling with an addiction professional is the best means to obtain improved coping skills. However, this type of counseling is not available in some communities, and where it is available, some patients may be unwilling or unable to access it. The buprenorphine clinician should be prepared to use brief counseling and/or role-play to ensure that patients have ways to cope with the normal exigencies of life without resorting to drug use. Counseling in this context involves brainstorming and problem solving with the patient regarding how he or she plans to manage high-risk situations, moods, craving, and slips. In this regard, useful lines of inquiry include the following:

- "In what kinds of situations (do/did) you use (drugs)?"
- "What (are/were) your triggers for using?"
- "During previous abstinent periods, what set you off to use again?"
- "How do you plan to cope with these situations this time?"
- "How do you plan to cope with major life crises or peer pressure to use?"
- "Do you feel confident that you can manage these situations without using?"
- "What would you do if you had a slip?"

The clinician should instruct the patient to write an emergency plan of responses. The plan should formalize any specific coping mechanisms identified by the patient. If the patient cannot identify any coping mechanisms, suggest simple strategies such as the following:

- Talk through the situation with a sponsor, another recovery group member on the patient's telephone list, or a supportive family member or friend—or call the AA hotline
- Go to an AA or other recovery group meeting
- Get involved in a distracting activity, such as reading, a hobby, going to a movie, or exercising
- Engage in prayer or meditation
- Employ behavioral methods learned in a treatment or aftercare program
- The plan should specify that the patient will leave the situation and, if necessary, seek help immediately

The social relationships of drug users revolve around substances. Their peer group has been populated with others who support and reinforce drug use. Being with drug-using friends, family members, or associates increases the risk of relapse through indirect social pressure; the result of the availability of drugs; the conditioned craving and feelings associated with people, places, and things; and direct social pressure to use, as when someone offers the individual drugs or alcohol (Kadden et al. 1995; McKay 1999). Thus, patients must be able to fend off pressure to use as quickly and convincingly as possible (Monti et al. 1989). For patients facing the likely prospect of peer pressure to use or high-risk social environments such as parties, the clinician can help the patient role-play what he or she would say to refuse the offer. At the very least, the clinician can ask the patient how he or she would respond if offered drugs. The patient should be clear that he or she is in recovery and avoid excuses (e.g., saying "I'm on medication") or vague answers (e.g., "not tonight") that imply that he or she might use in the future. Patients should be asked to consider how someone might react to such a refusal and be advised that they are not hurting anyone by not using drugs, so they should not feel guilty.

Despite their best efforts, many recovering persons do use again. After an initial return to use, the individual may experience guilt and shame. These negative feelings can lead to an attitude that there is nothing more to lose, resulting in a return to heavy substance use to assuage the negative feelings. Patients should be urged not to beat themselves up after initial use and to understand the potential for negative feelings to lead to even more drug use. Marlatt and Gordon (1985) have described this as the *abstinence violation effect.* The clinician should remind the recovering person that craving and slips are expected parts of the recovery process and present opportunities for patients to learn about their triggers and to practice their coping plan. The clinician can facilitate a positive approach to recovery as a learning process, with slips providing valuable lessons. That said, the clinician should be mindful of a fine line between helping patients see relapse as a learning opportunity and conveying the message that some use is acceptable. The clinician must make it clear that abstinence is the goal for the majority of patients and that continued use will likely require more intensive treatment (e.g., more counseling, more monitoring, referral to a more intensive level of care). However, because of the guilt and/or shame that could result if the patient were to interpret any use as failure, the goal of abstinence should not prevent the patient from returning to see the clinician or seeking help following a slip (Monti et al. 1989).

If the patient needs or desires other ways to cope with urges and craving, refer the patient to a relapse prevention therapist, an expert in CBT, or a CBT group, if these options are available and acceptable. CBT is based on the premise that substance abuse is a functional problem related to deficits in coping skills. Typically, CBT is provided in the form of group or individual, manual-guided therapy that aims to build cognitive and behavioral skills that support recovery. As originally conceived, it comprises 12 sessions, each of which focuses on specific skill sets such as anger management, coping with craving, and resisting peer pressure. A very useful resource for clinicians is the CBT manual developed by NIAAA (Kadden et al. 1995), which can be obtained free of charge as part of the Project MATCH Series.

Computer-Based Treatments

Two computer-based treatments for patients receiving opioid maintenance treatment have been tested. The first, Therapeutic Education System (TES; http://sudtech.org), is an Internet-based psychosocial intervention based on CRA. TES consists of 65 computerized self-directed modules that involve skills training (e.g., effective problem solving, drug-refusal training), interactive exercises, and homework. CRA was originally developed for the treatment of alcohol use disorder and aims to help patients learn about and adopt healthier lifestyle choices and use them as incentives to stop substance use. CRA is efficacious as a stand-alone treatment and when paired with contingency management (CM) for substance use disorders (Meyers et al. 2011). Patients taking buprenorphine had more weeks of abstinence from cocaine and opioids than did patients receiving standard treatment, and abstinence was comparable with that of patients who received therapist-delivered CRA (Bickel et al. 2008). CM plus TES increased days of abstinence compared with CM alone (Christensen et al. 2014).

The second treatment, Computer-Based Training for Cognitive Behavioral Therapy (CBT4CBT; http://www.cbt4cbt.com), is a computer-based version of CBT. It consists of seven 1-hour modules that teach patients skills to help reduce substance use through videos and interactive exercises. Lessons include learning about patterns of substance use, dealing with cravings, and addressing thoughts that trigger substance use. Cocaine-dependent methadone maintenance patients who received CBT4CBT were more likely to have 3 or more consecutive weeks of abstinence from cocaine than did patients receiving standard methadone maintenance treatment (Carroll et al. 2014).

Conclusion

Psychosocial counseling can be an essential part of office-based treatment with buprenorphine, but it is not effective for everyone. Certainly, the evidence does not support denying access to office-based buprenorphine treatment because a patient is unwilling to engage in psychosocial counseling.

Overall, few psychosocial approaches have been evaluated, and it remains unclear whether certain subgroups of buprenorphine patients benefit more from psychosocial treatment than do other subgroups. Computer-based approaches grounded in the community reinforcement approach currently have the best evidence of efficacy as an adjunctive psychosocial treatment. However, several studies suggest that many patients will do well with standard medical management, perhaps combined with referral to 12-step groups.

When a patient seeks formal counseling, the clinician should ask knowledgeable colleagues, patients, and their families to suggest therapists or programs that are supportive of pharmacological approaches to recovery and include a longitudinal approach across the entire continuum of care, case management, a comprehensive array of psychosocial services, and a patient-centered approach that recognizes the importance of evening hours and transportation to facilitate access. In making the referral, the clinician should coordinate with local treatment providers to ensure quality care; signed release of information forms are essential for enabling communication among treatment providers.

Buprenorphine clinicians should also facilitate patients' involvement with recovery groups. Recommendations for counseling and 12-step involvement should be made in a motivational style that recognizes that resistance is common and expected. For the resistant patient, a menu of possible options should be presented, and the clinician should negotiate a solution that is acceptable to both parties. In general, patients need to develop new drug-free social networks, and participation in 12-step groups should be encouraged as a way for patients to establish these relationships. Although formal relapse prevention counseling is the best means for developing coping skills, buprenorphine clinicians also should be prepared to help patients identify triggers and develop a coping plan as part of their routine medication supervision visits.

Clinical Pearls

- Counseling can be an essential component of quality buprenorphine treatment.

- A basic understanding of the dimensions of assessment and available treatment options will help ensure that the buprenorphine patient receives the appropriate intensity of care.

- Getting to know the competent therapists and quality programs in your community is no different from getting to know quality specialists in other arenas. Inquiries to knowledgeable colleagues and patients can help. Clinicians should locate therapists and programs that are supportive of addiction medication.

- Release of information and care coordination with treatment counselors are essential for quality buprenorphine treatment.

- Twelve-step groups such as AA and NA are cost-effective and widely available. Clinicians should encourage patients to seek groups that are supportive of addiction medication.

- Resistance to counseling and 12-step groups is common and to be expected. It should be addressed by counseling in a motivational style.

- The buprenorphine clinician should encourage patients to develop a plan to cope with high-risk situations, craving, and relapse.

CASE 6

Martha is a 35-year-old stay-at-home mother who started buprenorphine therapy 4 months ago after years of taking oral opioids for back pain related to a herniated disc. She has been a "perfect patient" in many respects but now reports that her AA sponsor insists she "isn't clean." She is confused—you had suggested mutual support groups as a reliable support system. She feels that she has benefited from "working the steps" but now doesn't know where to turn. She says, "I'll just stop going. I don't need the stress. I can get sober on my own."

1. How would you respond to this patient's last statement?

2. How important is a sponsor in a mutual support program?

3. What is AA's stance on prescribed medicines and psychiatric treatment?

4. How do you get a sense of your patient's involvement in AA?

5. Are there other mutual support groups available? Are there other treatment options?

References

Allen JP, Mattson ME, Miller WR, et al: Matching alcoholism treatments to client heterogeneity: Project MATCH posttreatment drinking outcomes. J Stud Alcohol 58(1):7–29, 1997 8979210

Amato L, Minozzi S, Davoli M, et al: Psychosocial combined with agonist maintenance treatments versus agonist maintenance treatments alone for treatment of opioid dependence. Cochrane Database Syst Rev (10):CD004147, 2011 21975742

American Psychiatric Association: Diagnostic and Statistical Manual of Mental Disorders, 5th Edition. Arlington, VA, American Psychiatric Association, 2013

Barnes HN, Samet JH: Brief interventions with substance-abusing patients. Med Clin North Am 81(4):867–879, 1997 9222258

Bickel WK, Marsch LA, Buchhalter AR, et al: Computerized behavior therapy for opioid-dependent outpatients: a randomized controlled trial. Exp Clin Psychopharmacol 16(2):132–143, 2008 18489017

Carroll KM, Kiluk BD, Nich C, et al: Computer-assisted delivery of cognitive-behavioral therapy: efficacy and durability of CBT4CBT among cocaine-dependent individuals maintained on methadone. Am J Psychiatry 171(4):436–444, 2014 24577287

Christensen DR, Landes RD, Jackson L, et al: Adding an Internet-delivered treatment to an efficacious treatment package for opioid dependence. J Consult Clin Psychol 82(6):964–972, 2014 25090043

Connors GJ, Longabaugh R, Miller WR: Looking forward and back to relapse: implications for research and practice. Addiction 91(suppl):S191–S196, 1996 8997792

Cutter CJ, Moore BA, Barry D, et al: Cognitive behavioral therapy improves treatment outcome for prescription opioid users in primary care based buprenorphine/naloxone treatment. Drug Alcohol Depend 146:e255, 2015

Dugosh K, Abraham A, Seymour B, et al: A systematic review on the use of psychosocial interventions in conjunction with medications for the treatment of opioid addiction. J Addict Med 10(2):93–103, 2016 26808307

Fiellin DA, Pantalon MV, Chawarski MC, et al: Counseling plus buprenorphine-naloxone maintenance therapy for opioid dependence. N Engl J Med 355(4):365–374, 2006 16870915

Fiellin DA, Barry DT, Sullivan LE, et al: A randomized trial of cognitive behavioral therapy in primary care-based buprenorphine. Am J Med 126(1):74.e11–74.e17, 2013 23260506

Finch JW, Kamien JB, Amass L: Two-year experience with buprenorphine-naloxone (Suboxone) for maintenance treatment of opioid dependence within a private practice setting. J Addict Med 1(2):104–110, 2007 21768942

Friedmann PD, Saitz R, Samet JH: Management of adults recovering from alcohol or other drug problems: relapse prevention in primary care. JAMA 279(15):1227–1231, 1998 9555766

Kadden R, Carroll K, Donovan D, et al: Cognitive-Behavioral Coping Skills Therapy Manual: A Clinical Research Guide for Therapists Treating Individuals With Alcohol Abuse and Dependence. Project MATCH Monograph Series, Vol 3 (NIH Publ No 94-3724). Rockville, MD, National Institute on Alcohol Abuse and Alcoholism, 1995. Available at: http://pubs.niaaa.nih.gov/publications/MATCHSeries3/index.htm. Accessed May 3, 2010.

Keen J, Oliver P, Rowse G, Mathers N: Residential rehabilitation for drug users: a review of 13 months' intake to a therapeutic community. Fam Pract 18(5):545–548, 2001 11604381

Ling W, Hillhouse M, Ang A, et al: Comparison of behavioral treatment conditions in buprenorphine maintenance. Addiction 108(10):1788–1798, 2013 23734858

Marlatt GA, Gordon JRE: Relapse Prevention: Maintenance Strategies in the Treatment of Addictive Behaviors. New York, Guilford, 1985

McKay JR: Studies of factors in relapse to alcohol, drug and nicotine use: a critical review of methodologies and findings. J Stud Alcohol 60(4):566–576, 1999 10463814

McLellan AT, Arndt IO, Metzger DS, et al: The effects of psychosocial services in substance abuse treatment. JAMA 269(15):1953–1959, 1993 8385230

Meyers RJ, Roozen HG, Smith JE: The community reinforcement approach: an update of the evidence. Alcohol Res Health 33(4):380–388, 2011 23580022

Miller WR: What is a relapse? Fifty ways to leave the wagon. Addiction 91(suppl):S15–S27, 1996 8997778

Miller WR, Rollnick S: Motivational Interviewing: Helping People Change, 3rd Edition. New York, Guilford, 2012

Miller WR, Wilbourne PL: Mesa Grande: a methodological analysis of clinical trials of treatments for alcohol use disorders. Addiction 97(3):265–277, 2002 11964100

Miller WR, Zweben A, DiClemente CC, et al: Motivational Enhancement Therapy Manual: A Clinical Research Guide for Therapists Treating Individuals With Alcohol Abuse and Dependence. Project MATCH Monograph Series, Vol 2 (NIH Publ No 94-3723). Rockville, MD, National Institute on Alcohol Abuse and Alcoholism, 1995

Monti P, Abrams D, Kadden R, et al: Treating Alcohol Dependence: A Coping Skills Training Guide. New York, Guilford, 1989

National Institute on Drug Abuse: Therapeutic Community (NIDA Research Reports Series, NIH Publ No 02–4877). Rockville, MD, National Institute on Drug Abuse, August 2002. Available at: www.nida.nih.gov/PDF/RRTherapeutic.pdf. Accessed July 18, 2008.

Nowinski J, Baker S, Carroll K: Twelve Step Facilitation Therapy Manual: A Clinical Research Guide for Therapists Treating Individuals With Alcohol Abuse or Dependence. Project MATCH Monograph Series, Vol 1 (NIH Publ No 94-3722). Rockville, MD, National Institute on Alcohol Abuse and Alcoholism, 1995. Available at: http://pubs.niaaa.nih.gov/publications/match.htm. Accessed April 15, 2016.

O'Farrell TJ, Fals-Stewart W: Behavioral couples and family therapy for substance abusers. Curr Psychiatry Rep 4(5):371–376, 2002 12230966

Weiss RD, Potter JS, Fiellin DA, et al: Adjunctive counseling during brief and extended buprenorphine-naloxone treatment for prescription opioid dependence: a 2-phase randomized controlled trial. Arch Gen Psychiatry 68(12):1238–1246, 2011 22065255

Zhang Z, Friedmann PD, Gerstein DR: Does retention matter? Treatment duration and improvement in drug use. Addiction 98(5):673–684, 2003 12751985

8

Referral, Logistics, and Diversion

Joji Suzuki, M.D.
Claudia P. Rodriguez, M.D.

OFFICE-BASED opioid treatment with buprenorphine-naloxone (BUP/NX) is an effective treatment for opioid use disorder (OUD; McNicholas 2004). The practice itself is relatively straightforward, but prescribers should be aware of the various logistical elements necessary for establishing a successful office-based treatment program. As long as the basic components of the practice are in place, there is a considerable amount of flexibility in meeting the recommendations set forth in various clinical guidelines. Office-based treatment, therefore, can be structured in a wide variety of primary care and psychiatric practice settings. In this chapter, we outline the logistics of setting up an office-based treatment program. Referral sources, staffing needs, office needs, documentation requirements, and models of care will be discussed. Finally, diversion and a variety of ways to minimize the risk of diversion are outlined.

Referral Sources

Referral sources should be identified prior to initiating treatment. Depending on the capacity of each particular practice, the need for referral sources will vary. A private practice physician who is interested in treating only his or her patients with OUD will have different needs compared with a substance use disorder treatment clinic with multiple BUP/NX prescribers. The following subsections provide examples of sources that will facilitate referral of a pool of potential patients for treatment.

INTERNET LISTINGS

Online listings are an important source of patient referrals. Nonwaivered physicians, substance use disorder treatment centers, and other sources of referral will use these listings to identify possible prescribers. Therefore, appearing in online listings will significantly increase the likelihood of a prescriber reaching potential patients. Conversely, if a prescriber wishes to limit the number of patients contacting the office, he or she may choose to remain off online lists or to remove his or her name after a certain period of time.

After completing the requirements for obtaining a BUP/NX prescribing waiver, a prescriber can choose to be listed as a BUP/NX prescribing physician on a Web site maintained by the Substance Abuse and Mental Health Services Administration (SAMHSA; https://www.samhsa.gov/medication-assisted-treatment/physician-program-data/treatment-physician-locator). The Web site allows patients to search providers by area, zip code, or name and identifies the office address of each provider. If prescribers do not wish to be on this list or later decide to be listed or to remove their names from the list, they can call (866) BUP-CSAT (287-2728) or e-mail info@buprenorphine.samhsa.gov with a request to change their listing.

Prescribers can also register their practice with the National Alliance of Advocates for Buprenorphine Treatment (NAABT) at http://www.naabt.org and join the physician-patient matching system. This matching system allows providers to connect with potential patients by matching characteristics that the provider can specify. Further instructions on how to use the system are provided on the Web site.

LOCAL PHYSICIANS AND CLINICIANS

Frequently, potential patients will be identified by physicians who are not waivered to prescribe BUP/NX themselves. These clinicians may appreciate being able to refer patients for BUP/NX maintenance while continuing to provide general medical or psychiatric care. In addition, some BUP/NX prescribers may choose to treat patients through referrals only from nonwaivered physicians within their own practice settings and may choose not to appear in any online listings at all. Therefore, it is important for the office to notify physicians or therapists within the practice that referrals for BUP/NX treatment are being accepted.

TREATMENT FACILITIES

Another source of referrals will be from medical, psychiatric, or other substance use disorder treatment facilities. For example, a patient who has been admitted to an inpatient facility for medically supervised withdrawal may request help in locating a prescriber. Treatment staff at such facilities should keep a listing of BUP/NX prescribers, which can be provided to care coordinators or directly to the patients. Prescribers can form particular alliances with a facility from which potential patients may be screened. Alternatively, patients can use online resources, if available, so that the process of locating a prescriber can begin before discharge.

Staffing Needs

Although office-based opioid treatment requires some common elements to be successful, staffing will vary with each practice setting. A private practitioner, for example, may decide to perform all the necessary clinical and administrative duties, including urine toxicology, while using community resources for psychosocial treatment. In larger practices, prescribers may choose to rely on clinical or administrative personnel to provide coordination of care as well as provide group counseling on site. The recommendations for staffing are described in the following subsections.

PRESCRIBER

Physicians must meet one of the following criteria: 1) be board certified in addiction medicine or addiction psychiatry by the American Board of Addiction Medicine (ABAM) or the American Board of Medical Specialties, 2) be certified by the American Society of Addiction Medicine (ASAM) or the American Osteopathic Academy of Addiction Medicine (AOAAM), or 3) complete 8 hours of required training in order to apply for a U.S. Drug Enforcement Administration (DEA) waiver to prescribe BUP/NX (see Chapter 1, "Opioid Use Disorder in America"). Resident physicians are eligible to obtain the waiver as long as the resident is able to obtain his or her own federal DEA license. Legislation passed in 2016 allows the buprenorphine patient limit to be increased ultimately to 275 patients for some prescribers. These prescribers must have had the waiver to prescribe to up to 100 patients for at least 1 year and have board certification, as described above and/or practice in a qualified practice setting (Table 8–1). For more detailed information, refer to http://www.samhsa.gov/medication-assisted-treatment/buprenorphine-waiver-management.

NONPHYSICIAN PRACTITIONERS

Beginning in 2017, nurse practitioners and physician assistants can prescribe BUP/NX for the treatment of OUD by completing 24 hours of required training (see Chapter 1 for details). This expansion of the categories of waivered clinicians will help address the need for additional buprenorphine providers and

TABLE 8–1.   **Requirements of providers in a qualified practice setting**

Provide professional coverage for medical emergencies during hours when the practice is closed

Provide access to case management services for patients, including referral and follow-up services for psychosocial, medical, and other related issues

Use health information technology systems if already required in the practice setting

Register for the state prescription monitoring program where operational and in accordance with applicable laws

Accept at least one form of third-party payment

will permit the development of interprofessional models of collaborative care with greater flexibility in office staffing.

Nurses, Psychologists, Social Workers, Counselors, and Peer Recovery Specialists

Registered nurses are currently not eligible to obtain the waiver to prescribe BUP/NX (McNicholas 2004). However, nonphysician clinicians can play an important role in the evaluation and ongoing care of patients. These clinicians can perform the initial telephone screens and the initial evaluations. Nurses can help with carrying out in-office BUP/NX inductions or supervised administrations if necessary. Ancillary staff also can play a role in providing individual psychosocial support and assisting with strategies implemented in treatment, including performing pill counts, obtaining releases of information, and making follow-up phone calls. Regardless of the structure of ongoing care, nonphysician practitioners and peer recovery specialists (recovery coaches) can be important members of the office-based opioid treatment program.

Program Coordinator or Case Manager

Unless the prescriber has the capacity to coordinate care for patients, as in a private practice with a limited number of patients, clinical or administrative staff should be identified to help manage the flow of patients through the practice. Depending on the circumstance, a nurse, a social worker, a case manager, or an administrative staff member may be able to play this role. Depending on staffing availability, these duties can be delegated to more than one individual. Adequate and ongoing training and regular feedback are imperative because many of the duties performed by the coordinator are critical to the operation of the practice. The coordinator might perform the following duties:

- Answer general questions about BUP/NX from patients, families, or other providers seeking to refer a patient
- Manage the initial phone screening of potential patients for BUP/NX treatment
- Help organize the required forms and ensure that each patient chart contains the necessary documentations
- Manage and schedule office visits for inductions and follow-up visits
- Generate templates to organize individual, group, and medication management appointments
- Review prescription monitoring programs to monitor controlled substance prescriptions and compliance or consistency with BUP/NX treatment
- Complete prior authorizations as needed
- Send no-show letters and discharge paperwork with list of appropriate referrals

REFERRAL TO PSYCHOSOCIAL TREATMENT

Ideally, psychosocial treatment is offered on site as an integral component of treatment. Availability of psychosocial treatment on site will improve adherence to treatment as well as outcomes (McLellan et al. 1993).

If psychosocial treatment is offered on site, one or more clinicians with experience in the treatment of substance use disorders will need to be identified. Motivation enhancement therapy, relapse prevention, cognitive-behavioral therapy, and contingency management are examples of individual therapies that may be offered (Strain and Lofwall 2008). Group therapy is also an effective method that is widely used and popular among patients (Brook 2008). Groups can be further subdivided to treat specific patient populations such as women, young adults, men, and patients with dual diagnosis (Brook 2008). Peer support plays an important role in recovery and can be used in group therapy.

If psychosocial treatment is not offered on site, it is recommended that appropriate therapists and counselors be found prior to prescribing BUP/NX. Ideally, these clinicians will provide treatment in multiple modalities so that treatment can be tailored to meet the needs of individual patients. A list of off-site providers and facilities should be kept and made available to patients. SAMHSA maintains a Web site (https://findtreatment.samhsa.gov/) that can be helpful in identifying such therapists at local substance use disorder treatment facilities. A collaborative approach and open communication about the clinical progress of patients will help improve patient care. In addition, feedback from patients about the services offered by outside providers and facilities will be helpful in evaluating the quality of such services.

Finally, all patients should be encouraged to attend and participate in 12-step or other mutual-support groups, such as Alcoholics Anonymous (AA) or Narcotics Anonymous (NA). Evidence is clear that patients involved with 12-

step or other mutual-support groups experience better outcomes (Moos and Timko 2008). Telephone directories in all areas of the United States will usually list local AA and NA groups, and these local central service offices (sometimes referred to as *intergroups*) will be able to direct patients to ongoing meetings. Patients also can contact the general service office of AA directly at (212) 870-3400 to obtain information about local offices. Finally, patients can look up local meetings by going on to the Web site http://www.aa.org/pages/en_US/find-local-aa. It is important to recognize that AA and NA meetings and members have varying levels of acceptance of BUP/NX treatment. As such, clinicians should discuss with patients in advance about the need to carefully consider if and to whom the use of BUP/NX should be disclosed.

REFERRAL TO GENERAL MEDICAL OR PSYCHIATRIC CARE

General medical practitioners should have the ability to refer buprenorphine patients for psychiatric assessment and treatment when indicated because psychiatric diagnoses are common in patients with OUD (Kessler et al. 2005). Conversely, psychiatrists should have the ability to refer patients for medical assessment (e.g., physical exams, baseline laboratory testing) if unavailable in the clinic and treatment as well as screening and treatment for infectious diseases (e.g., HIV or hepatitis C). Monitoring of liver function at onset of treatment and periodically during maintenance treatment is important because transaminitis has been reported in hepatitis C–positive patients (Berson et al. 2001).

TRAINING

Ongoing training and mentoring of prescribing physicians as well as of office staff are important considerations. Experienced BUP/NX prescribers in the local area can help less experienced prescribers navigate the various clinical and administrative issues that may arise during the course of treatment.

Additionally, or when no local expertise can be found, a SAMHSA-funded online network of experts called Providers' Clinical Support System for Medication Assisted Treatment (PCSS-MAT) is available at www.pcssmat.org. This network is available at no charge and is composed of experts from across the United States from medical and psychiatric specialties who have agreed to act as mentors. In addition, the PCSS-MAT Web site contains resources such as BUP/NX trainings, clinical tools for BUP/NX prescribing, and a wide range of free live and archived modules and educational activities. Another useful tool for providers is a mobile application created by SAMHSA to support medication-assisted treatment for OUD (see http://store.samhsa.gov/apps/mat/index.html?WT.ac=AD_20161021_MATx).

Another resource for ongoing training for prescribers can be found at http://buppractice.com, a Web site sponsored by the National Institute on Drug

Abuse. This site contains links to training guides and courses for clinical and administrative staff.

Training for staff should include the following topics:

- Role of pharmacological and psychosocial treatments in management of OUD
- Rationale of policies outlined in the treatment contract
- Patient confidentiality
- Responding to aberrant drug behaviors, positive urine toxicology screens, and reported relapses
- Professionalism

COVERAGE DURING ABSENCES

Coverage for the prescriber will need to be arranged during periods of absence. Ideally, the covering physician should have a waiver to prescribe BUP/NX if needed in an emergency. If this is not possible, a nonwaivered physician may also provide coverage to answer general questions or address minor needs, including such issues as need for prior authorizations or management of BUP/NX side effects, as long as the covering physician has sufficient basic knowledge of BUP/NX. Patients should be warned that the nonwaivered covering physician cannot prescribe BUP/NX, and prescription issues or sudden withdrawal may require going to the emergency department for guidance. Policies regarding early refills, lost medications, or benzodiazepine prescriptions, for example, should be agreed on in advance among covering physicians. The coverage system should be communicated clearly to the patient.

Office Needs

It is usually quite simple to incorporate BUP/NX practice into existing programs. However, consideration should be given to the following areas.

PHYSICAL SPACE

During the induction visit, patients may be required to wait in the waiting room for the duration of the visit, or they may be allowed to go off site and return at a prearranged time. If the patient is going to remain on site, comfortable seating, reading material, or a television may help pass the time. A waiting room specifically reserved for patients undergoing induction may be created to provide privacy.

If psychosocial treatment is being offered on site, rooms for individual and/or group therapy will need to be available. Efforts should be made to assure confidentiality, such as using white noise machines to prevent conversations from being heard outside the room.

If the prescriber chooses to dispense BUP/NX directly to patients for purposes of induction, the medication can be obtained from pharmacies or medical suppliers. The medications must be kept in a secure location (i.e., stored on site in a locked safe within a locked room, with limited access). The DEA recommends installing an electronic alarm to provide further security. A written log of all doses dispensed must be maintained and kept up to date. Additional state regulations may apply, and prescribers should ensure compliance by contacting their state substance use disorder agencies.

PHARMACY

If the prescriber chooses not to dispense BUP/NX during the induction phase of treatment, it is important to identify a pharmacy that will provide the necessary medications. Ideally, the pharmacy will be located close to the office, have a reliable supply of BUP/NX, and have business hours that are convenient for the purposes of induction; pharmacists should understand that patients may need to return frequently during or following an induction. If prescriptions will be faxed to the pharmacy, the patient will need to sign a release of information between the pharmacy and the office. This is specifically relevant to clinics operating under the Code of Federal Regulations, Title 42, Part 2 (42 CFR Part 2), which provides regulations about patient confidentiality relative to substance abuse treatment records. Generally, if a patient will always have a paper prescription to present to the pharmacy, a release of information is not necessary. However, exchanging information regarding the patient's treatment or changes in dosing or information for prior authorizations warrants a signed release of information.

The prescriber should decide prior to induction whether the patient will pick up the medications before the induction visit or arrive at the office first. If the former, the prescriber should specify that the prescription be filled only on the day of induction, or at most the day prior to induction. If the latter, prescribers should be aware of the possibility that during busy hours, pharmacies may require more time to fill the prescriptions, thus prolonging the distress and discomfort patients experience. Some pharmacies, however, allow for delivery, which will eliminate the need for prescriptions to be picked up.

URINE TOXICOLOGY TESTING

Assessing treatment efficacy through biological markers is an important component of substance use disorder treatment. Most commonly, urine toxicology testing is the preferred method because of its reliability, ease of administration, and low cost (Strain and Lofwall 2008). However, some practices may choose to incorporate breath, oral fluid, or serum testing. Hair, sweat, or oral fluid testing should not be required as long as adequate urine or serum testing is conducted. Various products intended for office-based testing with good reliability are available commercially at low cost (McNicholas 2004).

If on-site urine testing is done, a suitable bathroom facility is needed. For the majority of BUP/NX practices, unobserved urine testing is sufficient. Observed urine testing should not be a routine requirement unless there are reasons to believe that urine specimens are being tampered with or adulterated or that a patient is attempting to circumvent the testing by using, for example, a prosthetic device worn under the clothing. If testing is done off site, inquiries should be made about how the specimen is obtained, tested, and reported. Additionally, the testing facility should have the ability to detect tampered or adulterated samples.

The testing, whether on site or off site, should include buprenorphine along with common classes of misused substances—opioids, amphetamines, cocaine, cannabis, benzodiazepines, and barbiturates. Breath, serum, or urine tests for alcohol should be available if indicated. Testing specifically for heroin metabolites (6-monoacetylmorphine), oxycodone, fentanyl, and methadone also should be considered because routine toxicology testing assays are not sensitive to semisynthetic and synthetic opioids (Strain and Lofwall 2008). Ideally, urine specimens should be obtained both routinely and randomly because tests can identify only recent drug use, except cannabis, which is detectable for a longer period after cessation.

Finally, the prescriber and other clinical staff should have an agreement about how to respond to aberrant urine tests. The substance that tested positive, the phase of treatment, frequency of positive results, and status of other comorbid illnesses should all be included in determining the response to such positive results.

FORMS

Having standardized forms will be very helpful in assuring full compliance with all documentation requirements. The following is a suggestion of forms to be stocked and made available as needed:

- *Telephone screening forms.* Each practice will need to decide the appropriate criteria for entry into treatment. For practices without psychiatric expertise, for example, severe psychiatric illness may be an exclusion. Another reason for exclusion may be active comorbid alcohol or sedative/hypnotics use disorders. To facilitate making this decision, the initial telephone screening should be sufficiently structured so that all relevant information is obtained.
- *Treatment contract.* A clearly written treatment contract should be reviewed with every patient. Suggestions for the treatment contract are described later in this chapter in the subsection "Treatment Contract and Informed Consent."

- *Release of information.* Signed consent must be obtained before disclosing any individually identifiable addiction treatment information to any third party. Patients should be advised that signed releases to communicate with previous and current providers as well as the pharmacy may be a requirement prior to entry into treatment. A sample release is presented later in this chapter in the subsection "Confidentiality."
- *DSM-5 criteria for OUD.* Diagnosis of OUD based on DSM-5 (American Psychiatric Association 2013) criteria is a requirement for entry into office-based opioid treatment.
- *Clinical Opioid Withdrawal Scale (COWS).* COWS is a reliable and widely used clinician-administered scale to assess the severity of opioid withdrawal. The scale is helpful in assessing withdrawal symptoms during the induction phase of treatment.

INFORMATION FOR PATIENTS

Patient handouts should be made available in waiting rooms or given directly to patients during office visits. Helpful patient materials are available from Indivior, the manufacturer of Suboxone (BUP/NX sublingual film) at http://www.suboxone.com/treatment. Additional printable material is available on other sites, such as the national Alliance of Advocates for Buprenorphine Treatment (https://www.naabt.org/education/literature.cfm).

Suggestions for patient handouts include the following:

- *Information about buprenorphine.* Patients may find basic pharmacology of buprenorphine helpful. The ceiling effect and the blocking effect of buprenorphine should be included. Side effects, notably precipitated withdrawal, as well as the dangers of injection use of buprenorphine also should be included.
- *Explanation of the induction visit.* A written reminder should be provided, clearly explaining the procedure for the induction visit, including information on where and when to pick up the initial prescription if the medication is not available for administration in the office and the need to arrive in mild to moderate withdrawal and spend several hours at the clinic for monitoring of symptoms after first dose delivery. An alternative to an in-office induction is a home induction in which the patient initiates BUP/NX at home with the provider's guidance. Home inductions may be appropriate for patients who have had past experiences with BUP/NX; who have someone who can oversee the induction at home; or who have not been actively using opioids, thus decreasing the risk of precipitated withdrawal. Ancillary staff can assist in contacting the patient via telephone to discuss initiation of treatment and follow up throughout the day to ensure successful induction. Patients and their family members who help oversee the process can

be provided with written information that will help guide them through the induction. During home inductions, treatment staff should be available for contact in the event of an adverse event, such as precipitated withdrawal.

- *Psychosocial treatment resources in the local community.* If off-site psychosocial treatment is offered, patients should be given a list of local treatment providers and facilities, including information about AA and NA meetings.
- *Privacy rights.* Patients should be provided with a written summary of confidentiality provisions and a notice that federal regulations protect substance use disorder treatment records from unnecessary disclosure.

CONFIDENTIALITY

Patients entering substance use disorder treatment are justifiably concerned about privacy issues. Privacy rules, therefore, have been enacted to protect patient privacy but also to provide reassurance to patients that their information will not be disclosed unnecessarily.

The physician must adhere to the privacy requirements outlined by the confidentiality regulation 42 CFR Part 2. This regulation, which applies to office-based opioid treatment with BUP/NX, prohibits the prescriber from releasing individually identifiable addiction treatment information without a signed consent by the patient. However, if BUP/NX is being prescribed in the context of primary care or general psychiatric care, the records may not be subject to 42 CFR regulations. Prescribers are strongly encouraged to seek legal counsel if there is ambiguity about the need to adhere to 42 CFR regulations.

Release of information for the pharmacy is required for BUP/NX prescriptions to be faxed. However, consent for disclosure is not required for medical emergencies and mandated reporting. Additional information and sample forms can be obtained from PCSS-MAT at http://pcssmat.org.

The consent form authorizing the release of information must contain the following elements:

1. The name of the patient
2. The name or general designation of the program making the disclosure
3. The recipient of the information
4. The purpose of the disclosure
5. The information to be released
6. A statement of acknowledgment that the patient understands that he or she may revoke the consent at any time, orally or in writing
7. The date or condition on which the consent expires, if it has not been revoked earlier. This may be state dependent, as some state regulations provide automatic expiration of consents after a certain period of time
8. The date the consent form is signed

TABLE 8–2.   **Patient consent for the release of confidential information**

I, (name of patient) authorize (name or general designation of program making disclosure) to disclose to (name of person(s) or organization to which disclosure is to be made) the following information:

(Nature of the information, as limited as possible).

The purpose of the disclosure authorized herein is to (purpose of disclosure, as specific as possible).

I understand that my records are protected under the Federal regulations governing Confidentiality of Alcohol and Drug Abuse Patient Records, 42 CFR Part 2, and cannot be disclosed without my written consent unless otherwise provided for in the regulations. I also understand that I may revoke this consent at any time except to the extent that action has been taken in reliance on it, and that in any event this consent expires automatically as follows:

(Specification of the date, event, or condition on which this consent expires).

(Date) (Print name) (Signature of participant)

(Date) (Print name) (Signature of parent, guardian, or authorized representative when required)

Source. Providers' Clinical Support System for Medication Assisted Treatment, "Summary of the Rule (Title 42 CFR Part 2—Confidentiality Alcohol and Drug Use Patients Records)." Available at: http://pcssmat.org/wp-content/uploads/2015/03/Sample-Consent-for-Release-Information.pdf.

---

9. The signature of the patient or parent, guardian, or authorized representative as deemed appropriate
10. 42 CFR Part 2 notice

Note that one form may be used for multiple recipients, but it is important that the purpose of disclosure and information disclosed are the same for all recipients listed on a single form. See Table 8–2 for a sample release of information.

BILLING

Currently, there are no special addiction medicine or psychiatry codes for billing office-based OUD treatment. Prescribers should be aware that insurance reimbursements vary.

Primary Care

Primary care physicians should use *evaluation and management* Current Procedural Terminology (CPT) codes based on either complexity of service or time.

Coding based on time is used if counseling or coordination of care takes up more than 50% of the visit. Counseling is defined as face-to-face time spent with the patient, family members, or other caregiver discussing such topics as diagnostic results, impressions, prognosis, risks and benefits of treatment, or instructions for treatment. If billing is time based, the total time for the visit, total time spent counseling, and the content of the counseling must be included in the documentation.

For the induction visit, the usual evaluation and management codes are used, but additional prolonged visit codes also can be used. However, only face-to-face time with the patient, continuous or not, beyond the average time required for the visit can be billed. Home inductions are not typically billable, although some clinics allow billing of telephone calls, which may be a part of the home induction process depending on length of phone call.

Psychiatry

Psychiatrists should use *behavioral health* codes. These codes are time based and do not involve any complexity-based requirements. There are no special codes for prolonged visits. Refer to Table 8–3 for specific CPT codes.

Billing Without Insurance

Accepting cash for office-based treatment is an acceptable arrangement. In fact, because of privacy concerns, some patients may seek out providers who accept cash. Nevertheless, ethical billing practices should be followed when determining fees. It should be noted that if a prescriber has a contract with an insurer, the contract may prohibit the acceptance of cash for covered services, even if those services are provided in a different practice setting. Prescribers are advised to check with each insurer to confirm that accepting cash is permitted and, if not, whether accepting cash is allowed if the patient signs a specific waiver.

DOCUMENTATION

The recommendations for documentation of office-based opioid treatment are outlined in guidelines set by the Federation of State Medical Boards. The documentation should remain current and should be easily accessible and available if there is a need for review by regulatory agencies. Specifically, the physician should include the following components: summary of initial evaluation; treatment plan; treatment contract and informed consent; diagnostic, therapeutic, and laboratory results; referrals (if any); list of medications prescribed; review of the prescription monitoring program (if required); and inventory of controlled substances (if dispensed in the office).

TABLE 8–3.   **CPT codes for various practices**

Type of visit	Primary care CPT codes	Psychiatry CPT codes
Assessment visit		
New patient	99202–99205	90792 (with E/M)
Established patient	99212–99215[a]	99212–99215[a]
Induction visits		
Established patient E/M	99211–99215[a]	99211–99215[a]
Add-on prolonged service codes	99354–99355[b]	
Outpatient consultation		99241–99245
Maintenance visits		
Established patient	99211–99215	
Outpatient medication management		99212–99214
Add on therapy codes		
16–37 minutes		90833
38–52 minutes		90836
53+ minutes		90838
Group psychotherapy		90853

Note.   CPT=Current Procedural Terminology; E/M=evaluation and management.
[a]Code 99215 requires documentation that physician spent 60 minutes with patient in a combination of medical care and counseling.
[b]These codes are used for a patient who remains under care beyond the hour covered by code 99215.
Source.   www.buppractice.com/node/1437.

Summary of Initial Evaluation

At the time of the initial evaluation, a medical history and physical examination should be completed and documented. Evaluation of the medical history should include the following components:

- Nature of the patient's substance use disorders
- Underlying or comorbid medical conditions
- Physical and psychological dysfunction caused by the drug use
- History of substance use and prior treatments
- Suitability of patients for BUP/NX maintenance based on the diagnosis of OUD using the DSM-5 criteria

Refer to http://pcssmat.org/wp-content/uploads/2015/03/Sample-intake-questionnaire.pdf for a sample intake questionnaire.

Treatment Plan

The treatment plan should include clear objectives that can be documented and monitored throughout the course of treatment. Objective measures for treatment may include abstinence from substances of misuse, attendance at psychosocial treatments, and improved psychological and physical functioning. Referral to psychosocial interventions and the involvement of family and significant others should be recommended and documented in the treatment plan. Finally, the treatment plan should include responses to treatment failure.

Treatment Contract and Informed Consent

Patients must provide written informed consent to enter treatment. If indicated, family members and significant others should be included in the discussion, with appropriate release of information. The following issues, if indicated, will need to be discussed and included in the signed treatment contract:

- Risks and benefits of treatment with BUP/NX, including precipitated withdrawal and interactions with benzodiazepines
- Receipt of BUP/NX from one prescriber and pharmacy
- Treatment options other than BUP/NX
- Policies regarding urine toxicology and pill counts
- Policies regarding the number and frequency of refills for BUP/NX
- Policies regarding the discontinuation of BUP/NX
- Policies regarding no-shows and cancellations
- Responsibility for safe storage of medications
- Prohibition against diversion of prescriptions
- Expectations for psychosocial treatment
- Procedures for contacting the office during off hours
- Expectations of payment

Diagnostic, Therapeutic, and Laboratory Results

The medical record should contain the results of any tests that are conducted as part of the evaluation or ongoing monitoring. Baseline laboratory evaluation such as complete blood count, liver function tests, electrolytes, and urine toxicology, as well as assessments by mental health providers, all should be documented.

Referrals

The medical record should include documentation of referrals to consultants for additional evaluation and treatment, if indicated clinically. The results of such consultations should be included in the medical record.

List of Medications Prescribed

Documentation is required for all prescriptions provided to patients, which should include the date, name, dosage, quantity, and refills for each medication prescribed and/or dispensed. Including a photocopy of every prescription written will satisfy this requirement.

Review of Prescription Monitoring Program

Depending on the requirements in the state of practice, documentation of review of the prescription monitoring program prior to initiation of any controlled substance may be required. Some states require review of the prescription monitoring program prior to providing both initial and maintenance BUP/NX prescriptions. This should be documented and should include the date of review, with any pertinent information.

Inventory of Controlled Substances Dispensed

If the prescriber chooses to dispense BUP/NX directly to patients from supplies kept in the office, a physical inventory must be kept. The inventory should track and document the date, name, dose, and quantity of all medications dispensed (Figure 8–1).

Diversion and Nonmedical Use

As with other opioid medications, there is a risk of diversion and nonmedical use of BUP/NX. Diversion includes sharing or selling the medication, trading for other substances, or stockpiling the medication for later use.

NONMEDICAL USE

Nonmedical use of BUP/NX occurs when the medication is taken for reasons other than that for which it was prescribed—for example, taking more than prescribed or injecting to obtain a "high" or to self-medicate dysphoric moods. Studies have indicated that individuals most commonly report obtaining diverted BUP/NX in order to self-medicate withdrawal symptoms; using BUP/NX for the "high" is less frequently reported (Yokell et al. 2011). A survey found that factors associated with the use of diverted BUP/NX include an inability to access BUP/NX treatment, diagnosis of generalized anxiety disorder, and past 30-day use of OxyContin, methamphetamine, and/or alcohol (Lofwall and Havens 2012). The limited availability of prescribers in many areas is therefore a likely contributing factor to diversion of BUP/NX. As such, from a public health perspective, increasing access to treatment may be an important strategy for decreasing the rates of BUP/NX diversion.

Medication:

Physician Name:

Dose Form and Strength: 2/0.5 mg 8/2 mg

Dispensing Area:

Note: An inventory must be performed at the beginning and end of each day which can be performed by MD, nurse, or pharmacist.

Line No.	Date	Patient Name	Patient's ID No.	Dose	Quantity Dispensed or Received	Balance Forward / Balance	Manufacturer And Lot No.	Recorder's Signature (2 required if an inventory is performed)
1								
2								
3								
4								
5								

FIGURE 8–1. **Drug accountability record for stock buprenorphine supplies.**

Source. Providers' Clinical Support System for Medication Assisted Treatment, http://pcssmat.org/wp-content/uploads/2015/03/Bup-Stock-Drug-Accountability-Record.pdf.

PREVENTING DIVERSION

There are numerous strategies that should be considered to decrease the risk of diversion (Table 8–4). It is important to limit the medication supply by providing limited prescription, especially in early phases of treatment or when a patient exhibits aberrant behaviors. For patients who are early in treatment, weekly prescriptions should be the standard duration. Using the lowest necessary dose is also an important preventative measure.

Naloxone is minimally bioavailable if taken sublingually, but injection of the combination tablet results in a brief withdrawal reaction that dissuades injection use in an active user or delays the potential euphoria that can be experienced from buprenorphine in someone who is not actively using opioids. Therefore, the combination product should be used exclusively, except when the mono product (buprenorphine only) is the preferred agent because of pregnancy or confirmed allergy to or intolerance of naloxone.

Even though the therapeutic BUP/NX dosage can vary among individual patients, daily doses of 8 mg buprenorphine/2 mg naloxone to 16 mg buprenorphine/4 mg naloxone should be sufficient for most patients. Providers should be careful not to undermedicate or overmedicate, and doses above 16 mg/4 mg warrant evaluation of factors that may be contributing to the need for higher doses, such as comorbid mental illness, comorbid medical illnesses such as acute or chronic pain, cravings, diversion, nonmedical use of BUP/NX, and/or inappropriate administration leading to reduced effects. Observed sublingual ingestion may be helpful for first-time users (during induction) or in individuals who have symptoms of cravings or withdrawal despite daily use to ensure appropriate mode of administration.

Urine toxicology screening should be employed routinely to ensure adherence to BUP/NX. In individuals suspected of diversion or nonadherence, it may be helpful to obtain quantitative testing of buprenorphine and its metabolite norbuprenorphine and/or naloxone on the basis of laboratory availability. This practice can be effective in identifying patients who dissolve undigested tablets or films directly into their urine sample; high levels of buprenorphine paired with a low level or an absence of the metabolite, and/or the presence of high levels of naloxone, may indicate attempts at concealing diversion. Observed urine testing also may be necessary when tampering with urine samples is suspected or confirmed. Validity testing, such as testing for creatinine, color, temperature, and specific gravity, also should be performed where available.

Another strategy is to use random pill counts, in which individuals are contacted and given a specified amount of time (usually 24 hours) to come into the clinic with their remaining prescription. The state prescription monitoring program should be reviewed on a regular basis to ensure that patients are not obtaining multiple prescriptions from other providers. Some states require a

TABLE 8–4.   **Strategies for decreasing buprenorphine diversion and nonmedical use**

Use the combination (BUP/NX) product in nonpregnant patients without confirmed adverse reaction

Require weekly visits during early phase of treatment

Limit medication supply (provide a weekly supply in early phase of treatment)

Use lowest effective dose, avoiding underdosing or overdosing

Observe sublingual ingestion for first-time users or patients who find a stable dose ineffective

Conduct frequent urine toxicology screening, including qualitative and/or quantitative buprenorphine

Use a prescription monitoring program

Monitor for and respond to aberrant behaviors (e.g., random pill counts, increased frequency of treatment)

documented review of the prescription monitoring program. Observed daily or thrice weekly dosing may be considered for some patients before take-home doses are provided, although this may be beyond the resources of most programs. Finally, including the patient's family members and significant others in the treatment may help adherence to treatment.

Providers, support staff, and pharmacy staff should regularly monitor for behaviors that may signal diversion or nonmedical use, such as appearing intoxicated, requests for early refills, reports of lost or stolen prescriptions, increased frequency of urine toxicology screens positive for illicit drug use, or lack of adherence to appointments.

Ideally, the policies for addressing diversion and nonmedical use of BUP/ NX should be decided before patients are enrolled. Patients should be fully informed of these policies prior to treatment initiation, and discussions about diversion and nonmedical use should be conducted openly throughout treatment. Written information regarding different forms of diversion and potential response to diversion should be provided to all patients at initiation of treatment. This written information may also include reasons for administrative discharge as decided on by the clinic, such as selling opioids on site or aggressive treatment of patients or staff.

Responses to diversion or nonmedical use could include additional patient education about the importance of adherence to clinic policies; mandating observed dosing; increasing frequency of visits; referral to higher level of care that includes methadone maintenance; use of random pill counts; use of stricter urine toxicology screening procedures; and, in certain circumstances, termination from the practice. If patients are discharged from treatment, they should be provided with appropriate referrals to other programs, information regarding safe tapering of BUP/NX, and information on when the patient can be reconsidered for the program. However, as a general principle, every effort should be made to retain patients in treatment. Generally, lapses in use are an expected aspect of the process of recovery. Discharging patients prematurely may result in a missed opportunity to continue to learn from lapses, identify triggers, and implement better coping mechanisms in the future. Discharge should be a last resort rather than an immediate response to lapse in substance use.

Models of Care

Office-based treatment with BUP/NX can be provided in a variety of treatment settings and modified to match specific resource availability. For most primary care physicians and psychiatrists in the community, integrating office-based treatment into their current practice should not be difficult.

Several models of care are presented in the following subsections. Each of these models fulfills the basic clinical requirements and does so by using very different physical and staffing resources. Each of these models can be further customized according to the particular needs of the practice. Refer to Table 8–5 for information about each of the models of care.

Primary Care Models

Hub and Spoke Model

In the hub and spoke model, the comprehensive evaluation, care coordination, initial intake, induction onto BUP/NX, and stabilization are performed at an opioid treatment program (the *hub*). Either in-office inductions or home inductions can be used to initiate treatment of BUP/NX. Patients attend treatment as established by the hub, and once stable on a BUP/NX dose, they may be able to transfer to the spoke for ongoing medication management. The *spoke* typically consists of a primary care clinic, psychiatrist, or outpatient substance use disorder treatment provider. If necessary, patients can return to the hub for more intensive treatment or closer monitoring and then return to the spoke once they are stabilized. This allows for opioid treatment programs to manage complex patients and link with office-based BUP/NX providers in communities that may not have the higher level of treatment interventions (e.g., on-site therapy, case management, on-site laboratory testing).

TABLE 8–5. **Models of care**

Model	Staffing	Referral source	Urine toxicology	Psychosocial treatment
Hub and spoke	X-waivered physicians at hub and spoke; nonphysician prescribers, counselors, community providers	Self-referral; identified in primary or subspecialty clinic and other community health centers	Typically obtained at each visit or as directed by treatment program	On-site or off-site counseling, case management
Community-based primary care clinic	X-waivered physician, addiction counselor	Self-referral; identified in community health centers	Obtained at each visit, then as directed by treatment program	On-site counseling
Nurse care manager	X-waivered PCP, nurse care manager, addiction counselor (on site or by referral)	Self-referral; identified in primary or subspecialty clinic and other community health centers	Obtained at each visit initially, then randomly; for random testing or pill counts, patient must provide sample within 48–72 hours of contact	On-site or off-site individual or group counseling
Intensive outpatient	X-waivered psychiatrist and licensed social worker or psychologist at hospital-based dual diagnosis clinic; other staff may include case managers and nursing staff	Referrals accepted only from patients with a PCP at the affiliated hospital and a documented physical examination within 30 days of entry into treatment	Frequent on-site testing initially, then randomly	On-site intensive outpatient treatment for 2–4 weeks after induction (3 hours of group therapy per day, 3 days/ week±individual therapy); ongoing individual or group therapy on completion
Shared medical appointment (SMA)	X-waivered psychiatrist, licensed social worker; other staff may include case managers, nursing staff, and psychologists	Self-referral; referred from affiliated hospital providers or other community clinics	Urine testing coupled with group visits; varies in frequency depending on group appointment frequency	Coupled with SMA as group therapy appointments; can schedule individual therapy as appropriate

TABLE 8–5.   **Models of care** *(continued)*

Model	Staffing	Referral source	Urine toxicology	Psychosocial treatment
Private practice: psychiatry	X-waivered psychiatrist, on-site or off-site therapist	Self-referral; referred from other psychiatrist or community substance use disorder treatment program (e.g., facilities for medically supervised withdrawal, residential programs)	Obtained at every visit initially, then randomly	Off-site counseling
Emergency department (ED) initiation of BUP/NX	ED physician, X-waivered physician, social worker or care coordinator, nursing staff, affiliated clinic staff	Self-referral; identified by ED staff	Obtained prior to starting treatment and as determined by follow-up treatment staff	Brief intervention by physician within ED visit; ongoing interventions determined by OBOT affiliated with ED
Hospital initiation of BUP/NX	Multidisciplinary addiction consultation service	Identified by hospital staff	Obtained prior to starting treatment and as determined by follow-up treatment staff	During hospitalization, psychosocial interventions limited to supportive or motivational interviewing therapy; follow-up interventions as determined by treatment staff

Note.   X-waivered physicians are physicians who have completed the required buprenorphine training and have obtained a U.S. Drug Enforcement Administration waiver (X-waiver) to prescribe buprenorphine for the treatment of opioid use disorder.

Abbreviations: BUP-NX=buprenorphine–naloxone; OBOT=office–based opioid treatment; PCP=primary care provider.

Community-Based Primary Care Clinic

In community-based primary care, the primary care physician manages clinical care with the support of an on-site addiction counselor. Focus is on integrating primary care and substance use disorder treatment. After an initial telephone screening, the patient is evaluated face to face by a physician and separately by an addiction counselor. If appropriate, the patient is scheduled for the induction visit. The patient fills the prescription at the pharmacy before arriving for the induction, and the first dose is given in the office under direct observation. The patient returns 1–2 hours later to be reassessed to ensure improvement in symptoms. The patient is directed to take an additional dose at home if necessary for symptoms of withdrawal and may contact the clinic if he or she has additional questions regarding BUP/NX dosing. The patient is reassessed again in several days and returns to meet the prescriber weekly for the first month. If urine screens are negative and the dose is stable, the patient returns for monthly visits. Visits with the addiction counselor occur on a weekly basis.

NURSE CARE MANAGER MODEL: HOSPITAL-BASED PRIMARY CARE CENTER

In the nurse care manager model, the nurse care manager acts as the coordinator and is responsible for day-to-day clinical care, including initial screening, intake and education, induction, and ongoing maintenance visits. The nurse undergoes 8 hours of training similar in content to the training required for physicians to obtain the DEA waiver. Nurse care managers manage 100–125 patients alongside primary care physicians, often with assistance from a medical assistant. Focus is on providing coverage to large groups of patients effectively and efficiently in a primary care setting.

After the initial phone screening, the patient is scheduled to meet with the nurse for the initial evaluation visit. If appropriate, the patient returns for a second evaluation visit to meet the prescriber. The prescriber ultimately decides whether the patient will be allowed entry into treatment. If the patient is approved, a prescription for a 1-week supply of BUP/NX for induction is faxed to the pharmacy. The patient returns for the induction, which is supervised by the nurse. The patient remains at the clinic for several hours before being allowed to leave to complete the induction but remains in contact with the nurse by telephone. The patient meets the nurse frequently during the first week, then weekly for 1–2 months. If the patient is stable, the interval is gradually increased to every 2 weeks, then every 3 weeks, and then once a month. The patient meets with the prescriber at a minimum of every 6 months, and the prescription is faxed to the pharmacy with up to five refills. If patients are not adherent to treatment, the nurse can cancel any unused refills on the prescription.

Intensive Outpatient Model: Hospital-Based Dual Diagnosis Clinic

In the intensive outpatient model, psychiatrists and therapists work in an integrated dual diagnosis treatment clinic. The focus is on treating patients with comorbid psychiatric disorders and those who were not successful in a less structured program.

After the initial phone screening, the patient is scheduled to meet with a social worker for an initial evaluation visit. If appropriate, the patient returns for a second evaluation visit with a prescriber. The prescriber ultimately decides whether or not the patient will be allowed entry into treatment. If the patient is approved, a prescription for a limited supply of BUP/NX for induction is faxed to the pharmacy to be picked up on the day of induction. The patient is observed for the first induction dosing and then returns to the clinic every 2 hours as needed. The patient is reassessed within several days, then meets the prescriber weekly for 1–2 months. If the patient is stable, the interval is increased to every 2 weeks. After several months of stability, the interval may be increased to once a month.

Shared Medical Appointment Model

The shared medical appointment model combines medication management and education with group therapy consisting of a variety of treatment modalities (e.g., cognitive-behavioral therapy, motivational interviewing, relapse prevention, dialectical behavior therapy) (Suzuki et al. 2015). Up to 10 patients attend a group appointment with a BUP/NX prescriber and another health care provider, typically a licensed social worker. Patients are also seen individually before or after group for a brief session (up to 15 minutes) to review other medications, adherence to treatment, positive urine toxicology screens, and other concerns.

After the initial phone screening, the patient is scheduled to meet with a social worker for an initial evaluation visit. If appropriate, the patient returns for a second evaluation visit with a prescriber. The prescriber ultimately decides whether or not the patient will be allowed entry into treatment. If the patient is approved, a prescription for a limited supply of BUP/NX for induction is faxed to the pharmacy to be picked up on the day of induction. The patient is observed for the first induction dosing, then returns to the clinic in 1–2 hours for evaluation. Once the patient undergoes successful induction and an initial dose is established, the prescriber can then send a prescription for the remainder of the time necessary until a scheduled follow-up appointment. The patient attends an orientation appointment with a social worker to review program guidelines and regulations, receives information regarding the treatment model, and chooses a group to attend. The patient goes to weekly group for a predetermined time (e.g., 8 weeks), then transitions to every other week and then monthly treatment on the basis of stability. The patient meets with the provider in the group and briefly before or after the group during a shared medical appointment. If the patient wants to meet the provider for a longer period of time, individual appointments can be made in addition to the shared medical appointments.

PRIVATE PRACTICE MODEL: PSYCHIATRY

In the private practice model, a psychiatrist manages the treatment with support from off-site therapists. Focus is on integrating outpatient psychiatric care with substance use disorder treatment.

The patient is screened over the phone and then is scheduled for an initial evaluation visit. The patient is required to have a primary care physician and to meet with an individual therapist if not already connected to one. On day 1 of induction, a prescription for a 1-week supply is provided. The first dose is given under direct observation. The patient returns 1–2 hours later and again on day 2 or 3 for another assessment, and the dose is adjusted as needed. Treatment continues at a weekly frequency for 1 month. If the patient has no positive urine samples and the dose is stable, the visit interval is increased to every 2 weeks for 1–2 months before increasing to once a month.

EMERGENCY DEPARTMENT INITIATION OF BUP/NX

The emergency department (ED) initiation model involves the identification of OUD in patients in the ED, ED-initiated treatment with BUP/NX, and referral to a primary care office–based opioid treatment program for 10-week follow-up (D'Onofrio et al. 2015). Then, patients are transferred to office-based ongoing maintenance treatment and medication management.

Patients are screened in the ED, receive brief intervention by a physician, and are treated with BUP/NX if they are experiencing moderate to severe opioid withdrawal. Following consent to treatment and induction, the patient is provided with sufficient doses to take until his or her scheduled appointment at an opioid treatment program within 72 hours. Patients attend weekly or bimonthly medication management visits with physicians or nurses on the basis of their stability for 10 consecutive weeks. Thereafter, patients are transferred for ongoing maintenance treatment or medically supervised withdrawal if deemed appropriate (based on patient preference, stability, and other factors) either at a community program or with an independent BUP/NX prescribing physician.

Hospital Initiation of BUP/NX

The hospital initiation model encompasses identification of OUD in patients during medical hospitalization, initiation of BUP/NX treatment, and referral to office-based opioid treatment after discharge (Liebschutz et al. 2014). The patient is screened in the hospital for OUD and is offered the opportunity to discuss options for treatment of OUD with the addiction psychiatry or addiction medicine consultation/liaison (C/L) team. If the patient agrees, the C/L provider obtains complete drug use history, medical history, and psychiatric history as appropriate. If the patient is considered an appropriate candidate for BUP/NX treatment, he or she undergoes induction onto BUP/NX within the medical admission. Social work staff and care coordinators assist the patient in linking with a provider of office-based opioid treatment or alternative treatment, including those described above, for a follow-up appointment. The patient is discharged once his or her medical issues have resolved and the BUP/NX dose has been established for treatment, typically within 24 hours of BUP/NX induction. The patient is provided with sufficient medication until the scheduled follow-up appointment, which can vary on the basis of availability. Providing patients with prescriptions to fill prior to follow-up requires that one of the staff within the C/L team has a BUP/NX waiver. Some hospitals have established affiliations with specific providers of office-based opioid treatment, which facilitates disposition planning.

Conclusion

Office-based OUD treatment is an effective method of helping patients with OUD achieve recovery from illicit drug use. In this chapter, we reviewed the logistical requirements of setting up a successful office-based treatment program. Flexibility exists in how the necessary elements can be incorporated into existing programs. As long as the basic components as outlined in this chapter are present, various types of office-based treatment programs can be created to meet the needs of patients and the practice.

Clinical Pearls

- Necessary elements for office-based opioid treatment are not difficult to integrate with existing clinical programs.

- Providers should prepare in advance for on-site or off-site psychosocial treatments as well as referral to consultants.

- Office staff must receive adequate training regarding the treatment of patients with OUD, including confidentiality and office policy.

- Providers must ensure proper documentation.

- Urine toxicology is used to monitor treatment progress.

- There are a wide variety of implementation strategies to decrease the risk of diversion of BUP/NX.

References

American Psychiatric Association: Diagnostic and Statistical Manual of Mental Disorders, 5th Edition. Arlington, VA, American Psychiatric Association, 2013

Berson A, Gervais A, Cazals D, et al: Hepatitis after intravenous buprenorphine misuse in heroin addicts. J Hepatol 34(2):346–350, 2001 11281569

Brook DW: Group therapy, in Textbook of Substance Abuse Treatment. Edited by Galanter M, Kleber HD. Washington DC, American Psychiatric Publishing, 2008, pp 413–428

D'Onofrio G, O'Connor PG, Pantalon MV, et al: Emergency department-initiated buprenorphine/naloxone treatment for opioid dependence: a randomized clinical trial. JAMA 313(16):1636–1644, 2015 25919527

Kessler RC, Chiu WT, Demler O, et al: Prevalence, severity, and comorbidity of 12-month DSM-IV disorders in the National Comorbidity Survey Replication. Arch Gen Psychiatry 62(6):617–627, 2005 15939839

Liebschutz JM, Crooks D, Herman D, et al: Buprenorphine treatment for hospitalized, opioid-dependent patients: a randomized clinical trial. JAMA Intern Med 174(8):1369–1376, 2014 25090173

Lofwall MR, Havens JR: Inability to access buprenorphine treatment as a risk factor for using diverted buprenorphine. Drug Alcohol Depend 126(3):379–383, 2012 22704124

McLellan AT, Arndt IO, Metzger DS, et al: The effects of psychosocial services in substance abuse treatment. JAMA 269(15):1953–1959, 1993 8385230

McNicholas L (ed): Clinical Guidelines for the Use of Buprenorphine in the Treatment of Opioid Addiction. TIP Series 40 (DHHS Publ No SMA-04-3939). Rockville, MD, U.S. Department of Health and Human Services, 2004

Moos RH, Timko C: Outcome research on 12-step and other self-help groups, in Textbook of Substance Abuse Treatment. Edited by Galanter M, Kleber HD. Washington DC, American Psychiatric Publishing, 2008, pp 511–521

Strain E, Lofwall MR: Buprenorphine maintenance, in Textbook of Substance Abuse Treatment. Edited by Galanter M, Kleber HD. Washington DC, American Psychiatric Publishing, 2008, pp 309–324

Suzuki J, Zinser J, Klaiber B, et al: Feasibility of implementing shared medical appointments (SMAs) for office-based opioid treatment with buprenorphine: a pilot study. Subst Abus 36(2):166–169, 2015 25738320

Yokell MA, Zaller ND, Green TC, et al: Buprenorphine and buprenorphine/naloxone diversion, misuse, and illicit use: an international review. Curr Drug Abuse Rev 4(1):28–41, 2011 21466501

9

Methadone, Naltrexone, and Naloxone

Brad W. Stankiewicz, M.D.
Saria El Haddad, M.D.
Anna T. LaRose, M.D.

BUPRENORPHINE-NALOXONE (BUP/NX) is one of the first-line treatments for opioid use disorders (OUDs), and many patients will respond well to treatment with this medication. There will also be some patients who are not good candidates for treatment with BUP/NX, may fail treatment, experience adverse effects, or would like other options for treatment. In this chapter, we explore other medications useful in the treatment of OUD, specifically, methadone, naltrexone, and naloxone.

Methadone is an alternative option for patients who want maintenance treatment. Like BUP/NX, methadone is a first-line treatment for OUD that has distinct advantages and disadvantages. Naltrexone is an alternative to maintenance treatment that has less evidence for efficacy but is a good option for those patients who cannot be on maintenance treatments. Naloxone is not used for treatment of OUD relapse but is a medication that is used to reverse opioid overdoses and should be prescribed as a harm reduction strategy for patients who use opioids.

Methadone

BACKGROUND AND PHARMACOLOGY

The mid-1900s offered no pharmacotherapy options for the treatment of OUDs, with 1923 seeing the closure of the last clinics offering maintenance heroin or morphine treatment. By the early 1960s, heroin was a growing epidemic, with treatment failures approaching 100%. In 1963, Dr. Vincent Doyle, an internist working at Rockefeller University Hospital, was awarded a grant from the New York City Health Research Council to find an effective treatment for OUD. Alongside Marie Nyswander, he began to study methadone as a novel treatment in individuals with OUD. Their 1965 paper detailed their successful treatment of 22 participants with heroin addiction (Dole and Nyswander 1965). In the decades that followed, numerous studies supported the use of methadone in OUD, with reduction in both morbidity and mortality.

Methadone's efficacy is due in part to its pharmacology. It is a long-acting full opioid agonist, binding tightly to the μ opioid receptor. Its long half-life, averaging 24–36 hours, allows for it to be dosed typically as a single daily dose that offers relief from withdrawal symptoms and opioid cravings for 24 hours. Therapeutic doses of methadone lead to cross-tolerance for both short- and long-acting opioids, allowing methadone to effectively suppress withdrawal and cravings from a variety of opioids, including morphine and heroin.

Opioid treatment programs (OTPs) typically dispense the medication as an oral formulation that is 80% bioavailable. Serum levels peak 2–4 hours after dosing and then gradually decline. Although methadone typically provides only 4–6 hours of analgesic effect, it provides sustained activity at the μ opioid receptor and can provide sustained 24-hour relief from withdrawal symptoms and cravings.

Methadone is metabolized primarily in the liver by the cytochrome P450 (CYP) enzyme system, predominantly by CYP3A4 but also by CYP2B6 and CYP2D6. Metabolism rates can vary greatly among individuals because of genetic variations, pregnancy, protein binding, urinary pH, physical condition, age, and the use of other medications or supplements. Medications that lead to induction or inhibition of CYP enzymes can alter the metabolic rate and therefore increase or decrease serum concentration of methadone. Inducers of CYP enzymes, including rifampin, carbamazepine, phenytoin, phenobarbital, and some medications used to treat HIV, may increase the metabolism of methadone. Patients taking these medications may need increased doses of methadone to maintain stability. Conversely, inhibitors of CYP enzymes such as selective serotonin reuptake inhibitors, some antibiotics, and some antifungals may slow the metabolism of methadone. Drug interactions must be considered carefully in order to prevent excessively high or low serum methadone concentrations (Center for

Substance Abuse Treatment 2005). Table 2–2 in Chapter 2, "General Opioid Pharmacology," includes a list of medications metabolized by CYP3A4.

A variety of formulations are available, including tablets, diskettes, oral solution, and powder. The majority of methadone used in OTPs in the United States is administered as an orally ingested liquid. Tablets and diskettes are allowed under federal guidelines, but the liquid formulation provides several advantages, including greater flexibility of dosing (it is often dispensed with a computer-assisted dispensing pump) and less risk of diversion.

Early success with methadone maintenance in the 1960s led to a rapid expansion of OTPs. However, such rapid growth resulted in the advent of for-profit treatment programs often offering methadone maintenance without additional rehabilitation services. The early 1970s saw a regulatory response by the U.S. government with the Comprehensive Drug Abuse Prevention and Control Act. This legislation established early standards for the treatment of addiction with methadone. Regulations focused on admission criteria, dosing limits, and limits on take-home doses. Today, methadone treatment is still tightly regulated.

In the United States, methadone is classified as a Schedule II drug, and when it is used for the maintenance treatment of OUD, it can be ordered or dispensed only in a licensed OTP. OTPs are required to provide counseling and social services to patients, often in the form of mandatory group or individual counseling sessions. In order to be eligible for methadone maintenance in the United States, patients must be at least 18 years old and have a documented history of an OUD lasting at least 1 year.

TREATMENT WITH METHADONE

It is important to first obtain informed consent before initiating a patient on methadone maintenance therapy for OUD. The consenting process should include a discussion of the potential risks of treatment, relative contraindications, the availability of support services, and the expectations regarding compliance with treatment. Before a patient starts treatment, it is helpful to estimate the patient's opioid tolerance. Self-reported opioid use, pharmacy records, and data from state prescription drug monitoring programs can be helpful in this endeavor, but there is no direct way to measure the degree of a patient's tolerance. It is therefore best to initiate methadone at a low dose after first documenting opioid withdrawal and then to titrate on the basis of response.

Methadone induction comprises the first 2 weeks of treatment. The initial induction dose of methadone is typically 10–30 mg/day. If the patient continues to display withdrawal symptoms after 2–4 hours, when peak levels have been reached, an additional 5–10 mg can be administered. The dosage should not exceed a total of 40 mg on the first day of treatment. Given methadone's long half-life of 24–36 hours, serum methadone levels rise with each daily dose.

It typically takes at least 5–7.5 days to reach steady state (5 half-lives). For this reason, the daily dose should be titrated only every 5 days and in increments of 5 mg or less for the first 2 weeks of treatment (Baxter et al. 2013). It is important to assess the patient's response closely during this period, and assessment ideally should be performed at the time of peak effect to determine whether the patient continues to experience withdrawal or shows signs of intoxication. Patients frequently report early side effects of somnolence, insomnia, weight gain, sexual dysfunction, and constipation.

The third and fourth weeks of treatment are considered the early stabilization period. The goal of early stabilization is to reach a dose that allows the patient to be fully functional without signs of intoxication, sedation, withdrawal, or drug craving. During this period, the dose should be increased only by 5–10 mg every 3–5 days, provided the patient is receiving consecutive doses. If consecutive doses are missed during stabilization, it is difficult to determine the effect of a particular dose, and continued titration can be dangerous. As a precaution, the dose should be lowered or induction restarted if a patient misses 3–5 consecutive days of treatment (Baxter et al. 2013).

The late stabilization period is reached once the patient is stable on a therapeutic daily dose. Optimal daily dosing is indicated by freedom from opioid withdrawal symptoms for 24 hours, elimination of drug cravings, blockade of euphoric effects of self-administered opioids (due to cross-tolerance), and tolerance to the sedative effects of methadone. Some patients may continue on the same dosage of methadone for years. Others may require dose adjustments over the course of treatment because of changes in health, medication interactions, pregnancy, stress, or events that lead to cravings or relapse. Many patients do well on doses of 80–120 mg, but there is no uniformly recommended dosage range or upper dosage limit because of significant variation in patient response. Some patients do well at doses well below 80 mg, whereas others require doses much higher than 120 mg (Center for Substance Abuse Treatment 2005).

Most patients are able to be maintained on single daily dosing. However, if a patient experiences signs of overmedication at peak levels and/or withdrawal symptoms prior to the next dose, he or she may benefit from splitting the daily dose into two or three doses to provide for a more consistent serum methadone level. Splitting may be indicated in the case of fast metabolizers, pregnancy, or drug interactions. However, split dosing requires the medical director of the OTP to obtain a federal exception from the Substance Abuse and Mental Health Services Administration, and patients may be better served by transitioning to BUP/NX, with which there is no prohibition on split dosing.

At the beginning of methadone maintenance, patients are required to present to the OTP each day for dosing. After 90 days, federal regulations allow for take-home doses if a patient demonstrates stability of treatment. In order to qualify for take-home dosing, patients must maintain abstinence from unauthorized substances and demonstrate regular clinic attendance, absence of be-havioral problems or criminality, stability of home environment, and ability to safely store methadone. In stable patients, take-home doses can be gradually increased to a maximum of a 1-month supply after 2 years of consistent treat-ment (Substance Abuse and Mental Health Services Administration 2015).

EVIDENCE FOR METHADONE EFFICACY

Methadone is an effective treatment for OUD and is considered a first-line treatment (along with buprenorphine). A review found high retention rates for patients in methadone maintenance treatment, with retention ranging from 70% to 84% at 1-year follow-up (Garcia-Portilla et al. 2014). Methadone maintenance leads to a significant reduction in the use of heroin, nonprescribed methadone, benzodiazepines, cocaine, and alcohol by both self-report and urine drug screens. It also has been shown to lead to a significant reduction in intravenous drug use, high-risk sexual behavior, overall health problems, and criminal activities (including rates of incarceration, probability of arrests, illegal income, and frequency of crime).

All-cause mortality is severalfold lower in methadone-treated patients compared with untreated individuals with OUD. However, there are a number of adverse effects that necessitate caution when using methadone maintenance treatment. Common adverse effects include constipation, sweating, insomnia, early awakening, weight gain, and decreased libido. Many of these effects im-prove as tolerance to methadone develops, although constipation typically per-sists for the duration of treatment.

A more serious adverse effect is prolongation of the QTc interval, which can increase the risk for torsades de pointes, a potentially fatal arrhythmia. A screening electrocardiogram (ECG) should be obtained in patients with a his-tory of syncopal episodes, history of heart disease, or family history of long QT or who are taking medications that may interact with methadone. ECG should be repeated after 30 days and then annually. The risk of QTc prolongation is greater at doses of 100 mg or more. If QTc is greater than 500 ms, the metha-done dose should be decreased.

Methadone also carries the risk of fatal overdose. Among patients in OTPs, the vast majority of methadone-related overdose deaths occur within the first 2 weeks of treatment. Deaths most frequently occur when the initial dose is too high, the dose accumulates over the first few days, or methadone is combined with another drug (often a central nervous system [CNS] depressant such as benzodiazepines). For these reasons, OTPs follow the gradual dose induction protocol described above.

Despite these risks, methadone has a long history of safe use and positive out-comes. Its efficacy is similar to that of buprenorphine, and methadone maintenance may benefit patients who require an increased level of structure and more frequent interaction with providers. As with other medication-assisted treatments, outcomes are maximized when methadone is used as part of a comprehensive treatment program that includes counseling and psychosocial interventions.

In the next sections, we review the clinical use of commonly used opioid antagonists naltrexone and naloxone. We present a brief overview of the pharmacology of these compounds and some general considerations regarding clinical treatment.

Naltrexone

BACKGROUND AND PHARMACOLOGY

Opioid antagonists were developed initially to reverse the actions of opioids and later as possible treatments for OUDs. The first generation of opioid antagonists included nalorphine, naloxone, and cyclazocine. These antagonists had their limitations, including partial agonist activity, route of administration (many were not orally bioavailable), side effects such as dysphoria, and short half-life. The development of naltrexone led to the creation of a μ opioid antagonist that was orally available, highly potent, and longer acting than many other opioid antagonists. When naltrexone binds to the opioid receptor, it blocks the actions of opioid agonists and has virtually no other physiological effects, although some pupillary dilation has been observed (Martin et al. 1973).

Since its development, naltrexone has been studied extensively for both alcohol use disorder (AUD) and OUD. Currently, naltrexone is available in oral formulations as well as an extended-release (28-day) depot injectable formulation. The oral formulation gained approval for OUD from the U.S. Food and Drug Administration (FDA) in 1984, and it was approved for AUD in 1994. The extended-release injectable naltrexone formulation (XR-NTX) gained approval for AUD in 2006 and for OUD in 2010 (Center for Substance Abuse Treatment 2009). Implantable formulations of naltrexone have been developed but to date have been clinically approved for use only in Russia. The benefits of these formulations include that they last longer than a month, and most trials have shown decreased use of opioids in patients with OUD who are treated with these formulations. However, the data are limited, the cost of the implants can be high, and the safety of these implants needs to be further studied (Goonoo et al. 2014).

In AUD, the mechanism of action has not been fully clarified, but naltrexone is thought to act by affecting the dopaminergic mesolimbic pathway through blockage of endogenous opioids, which decreases the rewarding effects associated with the consumption of alcohol, thus decreasing alcohol use. Initial studies found that for AUD, naltrexone decreased cravings, drinking days, and heavy drinking. Predictors for response to naltrexone in individuals with AUD include a family history of AUD (Garbutt et al. 2014). There is also evidence that having the Asn40Asp polymorphism of the μ opioid receptor gene (*OPRM1*) can predict response to naltrexone. Genetic evidence is equivocal for this association, and although behavioral, pharmacological, and neuroimaging studies have found evidence that the polymorphism can predict response to naltrexone, more research is needed to determine the clinical applicability of genetic screening for *OPRM1* polymorphisms. (Ray et al. 2012).

For OUD, naltrexone works by competitively binding the μ opioid receptor and thus blocking the action of other opioids. Naltrexone has the benefit of not being a controlled substance and does not have the misuse and diversion potential of BUP/NX and methadone. In some countries where agonist treatment is not available, naltrexone is the only treatment option for patients with OUD.

Oral naltrexone has been found to have limited effectiveness in OUD because of poor adherence similar to the limited efficacy of disulfiram (Antabuse) in individuals with AUD. Depot and long-acting formulations were created to increase compliance.

The only current FDA-approved formulation of XR-NTX available is Vivitrol (Alkermes 2015). It consists of naltrexone encapsulated in biodegradable polymer microspheres that is slowly released after injection into the gluteal intramuscular region. Compared with the oral formulation, XR-NTX avoids first-pass metabolism and is theoretically less hepatotoxic than oral naltrexone. Until 2013, XR-NTX carried a black box warning for hepatotoxicity. Although the warning has been removed, the FDA does note that hepatitis and liver dysfunction occurred during clinical trials and that transient, asymptomatic transaminitis occurred in clinical trials and during the postmarketing period. Peak plasma times occur 1–2 hours after initial injection as well as 2 days after injection. At 14 days postinjection, the naltrexone concentration decreases in a log-linear fashion. Clearance occurs through renal excretion. (For information from the manufacturer, see www.vivitrol.com.)

EVIDENCE FOR NALTREXONE

Initial approval of XR-NTX for OUD was largely based on a 24-week double-blind, randomized placebo-controlled trial that took place in Russia (Krupitsky et al. 2011) as well as a subsequent 52-week open label extension of the original trial (Krupitsky et al. 2013). In addition to XR-NTX, the subjects received individual drug counseling. Weeks free from opioids as evidenced by urine drug tests for opioids were the main endpoint. Of the subjects in the original naltrexone arm, 66% were opioid free for at least half the weeks, versus 48% of the control group. Absolute abstinence was also higher in the naltrexone treatment group, and patients in the treatment group reported fewer cravings. In the open label extension, a reduction in cravings was also found, and 50.9% of subjects were completely opioid free during the trial.

Subsequent studies have looked at other populations, including health care professionals, incarcerated individuals, and adolescents. The use of naltrexone is important to study in these populations because often it is the only available treatment option other than psychosocial interventions. These smaller studies have found increased rates of abstinence as well as decreased cravings in individuals treated with XR-NTX (Syed and Keating 2013).

The studies looking at efficacy of naltrexone have their limitations. Many of the studies had a small number of subjects, were not blinded, were retrospective, or had high dropout rates. In a meta-analysis of naltrexone in OUD (Johansson et al. 2006), high dropout rates seemed to be the largest limiting factor in the trials, and the authors suggested using such interventions as contingency management to improve retention rates. There is also no evidence comparing naltrexone to opioid agonist treatment, although there is a U.S. trial currently under way comparing BUP/NX to depot injectable naltrexone. Another limitation is that many of the trials enrolled small numbers of women. Naltrexone is considered to be a pregnancy category C drug, and no trials are available in pregnant women. Generally, naltrexone is not considered to be a standard treatment in pregnant women and should be avoided in women who are breastfeeding. Patients with chronic pain are also likely not good candidates for naltrexone given its mechanism of action.

In general, there is far more evidence for use of agonist and partial agonist treatment for OUD than for naltrexone, and naltrexone cannot be recommended as a first-line treatment for OUD at this time. There is also no evidence comparing naltrexone with opioid agonist treatment, although a recent trial comparing BUP/NX with depot injectable naltrexone has been completed and results are pending (ClinicalTrials.gov identifier NCT02032433). However, naltrexone is a possible option for patients who cannot access methadone or BUP/NX. One issue to consider when treating patients with naltrexone is the time period necessary for induction; many patients would not be able to maintain the required period of sobriety from opioids in a nonstructured environment. Other important limitations to treatment with naltrexone are side effects. Naltrexone is associated with certain common side effects, including nausea, anxiety, depression, headache, gastrointestinal upset, dizziness, insomnia, and anorexia. Other less common but important side effects include hepatitis and decreased platelet counts. Naltrexone has been associated with hepatocellular injury and should not be given to patients with active hepatitis or liver function test (LFT) elevations above five times normal. In addition to the side effects of naltrexone itself, XR-NTX carries the added risk of injection site effects, including pain, tenderness, bruising, and swelling; there are also reports of patients developing cellulitis, abscesses, or necrosis requiring surgical interventions (see www.vivitrol.com).

Treatment With Naltrexone

A few key elements should be considered when deciding to induce patients on naltrexone. Baseline laboratory testing should include LFTs and expanded urine toxicology screens for opioids. LFTs should be repeated 1 month later, and then at least every 6 months if clinically indicated to monitor for transaminitis. In patients with LFTs greater than five times normal, naltrexone is contraindicated, although it is not contraindicated in those with chronic hepatitis C and has been used in patients with chronic illnesses, including hepatitis C and HIV. The FDA advises that patients should be abstinent from opioids for at least 7–10 days before receiving the first dose of naltrexone. This can be difficult to achieve with patients who have been on opioids for long periods of time, and longer-acting opioids such as methadone may take a longer period of abstinence to avoid precipitation of withdrawal. Because naltrexone can precipitate opioid withdrawal, many clinicians will perform either an oral naltrexone test dose or a naloxone challenge. The oral naltrexone test dose consists of 25–50 mg of naltrexone given orally the day or evening before the injectable depot. There are also protocols in which detoxification is linked with a low-dose naltrexone taper up so that patients can get the naltrexone injection before discharge from inpatient treatment. Naloxone challenge can be done in the following way:

1. Obtain a urine drug screen to confirm absence of opiates, oxycodone, buprenorphine, fentanyl, and methadone.
2. Obtain baseline vital signs
3. Confirm with participant that no use of methadone or buprenorphine has occurred in the past 10 days and no use of other opioids has occurred in the past 7 days
4. Remind participant that if opioid use has occurred, the administration of naloxone will result in severe opioid withdrawal that might last 1–2 hours
5. Proceed with naloxone challenge once negative urine screen and confirmation of no use are obtained from participant
6. Administer an initial naloxone test dose of 0.1 mg (1/4 mL) or 0.2 mg (1/2 mL) (intravenous, intramuscular, or subcutaneous per provider and patient preference and availability)
7. If no subjective discomfort or objective signs of withdrawal occur after a few minutes, give additional naloxone to bring total dose to 0.4 mg (1 mL)
8. If no subjective discomfort or objective signs of withdrawal occur after a few minutes, give additional naloxone to bring total dose to 0.8 mg (2 mL)

After 45 minutes, if no subjective discomfort or objective signs of withdrawal occur, the participant has passed the naloxone challenge test. XR-NTX can be administered at this point.

When patients are first started on XR-NTX, they may attempt to test whether the medication is working. There has also been concern that some patients may accidentally overdose in an attempt to override the naltrexone opioid antagonism. Accidental overdose has not been observed in clinical studies, but it should be discussed with patients, especially when high-potency opioids (such as fentanyl) are available in the illicit market. In addition, patients should be counseled that overdose may be more likely if they have been abstinent from opioids because they may have decreased physiological tolerance.

Another common issue is that some patients will complain that the anticraving effects of XR-NTX wane in the last week of treatment. In these patients, supplemental oral naltrexone (50 mg po daily) can be prescribed, or dosing can be shifted to every 3–3.5 weeks.

Finally, patients should be aware that naltrexone blockade can interfere with typical pain management in medical emergencies. Individuals who are treated with naltrexone should carry medication lists or medical alert identification or discuss with their next of kin or health care proxy their use of naltrexone so that health care professionals can treat them appropriately in cases where pain needs to be controlled. Typically, pain in patients who are taking naltrexone can be controlled with regional analgesia, non-opioid analgesics, or monitored anesthesia.

Overall, naltrexone does not have the evidence for efficacy that BUP/NX and methadone have, but in conjunction with psychosocial treatments it is a good alternative for patients who fail treatment, do not want agonist treatment, or cannot be on maintenance treatment. Naltrexone is generally well tolerated, but patients should be counseled on the side effects and risks unique to this medication, including precipitated withdrawal, injection site side effects, hepatitis, and opioid receptor blockade leading to pain control limitations.

Naloxone

BACKGROUND AND PHARMACOLOGY

Naloxone is a semisynthetic competitive opioid antagonist with short duration of action that is approved for opioid overdose treatment and reversal of respiratory depression with therapeutic opioid doses. It is also used off-label for treatment of opioid-induced pruritus. Naloxone is combined within the same pill with opioids such as buprenorphine or pentazocine to decrease the risk of misuse. Naloxone was patented in 1961 and is now available as a generic and is sold under various trade names, including Narcan, Nalone, Evzio, Prenoxad Injection, Narcanti, and Narcotan. Narcan as a sterile solution for intravenous, intramuscular, and subcutaneous administration was approved by the FDA in 1971, with intravenous being the recommended route.

Naloxone is on the World Health Organization's List of Essential Medicines, the most important medications needed in a basic health system. Naloxone typically requires a prescription but is not a controlled substance and has no abuse potential (World Health Organization 2015). Some states, such as California, Colorado, Kentucky, and Ohio, allow naloxone to be dispensed without a prescription. As of May 15, 2017, 40 states and the District of Columbia have implemented "Good Samaritan" laws, offering immunity from legal action for bystanders who use naloxone in case of emergency without prior approval from a doctor.

Naloxone hydrochloride is available in 0.02 mg/1 mL, 0.4 mg/1 mL, and 1 mg/1 mL vials; a 4 mg/10 mL multiuse vial; and 2 mg/1 mL, 2 mg/2 mL, and 2 mg/5 mL prefilled syringes for intravenous, intramuscular, or subcutaneous injection. Intravenous administration is essentially limited to trained health professionals and has been used for in-hospital opioid overdose reversal for more than 40 years. Endotracheal administration is the least desirable option and is supported only by anecdotal evidence. Off-label routes of administration include inhalation via nebulization and intraosseous administration.

Onset of action is 1–2 minutes following intravenous administration and 2–5 minutes following subcutaneous or intramuscular administration. The median time to peak naloxone concentration ranges from 15 minutes for intramuscular and subcutaneous administration to 19–30 minutes for intranasal administration. The bioavailability for intranasal and intramuscular naloxone is 4% and 35% of that for intravenous naloxone, respectively.

The mean serum half-life ranges from 30 to 81 minutes, which is shorter than the average half-life of some opioids. Therefore, repeat dosing might be warranted in the setting of opioid intoxication in order to prevent re-intoxication. Naloxone is metabolized primarily by the liver into its major metabolite, naloxone-3-glucuronide, which is excreted in the urine.

In April 2014, the FDA approved a handheld automatic injector naloxone product that delivers naloxone intramuscularly or subcutaneously and can be used in nonmedical settings (U.S. Food and Drug Administration 2014). It is designed for use by laypersons, including bystanders and family members of opioid users at risk for an opioid overdose. Similar to automated defibrillators, when the device is turned on, it provides verbal instructions on how to deliver the medication. This was followed in November 2015 by approval of a wedge device (nasal atomizer) attached to a syringe that creates a mist that delivers the drug to the nasal mucosa. Because distribution of naloxone to laypersons may reduce the time taken to give naloxone, the approval process of both new formulations was fast tracked as an initiative to reduce the death toll caused by opioid overdose (Wolfe and Bernstone 2004).

The availability of alternative routes of administration over injection has many benefits, which include earlier access to the medication in the prehospital setting, overcoming the difficulty in obtaining venous access under emergency conditions in the field, and eliminating the risk of needle stick injury of health care personnel working with patients who have high risk factors for HIV and hepatitis B and C. Nevertheless, intranasal administration can be suboptimal in certain cases. Nasal pathology or injury, such as nasal septal abnormalities, trauma, epistaxis, excessive mucus, or intranasal damage caused by the use of substances such as cocaine, may have a significant effect on the rate and amount of absorption of intranasal medications, making it difficult to achieve systemic drug levels rapidly and reliably. Individuals who misuse substances might be a population at higher risk for these nasal abnormalities.

Marketing of alternative needle-free naloxone delivery systems such as buccal and sublingual formulations is under consideration because they can facilitate wider naloxone access across the community and enhance treatment of opioid overdose emergencies. Such formulations do not require medical training; are acceptable for administration by nonmedical bystanders; provide adequate systemic drug concentration; and produce sufficiently rapid drug absorption, allowing for a rapid onset of action.

EVIDENCE FOR NALOXONE

Meta-analysis of randomized controlled trials comparing intranasal (initial dose 2 mg) with intramuscular (initial dose 2 mg) naloxone for opioid overdose reversal in the prehospital setting found no difference in the rates of overdose complications, overdose morbidity, opioid withdrawal reaction to naloxone, or time to opioid reversal (Kelly et al. 2005; Kerr et al. 2009). There are no studies comparing intravenous with intranasal or intramuscular naloxone in the prehospital setting.

TREATMENT WITH NALOXONE

Naloxone has almost no clinical action if administered in the absence of an opioid. The naloxone dose needed to achieve reversal of opioid overdose depends on multiple factors, including the opioid load (the amount of opioid present in the body and the potency of the specific drug) and the presence of other CNS depressants. According to guidelines from the manufacturer, Sankyo, the recommended dose for management of opioid overdose is 0.4–2 mg via intramuscular, intravenous, or subcutaneous injection, repeated as necessary, not to exceed 10 mg. The American Heart Association recommends calling 911 and initiating initial CPR rescue measures, followed by the administration of 2 mg intranasal or 0.4 mg intramuscular naloxone, with repeat dosing after 4 minutes. The British National Formulary advises 0.8–2 mg boluses, repeated as necessary up to 10 mg, for adults. Long-acting opioids such as methadone and potent opioids such as fentanyl typically require closer inpatient monitoring for 24–48 hours using a naloxone drip.

Use of higher doses of naloxone carries a risk of precipitating an acute opioid withdrawal syndrome characterized by agitation, nausea, vomiting, piloerection, diarrhea, lacrimation, yawning, and rhinorrhea. These symptoms generally are not life threatening and tend to dissipate in 30–60 minutes because of the relatively short half-life of naloxone. Reported rates of precipitated opioid withdrawal syndrome with 2–4 mg boluses vary widely from 7% to 46%. Tremor and hyperventilation associated with an abrupt return to consciousness has occurred in some patients receiving naloxone for opiate overdose.

Conversely, lower-dose approaches may result in an increased risk of reoverdose when naloxone levels drop. Therefore, a balance should be struck between rapidity of opioid reversal versus frequency and intensity of adverse reactions.

In 2014, the World Health Organization launched guidelines on the community management of opioid overdose. These guidelines state that naloxone is effective when delivered in various parenteral formulations and recommend that "people likely to witness an opioid overdose should have access to naloxone and be instructed in its administration" (p. 9). Studies have reported that many overdoses are witnessed by individuals who would be willing to intervene and provide assistance (World Health Organization 2014).

The community-based provision of naloxone rescue kits, or take-home naloxone (THN), to opioid users was first proposed in the 1990s. THN programs typically involve training opioid users and/or their family members or peers in overdose risk awareness, overdose emergency management, and naloxone administration (Wheeler 2012). During the past 15 years, THN programs have been implemented in Europe, North America, Asia, and Australia. To date, THN programs have been implemented in more than 15 countries worldwide.

Conclusion

Although BUP/NX is an excellent first-line medication for treatment of OUD, familiarity with other medications useful in treating OUD is important when working with patients with OUDs. When patients fail BUP/NX or when they are not good candidates for treatment with BUP/NX, methadone or the extended-release version of naltrexone (XR-NTX) can be good options. Methadone is a long-acting full opioid agonist that is a first-line treatment for OUD, and it can be especially useful for treatment of individuals who need more structure because it can be dispensed only through OTPs. Precautions that need to be taken with patients taking methadone include monitoring interactions with medication (such as hypnotics and tranquilizers) that can lead to changes in the metabolism of methadone or to oversedation; monitoring for QTc prolongation; and close monitoring for the potential of an overdose, especially earlier in treatment or if the dose is raised too quickly.

In addition to BUP/NX and methadone, naltrexone is the only other approved medication for OUD. XR-NTX has been studied, but it does not have as much evidence for efficacy as methadone or BUP/NX. The mechanism of action of naltrexone is very different from other medication-assisted treatment for OUD because naltrexone works by antagonism at the μ opioid receptor. Patients who cannot have access to methadone or buprenorphine or have contraindications to being on these medications may be good candidates for naltrexone. There can be difficulty with the induction of this medication because patients need to be free of opioid use for at least 7–10 days and because of other issues, including the potential of precipitation of withdrawal and blockade of opioids in emergency situations.

Finally, naloxone is an important medication to discuss when treating patients with OUD. Although naloxone is not approved as a medication-assisted treatment for OUD, it can be useful to prescribe as a harm reduction strategy to patients who are at risk for misuse and overdose of opioids.

Clinical Pearls

- Methadone is a first-line treatment for opioid use disorder (OUD) that can be considered in patients who need more structure and support in recovery.

- Methadone can be dispensed only out of federally regulated opioid treatment programs.

- Extended-release injectable naltrexone (XR-NTX) is an opioid antagonist that can be considered for patients with OUD who cannot take methadone or buprenorphine-naloxone.

- Induction on XR-NTX can be challenging because patients need to be abstinent from short-acting opioids for at least 7 days or long-acting opioids for at least 10 days before induction.

- A naloxone challenge can be used to test whether withdrawal will be precipitated before administering XR-NTX.

- Naloxone is a cost-effective, safe, and user-friendly life-saving medication that is a key element in harm reduction for OUD.

- Community distribution of parenteral naloxone formulations is an effective public health approach for reducing the toll of opioid-related overdose deaths.

CASE 7

Carl first began methadone treatment 9 months ago. He is a 26-year-old carpenter who has been doing well on 90 mg methadone. He currently gets three days of take-home doses a week and has not had a urine test positive for opioids or other illicit drugs for the last 5 months. Last week, his urine tested positive for marijuana. He admitted smoking a few joints a month and insisted that it was not a problem. Recreational marijuana recently became legal in your state.

1. Have you developed a policy on recreational marijuana use for your clinic?

2. Do you test regularly for marijuana?

3. Would you implement a testing policy if medical or recreational marijuana were legal in your state?

CASE 7 (CONTINUED)

Since marijuana use is now legal in your area, you decide to discuss Carl's test results with him but to continue treatment. One month later, his urine toxicology test is positive for both cocaine and marijuana. As per standard clinic policy, his take-home privileges are cut back to weekends only, and he is required to provide a random urine sample for testing each week and to attend a weekly group that focuses on the elimination of cocaine use. He has two more positive urine toxicology tests for both cocaine and marijuana over the next 6 weeks and misses two out of the six required weekly groups.

1. Would an increase in Carl's methadone dose be indicated at this time?

2. Would you consider terminating his methadone treatment?

3. In several double-blind, placebo-controlled trials, disulfiram has been demonstrated to reduce cocaine use. Would that be a reasonable option at this time?

4. Are there any psychological therapies that you would consider?

5. Do you think that Carl's marijuana use is related to the cocaine problem? Would you change your treatment plan to include a focus on the marijuana?

CASE 7 (CONTINUED)

Carl was able to eliminate both his cocaine and marijuana use after participating in the clinic's contingency management program for 6 months. For the next 2 years he continued to do very well. He is now married, is a foreman at his job, and is on biweekly medication pick-ups. He has been asked to take on the supervision of some out-of-town jobs, but he is worried that this will conflict with his clinic schedule. Because of his treatment progress, he feels that he is ready to taper off of methadone and asks for your advice.

1. Is Carl at any risk if he tapers off his methadone?

2. Are there other parameters of progress that you would like to see before he makes any changes?

3. Would he be a good candidate for XR-NTX?

4. What about a transfer to BUP/NX?

5. Would you prescribe a naloxone rescue kit under these circumstances?

References

Alkermes: Vivitrol prescribing information. Waltham, MA, Alkermes, 2015. https://www.vivitrol.com/content/pdfs/prescribing-information.pdf. Accessed February 7, 2017.

Baxter LE Sr, Campbell A, Deshields M, et al: Safe methadone induction and stabilization: report of an expert panel. J Addict Med 7(6):377–386, 2013 24189172

Center for Substance Abuse Treatment: Medication-Assisted Treatment for Opioid Addiction in Opioid Treatment Programs. Treatment Improvement Protocol (TIP) Series, No 43. HHS Publ No (SMA) 12-4214. Rockville, MD, Substance Abuse and Mental Health Services Administration, 2005

Center for Substance Abuse Treatment: Incorporating Alcohol Pharmacotherapies Into Medical Practice. Treatment Improvement Protocol (TIP) Series, No 49. HHS Publ No (SMA) 13-4389. Rockville, MD, Substance Abuse and Mental Health Services Administration, 2009

Dole VP, Nyswander M: A medical treatment for diacetylmorphine (heroin) addiction: a clinical trial with methadone hydrochloride. JAMA 193:646–650, 1965 14321530

Garbutt JC, Greenblatt AM, West SL, et al: Clinical and biological moderators of response to naltrexone in alcohol dependence: a systematic review of the evidence. Addiction 109(8):1274–1284, 2014 24661324

Garcia-Portilla MP, Bobes-Bascaran MT, Bascaran MT, et al: Long term outcomes of pharmacological treatments for opioid dependence: does methadone still lead the pack? Br J Clin Pharmacol 77(2):272–284, 2014 23145768

Goonoo N, Bhaw-Luximon A, Ujoodha R, et al: Naltrexone: a review of existing sustained drug delivery systems and emerging nano-based systems. J Control Release 183:154–166, 2014 24704710

Johansson BA, Berglund M, Lindgren A: Efficacy of maintenance treatment with naltrexone for opioid dependence: a meta-analytical review. Addiction 101(4):491–503, 2006 16548929

Kelly AM, Kerr D, Dietze P, et al: Randomised trial of intranasal versus intramuscular naloxone in prehospital treatment for suspected opioid overdose. Med J Aust 182(1):24–27, 2005 15651944

Kerr D, Kelly AM, Dietze P, et al: Randomized controlled trial comparing the effectiveness and safety of intranasal and intramuscular naloxone for the treatment of suspected heroin overdose. Addiction 104(12):2067–2074, 2009 19922572

Krupitsky E, Nunes EV, Ling W, et al: Injectable extended-release naltrexone for opioid dependence: a double-blind, placebo-controlled, multicentre randomised trial. Lancet 377(9776):1506–1513, 2011 21529928

Krupitsky E, Nunes EV, Ling W, et al: Injectable extended-release naltrexone (XR-NTX) for opioid dependence: long-term safety and effectiveness. Addiction 108(9):1628–1637, 2013 23701526

Martin WR, Jasinski DR, Mansky PA: Naltrexone, an antagonist for the treatment of heroin dependence. Effects in man. Arch Gen Psychiatry 28(6):784–791, 1973 4707988

Ray LA, Barr CS, Blendy JA, et al: The role of the Asn40Asp polymorphism of the mu opioid receptor gene (OPRM1) on alcoholism etiology and treatment: a critical review. Alcohol Clin Exp Res 36(3):385–394, 2012 21895723

Substance Abuse and Mental Health Services Administration: Federal Guidelines for Opioid Treatment Programs. HHS Publ No (SMA) PEP15-FEDGUIDEOTP. Rockville, MD, Substance Abuse and Mental Health Services Administration, 2015

Syed YY, Keating GM: Extended-release intramuscular naltrexone (VIVITROL®): a review of its use in the prevention of relapse to opioid dependence in detoxified patients. CNS Drugs 27(10):851–861, 2013 24018540

U.S. Food and Drug Administration: FDA approves new handheld autoinjector to reverse opioid overdose. FDA News Release, April 3, 2014

Wheeler E: Community-based opioid overdose prevention programs providing naloxone—United States, 2010. MMWR Morb Mortal Wkly Rep 61(6):101–105, 2012 22337174

Wolfe TR, Bernstone T: Intranasal drug delivery: an alternative to intravenous administration in selected emergency cases. J Emerg Nurs 30(2):141–147, 2004 15039670

World Health Organization: Community Management of Opioid Overdose. Geneva, World Health Organization, 2014

World Health Organization: Model List of Essential Medicines, 19th List. Geneva, World Health Organization, April 2015. Available at: www.who.int/medicines/publications/essentialmedicines/EML_2015_FINAL_amended_NOV2015.pdf?ua=1. Accessed September 12, 2017.

10

Psychiatric Comorbidity

Elie Aoun, M.D.
Elinore F. McCance-Katz, M.D., Ph.D.

MENTAL DISORDERS co-occur frequently in patients with opioid use disorder (OUD). Significant rates of co-occurring affective disorders, particularly major depression, anxiety disorders, posttraumatic stress disorder (PTSD), attention-deficit/hyperactivity disorder (ADHD), and antisocial personality disorder (ASPD), as well as other psychiatric disorders, occur in this population (Chen et al. 2011). In addition, substance-induced mental disorders are common in the patient presenting for treatment of OUD. Key to providing effective treatment is to accurately diagnose and implement appropriate treatment for these conditions.

In this chapter, we review how to differentiate substance-induced mental disorders from independent psychiatric disorders and how to determine which patients can be successfully managed in specific office settings. We also consider the complexities of pharmacotherapy and clinical management of co-occurring mental and substance use disorders in buprenorphine-treated patients and present recommendations for managing some of the more common clinical problems.

Epidemiology

The underlying etiology for the high rates of comorbidity in patients with OUD is likely to be multifactorial. As with the use of other substances with abuse liability, the use of opioids is associated with reactive increases in dopamine release and dopamine receptor activity and an increased affinity of dopamine receptors to endogenic dopamine in the nucleus accumbens. This is thought to be the mediator of the desired effects related to substance use reinforcing the associated euphoria. The chronic abuse of opioids leads to changes in the brain, including the nucleus accumbens, such that there is decreased ability to experience pleasure without the presence of opioids due to an impaired non-opioid-triggered endogenic dopamine production and release. Over time this may contribute to the depression that many patients complain of when presenting for treatment of OUD. Alternatively, those with vulnerability to developing a mental disorder such as depression may hasten onset of that disorder as a result of changes that occur with chronic exposure to opioids, although this mechanism has not been well defined to date.

There may be other neurophysiological changes that occur following chronic exposure to opioids that might render an individual vulnerable to the development of other mental disorders. It is also possible that individuals with disturbing psychiatric symptoms will attempt to self-medicate these symptoms with illicit drugs such as opioids. This can eventually lead to physical dependence and substance use disorders (SUDs). Unfortunately, substance use does not provide adequate relief of the target symptoms that the patient is attempting to medicate but instead can modify the patient's feelings to keep him or her from experiencing mood- and anxiety-triggered distress. This effect may ultimately aggravate the symptoms by keeping the patient from addressing the underlying psychosocial stressors leading to depression, anxiety, or other psychiatric symptoms, as well as by altering neurobiological substrates contributing to the development of co-occurring mental disorder(s). Given the complex etiologies of co-occurring mental illness in persons with OUD, it is clear that careful longitudinal evaluation is needed to fully understand the psychopathology of the patient in order to accurately diagnose the patient and provide appropriate treatment.

In evaluating the co-occurrence of psychiatric symptoms and syndromes in patients with histories of chronic substance use, it is important not to assume that all symptoms reported are related to an independent mental disorder, even in the presence of a history in which the patient states that such symptoms predated drug use. The symptoms associated with intoxication and withdrawal can mimic virtually any mental disorder. Patients often have a need to rationalize their substance use by attributing their use to another problem or disorder. Therefore, careful evaluation over time is required to fully understand the relationship between OUD and other reported psychiatric symptoms.

Anxiety and/or panic symptoms are frequent complaints in individuals with OUD and must be carefully evaluated. Anxiety is a common symptom of opioid withdrawal. Anxiety also may occur as part of a withdrawal syndrome from other substances (discussed in greater detail below). When evaluating a patient for co-occurring disorders, it is important for the clinician to understand that opioid withdrawal is ubiquitous in individuals with OUD, whether or not the patient endorses withdrawal signs and symptoms. It is simply a fact that OUD is characterized by the ongoing and frequent use of opioids, and withdrawal symptoms occur as blood levels of opioids decline, serving as a negative reinforcer driving continued use (and, as such, individuals continue using opioids to avoid withdrawal symptoms). Part of that constellation of withdrawal symptoms is anxiety. Further, patients frequently lack the insight to make the connection between the onset of opioid withdrawal and the temporal relationship of anxiety symptoms. Rather, patients often will ask for anxiolytic medication (usually benzodiazepines), which have abuse liability and can enhance the effects of prescribed opioids (methadone, buprenorphine)—certainly, unwanted effects in the treatment of such patients. The goal of opioid therapy is to stabilize the patient so that his or her life does not revolve around the misuse of opioids, including intoxication and withdrawal with constant drug seeking. Therefore, the use of anxiolytic medications, which enhance the effect of opioids and may contribute to intoxication, is not therapeutic and could be dangerous to the patient and to others. In addition, the presence and characterization of drug interactions between benzodiazepines and opioids such as buprenorphine have not been well defined as yet, but significant adverse events are possible. Although benzodiazepines are not absolutely contraindicated in patients with OUD, evaluation must be thorough and thoughtful prior to prescription of these medications for anxiety in opioid-addicted patients receiving opioid agonist therapy (OAT). Independent anxiety disorders may also occur in persons with OUD, and in such cases, pharmacotherapy for the anxiety will be necessary.

PTSD is also a frequently co-occurring mental illness in patients with OUD, particularly women. Up to 92% of women with OUD report trauma, either physical or sexual. Further, it has been reported that PTSD occurs in up to 53% of women with OUD (Ross et al. 2005). The drug-abusing lifestyle can be quite conducive to trauma, given the illegal activities related to drug procurement and abuse. Often, individuals engage in risky activities or will be victimized in the context of drug use. Intoxication also renders an individual more vulnerable to traumatic events. Such occurrences may lead to the onset of PTSD, which may be detected only when the person comes to treatment. As with other psychiatric disorders, untreated PTSD will negatively impact the overall response to drug use treatment.

ADHD is a diagnosis that has been made with increasing frequency over the past few years and is characterized by impulsivity, inattentiveness, and increased nonproductive activity levels. DSM-5 (American Psychiatric Association 2013) requires that some symptoms start prior to age 12. However, recent work indicates the validity of the diagnosis in adults who do not have a clear history of a childhood onset of symptoms and shows that we are still missing the diagnosis in up to 80% of cases (Ginsberg et al. 2014). It is estimated that 39%–68% of persons with OUD may have co-occurring ADHD and that opioid-addicted patients with ADHD are at increased risk for other psychiatric comorbidities, such as mood and anxiety disorders, as well as ASPD (Carpentier et al. 2012). Some studies have found that the development of an SUD in adolescence is less likely in a child with ADHD who receives appropriate pharmacotherapy in childhood (McCabe et al. 2016), underscoring the importance of accurate diagnosis and treatment. In patients with OUD, it is important to remember that impulsivity and inattentiveness often are directly related to the effects of the abused substances. A reasonable period of verified abstinence is suggested prior to making the diagnosis of ADHD in an individual with any SUD to help distinguish ADHD from subacute effects of substances of abuse.

Antisocial personality disorder is the most common personality disorder seen in patients with OUD (and SUD in general). Antisocial behaviors such as lying, cheating, and stealing are common in those who must support a costly drug habit. Such behaviors often resolve with appropriate treatment of addiction such as medication-assisted treatment (MAT) and counseling. The major differential in an individual with OUD with a history of antisocial behavior is whether there is true underlying ASPD or whether the behaviors were induced secondary to the addiction. Clues to this question often lie in the developmental history of the patient. For example, those exhibiting conduct disorder in childhood and adolescence prior to the onset of substance use are more likely to have ASPD. Further, a history of property destruction or cruelty to others or animals (diagnostic criteria for ASPD) is not generally associated with addiction but is more likely to occur in persons with ASPD. It is important to know that most individuals with OUD will not have true ASPD but rather will present with the symptoms of substance-induced sociopathy necessary to procure and use drugs. Such patients respond well to opioid therapies, including buprenorphine. Further, such patients can be treated effectively in office-based settings.

To conclude, mental disorders co-occur at significant rates in persons with OUD. These mental disorders can be either substance-induced or independent of the OUD. It is important to differentiate between substance-induced and independent disorders because the treatment is quite different. Substance-induced disorders will resolve with appropriate treatment of OUD (and other co-occurring SUDs when present). Independent mental disorders will not resolve and possibly may worsen as psychopathology is unmasked with treatment of the addiction. Individuals with these co-occurring conditions will require integrated treatment of both disorders to establish any meaningful recovery from their substance use. In the following sections, we provide guidance on how to evaluate and treat the opioid-dependent patient with co-occurring mental illness.

Evaluation

Evaluation of the patient with OUD requires attention to the history of opioid use and to the history of other substance use, medical illnesses, and psychiatric symptoms. The history is critical to arriving at the appropriate diagnoses and treatment plans. Patients with OUD may be uncomfortable answering some of these questions; therefore, the approach of the clinician will be important in determining how much of the relevant information can be gathered (see Chapter 4, "Patient Assessment," Chapter 6, "Buprenorphine Treatment in Office-Based Settings," and Chapter 7, "Psychosocial and Supportive Treatment"). A nonjudgmental approach, open-ended questions with follow-up questions to clarify responses as needed, and reassurance regarding confidentiality are all important parts of the interview. It is also important to obtain consent to speak with important significant others in the life of the patient who can provide additional history and progress reports over the course of treatment.

ASSESSING THE USE OF OTHER SUBSTANCES

Diagnosing OUD and assessing for the presence of other SUDs has been discussed in more detail in Chapter 4. It is worth reiterating, however, the importance of ensuring that the patient has OUD through history, medical records, signs on physical examination (e.g., needle track marks, signs of opioid withdrawal), and urine toxicology screen results. It is also important to ask about illicit opioids (e.g., heroin, opium) as well as prescription opioids (see Chapter 4, Table 4–1). Prescription opioid misuse has rapidly increased in the past 10 years and is characterized by aberrant drug-taking behavior, including compulsive use of opioid analgesics with unauthorized dose increases; using the drugs to get high, to relieve stress, or to get to sleep; obtaining prescriptions from multiple physicians; frequenting emergency departments to seek opioids; forging prescriptions; taking the drugs from friends and/or family; and buying or selling drugs. In 2015, the number of people with prescription OUDs (2,038,000) far exceeded the number of heroin-addicted individuals (591,000) in the United States. It is encouraging that the most recent numbers from the National Survey on Drug Use and Health (2015) show that heroin use has begun to drop, but it is too early to know the significance of this change. Past-year heroin use decreased by 9%, from 914,000 to 828,000, between 2014 and 2015 (Substance Abuse and Mental Health Services Administration (2015) (see Chapter 1, "Opioid Use Disorder in America"). These findings underscore the ongoing need for office-based treatment of OUD to increase access to treatment for the burgeoning numbers of opioid-addicted individuals.

It is also important to screen for other SUDs because the patient may require treatment for these as well. If the patient has an alcohol use disorder or benzodiazepine use disorder, he or she should be admitted to a facility for medically supervised withdrawal (detoxification) treatment. Such a patient may not be appropriate for office-based buprenorphine treatment because of the risk of adverse events (see section "Drug Interactions With Buprenorphine" below) if he or she re-initiates alcohol and/or benzodiazepine use. The use of stimulants such as cocaine or methamphetamine predicts a poor course for buprenorphine-treated individuals if they do not receive treatment specific to stimulant use disorders. There is now also evidence that cocaine use can adversely impact buprenorphine pharmacokinetics (McCance-Katz et al. 2010), adding another layer of complexity to the treatment. Tobacco use disorder is a common problem in patients with OUD, and cigarette smoking is strongly linked to relapse to other substance use. All patients should be strongly encouraged to stop tobacco use, and treatment for smoking cessation should be offered. Effective pharmacotherapies are available. It is important to query regarding other substance use as well, although the most common co-occurrence of substance use with opioids is alcohol, sedatives/hypnotics, stimulants, and nicotine. For a list of abused substances that should be queried in the evaluation of the patient with OUD and tested for by urine toxicology screening, see Table 5–2 in Chapter 5 ("Clinical Use of Buprenorphine").

Evaluating for medical illnesses is an important component of the overall evaluation of patients with OUD. These persons often have co-occurring medical illness as a result of risky behaviors related to the development and maintenance of opioid addiction. Individuals who inject opioids are at high risk for HIV, hepatitis B and C, cellulitis, abscesses, sepsis, endocarditis, and other medical problems that will require acute and possibly ongoing medical care (see Chapter 11, "Medical Comorbidity"). The medical needs of a patient with OUD are an important consideration when determining the most appropriate setting for office-based treatment with buprenorphine-naloxone (BUP/NX).

Assessing Co-occurring Psychiatric Disorders

Evaluation for the presence of co-occurring psychiatric disorders is critically important in instituting effective treatment for OUD in any clinical setting, but it can take on special importance when treatment will be provided from an office-based setting. It is imperative that the treating clinician understand the patient's mental health history and current problems and determine a prognosis because all of these factors are important to determining whether the patient is appropriate for office-based treatment of OUD with buprenorphine.

Specific current psychiatric symptoms as well as past psychiatric history must be reviewed prior to the decision to begin BUP/NX treatment because these issues are a significant part of the decision as to whether an opioid-dependent patient is a good candidate for office-based treatment of OUD. Table 10–1 provides an outline for obtaining the most important parts of the mental health history, both current and past. Obtaining the information outlined in Table 10–1 and following up in other relevant areas brought up by the patient should provide the necessary information to assist the clinician in determining whether this is a patient who could be appropriately managed in the clinician's practice. For example, the primary care physician may be less comfortable taking a patient with OUD with significant mental illness, whereas a psychiatrist offering office-based treatment of OUD may judge this patient to be a good fit for his or her practice. Alternatively, a primary care physician might find appropriate for his or her practice a patient with a history of co-occurring HIV/AIDS and OUD, whereas a psychiatrist may refer such a patient to a physician with expertise in the treatment of HIV infection and treat only the OUD or may refer the patient to an addiction specialist who can offer treatment for both conditions.

Patients should be informed that the evaluation does not guarantee acceptance into the physician's practice, but the evaluating physician will provide appropriate referrals for treatment if he or she does not believe the patient's condition to be a good fit for his or her practice. It is also important not to rely on information gleaned from a telephone screening done by an office staff member. Although it may be beneficial to have an office staff member do a cursory initial screen to exclude patients requiring services not available through the clinician's practice (e.g., the opioid-addicted patient with a long-standing history of schizoaffective disorder and nonadherence to psychotropic medications who calls a primary care doctor requesting office-based treatment of OUD), it is imperative that the clinician take a thorough history to evaluate the patient. Support staff may not have the expertise to ask the questions that would be likely to clarify a complicated history.

As previously mentioned, the most frequently occurring psychiatric disorders in this population are depression, anxiety, PTSD, ADHD, and personality disorders. Knowledge of the status of any patient regarding these disorders is essential in determining appropriateness for office-based treatment. Certain mental conditions render some individuals poor candidates for office-based treatment using buprenorphine (Table 10–2). Any patient showing signs of active psychosis, including hallucinations (either auditory or visual) or delusions, should not be inducted onto BUP/NX. Any individual who endorses active suicidal or homicidal ideation is a poor candidate for office-based treatment. Any individual who appears to have significant cognitive impairment or dementia is also not a candidate for office-based treatment. All these patients may require a higher level of care than is customarily available in most office-based settings.

TABLE 10–1.   **Taking the mental health history**

History of substance use

Opioids, including prescribed analgesics and heroin

Alcohol

Benzodiazepines

Cocaine

Methamphetamine

Other synthetic stimulants (e.g., "bath salts")

Cannabis

Synthetic cannabinoids

Tobacco

Steroids

Other street drugs

Other prescription drugs

History of mental health problems

Depression

Anxiety

Psychosis

Trauma

Attention-deficit/hyperactivity disorder

Antisocial behavior, including property damage, truancy, aggression toward other people or animals, and violent behavior

History of mental health treatment

Has the person ever been under the care of a psychiatrist or therapist?

Was a diagnosis ever given?

Was there ever a referral for psychotherapy? What type?

Was medication treatment ever recommended?

What medications have been prescribed in the past? Currently?

What do the medications help with?

Are the medications effective?

Are the medications taken as prescribed?

Has there been a hospitalization for a psychiatric condition?

Are there current symptoms of mental illness?

Ask about current depression, anxiety, and psychotic thinking

Assess cognition (orientation, memory, concentration, abstracting ability, fund of knowledge, judgment, insight)

TABLE 10–1.   **Taking the mental health history** *(continued)*

Suicidality

  Current plans

  Means available to act (e.g., guns in the home, medications to overdose)

  Past attempt(s) made and description (assess lethality)

  Planned or impulsive?

  Current support system

Homicidality

  Current plans

  Specific target?

  Past events

  Means available to act

  Planned or impulsive?

TABLE 10–2.   **Psychiatric contraindications to office-based treatment of opioid use disorder**

Psychiatric contraindications

  Active psychosis

  Active suicidal/homicidal ideation

  Cognitive impairment/dementia

Relative psychiatric contraindications

  Psychosis (if not well controlled on medication)

  History of suicidality

  History of homicidality

In addition to eliciting current history of such issues, the clinician should review the past history of such problems. For example, a patient who is not currently suicidal but who has a history of suicide attempts may be more appropriate for methadone maintenance treatment because of the additional structure and observation available in that setting.

What are the options for patients with OUD who are not good candidates for office-based treatment? Depending on the setting in which the patient is evaluated, several options are available. For the patient with significant psychiatric symptoms who is evaluated in a primary care setting, the options include referral to a psychiatrist who may be more comfortable providing buprenorphine treatment in an office-based practice setting or to a program capable of providing treatment for both OUD as well as other mental disorders. Some opioid treatment programs can provide these services. Referral of such patients to community- or clinic-based SUD/mental health services may be appropriate in some cases. In these settings, choices for treatment of OUD may include methadone maintenance or medically assisted withdrawal and treatment with injectable naltrexone. Another possibility is referral to a program that can administer buprenorphine on site, thus eliminating the need to provide take-home medication. Because of buprenorphine's long half-life and the even longer half-life of its active metabolite, norbuprenorphine, this medication can be dosed thrice weekly for treatment of OUD. If the community in which the clinician is practicing has good, supportive treatment services as described earlier, it may be possible for the clinician to provide office-based treatment of OUD with BUP/NX while the patient also attends another appropriate psychiatric treatment facility. The patient with severe psychopathology who is judged not to be a good candidate for office-based treatment of OUD should be referred to an opioid treatment program that can offer greater structure and individual attention.

Differential Diagnosis

Differentiating substance-induced mental disorders from independent mental disorders can be a challenge even for very experienced addiction psychiatrists. Important to this differentiation is the patient's history and family history and the course of symptoms following cessation of substance use.

Obtaining an accurate history regarding the temporal relationship of psychiatric symptoms to the substance use can be very illuminating. A patient who describes anxiety and/or depression but only since the onset of substance use is more likely to have a substance-induced disorder. Similarly, the individual whose symptoms abate as the length of sobriety increases also has a substance-induced disorder. As a general rule, substance-induced disorders resolve fairly rapidly following cessation of substance use. Improvement can be seen in days to weeks following completion of medical withdrawal or stabilization on OAT. If symptoms worsen with abstinence or do not abate after 30 days, it is more likely that the individual has an independent mental disorder, and appropriate treatment should be instituted.

Patients with a family history of major mental disorders or with a documented history of onset of a mental disorder prior to the onset of substance use are more likely to have an independent mental disorder. It is also important to determine when psychiatric symptoms occurred after initiation of SUDs. For example, the patient with a history of mental illness occurring during extended periods of sobriety has an independent psychiatric disorder. Review of the patient's medical records is important in determining the relationship of psychiatric symptoms to the cessation of substances and abstinence. It is also important to know all the substances being misused by the patient. For example, a patient with OUD may have had several episodes of medical withdrawal followed by periods of opioid abstinence. However, if that patient also abused other substances (e.g., alcohol, stimulants) and these issues were not treated or if he or she did not abstain from use of all abused substances, then a diagnosis of an independent mental disorder would not be appropriate. It is often difficult to be certain whether all SUDs were identified and treated. Unfortunately, some substance use treatment facilities focus primarily on the identified primary substance use disorder and ignore other substance problems. Similarly, when a substance-abusing patient enters the mental health system, substance use may be neither identified nor treated in favor of a focus on other mental disorders. The more conservative approach of delaying the treatment of mental disorders until they can be observed independent of substance use is often the best approach.

Reevaluation

In the previous section, we emphasized the need to do a thorough initial evaluation to determine immediate diagnoses and to initiate appropriate treatment. The prevalence of symptoms of mental illness in patients with OUD is quite high. Clearly, the use of substances produces psychiatric symptoms outside of the presence of an independent mental disorder. By diagnostic definition, individuals with SUD have had their lives significantly impacted by their substance use. Problems with significant others, children, and other family members and problems with employment, finances, and legal issues are common. Such issues would be expected to produce depression and anxiety. These responses would be normal, and lack of concern about such issues also could be indicative of a current mental disorder. Therefore, it is important not to make the diagnosis of a mental disorder prematurely or to immediately initiate treatment with psychotropics. In such circumstances, it is prudent to follow the symptoms over time. These patients should be reevaluated again after being stabilized on buprenorphine; change of symptoms over time, partial or full resolution, or worsening despite abstinence from illicit substances will provide the data needed to make the appropriate diagnosis and to institute treatment.

A WORD TO THE WISE: DO NOT EVALUATE INTOXICATED PATIENTS OR INDIVIDUALS IN WITHDRAWAL

Patients who come to the office for evaluation and appear to be intoxicated more than likely are intoxicated and are not capable of giving accurate history or providing informed consent for the treatment. Essentially, evaluation of such patients (or speaking to them on the telephone, as office staff frequently will) may not provide reliable information. This type of presentation suggests that the patient requires a higher level of care than that available in the office-based setting.

Office staff may wonder if a patient with an OUD might be intoxicated constantly and therefore be unable to come to an appointment prior to initiating BUP/NX at a time when he or she is not intoxicated. The answer is that a patient who is physiologically dependent on opioids and therefore has substantial tolerance to the effects of opioids is quite able to come to an appointment when he or she does not show obvious signs of intoxication. Once they have become physically dependent, individuals with OUD will experience opioid intoxication for only a brief period (hours or less) after use. They spend far more time trying to find the next dose of heroin or pain pills and experiencing the onset of withdrawal symptoms than they do experiencing actual intoxication.

Often, patients with OUD abuse other drugs in combination with heroin and/or opioid analgesics to potentiate the euphoric effects of the opioids. Maintaining their desired level of euphoria becomes increasingly difficult as they become increasingly tolerant to the effects of the opioids. Therefore, it is very important to evaluate for other SUDs in this population and, for effective treatment, to focus on discontinuation of all substances of abuse. Patients should be told that they must not come to office appointments intoxicated and that if they show evidence of intoxication, the appointment will be terminated (after a brief evaluation as described below).

This brings up another important issue in the assessment of an individual who misuses alcohol or other drugs. If the patient appears to be intoxicated (e.g., appears to have altered cognition, has slurred or slowed speech, gives answers that do not make sense or are not appropriate to the question asked, shows evidence of sedation or motor incoordination), an intervention must be made to protect both the patient and the public. There is liability for the clinician who does not intervene if the patient drives away and has an accident that harms self or others. The following procedure is recommended if the clinician suspects that the patient is intoxicated:

- Ask the patient when he or she last used drugs or alcohol. If the patient endorses drinking alcohol, a breath alcohol test should be obtained with a breathalyzer.
- Ask the patient if he or she wishes to be referred for medical withdrawal treatment; if so, arrange for an admission.
- Inquire about suicidal or homicidal ideation. If an intoxicated individual admits to such thoughts, he or she must be assessed carefully (see below) and hospitalized if necessary.
- If the patient denies any suicidal or homicidal ideation and does not wish to be hospitalized for medical withdrawal, ask how he or she arrived at the

appointment. If another person brought the patient, nothing further need be done except to document that you ascertained that the patient would not be driving. Ensure that the patient has a means of getting home with the person who brought him or her to the appointment. If arriving by public transportation, the patient can use that means to leave the appointment and should be encouraged not to leave until sober enough to manage safely on his or her own.

- If the patient drove to the appointment, tell the patient that it is not safe for him or her to drive away from the appointment. Ask the patient to identify someone who can be called to come to pick him or her up or offer the patient a quiet space in which to wait until he or she is no longer intoxicated.
- If the patient insists on driving while still moderately intoxicated, if possible, have a staff member escort him or her out and observe what car the patient drives. This should be reported to the police. This is not in violation of the Code of Federal Regulations, Title 42, part 2 (42 CFR Part 2) because you are not telling the police why the individual was at your office, only that he or she may be intoxicated while driving. No other information should be given out regarding the patient's history.
- If the patient is grossly intoxicated, hospitalization may be required, even on an involuntary basis depending on local statutes for involuntary hospitalization. You can be held responsible for permitting a grossly impaired individual to leave before he or she is deemed sober enough to manage safely on his or her own.
- Document the interaction thoroughly.

Having said all of this, it should be noted that the recommendations above are primarily precautionary. Situations in which police are informed of a possible intoxicated driver are quite rare. Furthermore, patients who wish to obtain BUP/NX for treatment of OUD are generally quite cooperative, eager to get treatment, and cooperative with office procedures. The information above is detailed only because it is a potential liability for the clinician should it occur, and how these situations will be handled should be considered *before* a decision to provide this form of treatment.

MANAGING PATIENTS WHO SHOW UP IN ACUTE WITHDRAWAL

It is also possible that a patient with OUD will show up to the first appointment in withdrawal, expecting treatment to begin with the first visit. This generally can be avoided by informing the patient prior to the first appointment that he or she will not receive medication treatment on the first visit. The clinician should ensure that staff explain that the first visit is to determine whether the patient should be treated with BUP/NX (or whether another form of treatment for OUD would be more appropriate) and whether the patient has any other health or mental health problems that might need a higher level of care than can be provided in the clinician's office. If the patient is not appropriate for the services that are offered by the clinician, the patient should be given a referral to another provider in the community. The patient also should be given a copy of any laboratory results to take to another provider. This can help to inform the next provider about the patient and reduce the cost of care by avoiding a repeat of laboratory testing.

If a patient does show up in withdrawal, it should be reiterated that treatment will not occur on that visit because the assessment to determine if the patient is an appropriate candidate for buprenorphine must be completed first. An adequate, comprehensive evaluation cannot be completed when a patient is either intoxicated or in severe withdrawal. Such patients can, at the discretion of the clinician, be started on BUP/NX if the clinician believes them to be in opiate withdrawal and otherwise are appropriate candidates for BUP/NX. However, the physician also can advise use of comfort medications (e.g., clonidine) and schedule the patient for an induction time on another date. The patient then should be rescheduled to come back at a time when he or she can be assessed more appropriately.

Management of Co-occurring Psychiatric Disorders in Patients Treated With Buprenorphine

GUIDELINES

1. Do not assume that a patient with an independent psychiatric disorder cannot be treated in an office-based practice setting or is not a candidate for buprenorphine treatment.
2. Determine the severity of the psychiatric disorder and treatment needs to determine whether office-based treatment of OUD is in the best interest of the patient.
3. Always insist on psychosocial therapies in conjunction with BUP/NX treatment.
4. For nonpsychiatrists, have a psychiatry colleague with experience in addiction psychiatry assist with the evaluation as needed.
5. Refer the patient for any other indicated mental health services that can be given in the most appropriate treatment setting. Make sure that releases are obtained to ensure that both treatment providers are aware of the patient's condition at any point in time.

Use of the above guidelines will help clinicians think through which patients with independent psychiatric disorders can be managed in their practice and under what conditions such patients should be treated. Not all independent psychiatric disorders dictate treatment by a psychiatrist. An uncomplicated major depression, for example, might be managed by a primary care physician, but a clear history of bipolar disorder would be an indication for treatment by a psychiatrist with experience in the treatment of SUDs and co-occurring disorders. The history will help the clinician develop the best treatment plan for these patients. It must be strongly emphasized that all patients (with or without co-occurring mental disorders) who receive office-based treatment of OUD with BUP/NX require ancillary counseling (see Chapters 6 and 7).

Counseling is an important part of addiction treatment, as is treatment for other mental disorders. Although Weiss et al. (2011) reported that medical management (consisting of regular office visits with the buprenorphine prescriber assessing treatment response and recommending abstinence and self-help participation) with pharmacotherapy was as effective as BUP/NX treatment with intensive counseling services, the physician contact in the medical management arm of the study included significant time with the patient, who was provided support and encouragement by the physician. This study makes the case for the value of a range of therapeutic interactions from relatively brief, supportive interventions to more intensive psychotherapies. For uncomplicated addiction, group therapy addressing addiction and recovery issues should be considered. If no group therapy is available in the clinician's community, then individual counseling must be required. For patients with additional psychopathology, individual therapy is generally indicated, and specialized group therapy for those with co-occurring disorders is beneficial. Many patients will benefit also from referral to 12-step or other mutual-support groups, although some mutual-support groups may be more or less accepting of medication therapy for addiction. Groups that do not accept the concept of medication treatment for SUD (and/or psychiatric disorders) can be detrimental to the individual's recovery by discouraging adherence to needed treatment. The clinician should attempt to identify groups in the community that are supportive of patients on medication and should encourage patients to participate actively.

Office-based treatment of OUD should not be started in any patient who is unwilling to obtain ongoing counseling. The aberrant behaviors that characterize addiction are not adequately treated by medication alone and require ongoing counseling to help patients to gain insight into their disease.

Patients with more severe mental disorders should be considered for treatment programs that provide greater structure, at least initially. There are a few possibilities that will be discussed briefly. First, for a patient who does not appear to be a good candidate for office-based treatment of OUD but who is felt to need OAT, referral to methadone maintenance will be the best option. Opioid treatment programs provide more structure than office-based treatment. Federal regulations limit the amount of take-home medication that can be provided by opioid treatment programs, with relatively few doses available in the early treatment period. Many methadone programs provide medical and psychiatric care for patients with co-occurring disorders and thus make it possible for a patient to obtain treatment for multiple problems in one treatment setting. Methadone maintenance programs provide for observed methadone dosing and may also provide observed dosing for other prescribed medications (e.g., psychotropic medications, antiretroviral medications, tuberculosis medications), making methadone maintenance potentially a better placement for patients with a history of difficulty adhering to prescribed regimens. BUP/NX also may be administered from some intensive outpatient programs, eliminating the need for take-home medication. Thrice-weekly dosing of BUP/NX has been shown to be effective in the treatment of OUD (Schottenfeld et al. 2000) and can provide a means of delivering both substance use treatment and psychiatric treatment to patients. These programs will require dispensing of BUP/NX at the program itself; prescribed BUP/NX cannot be kept at the program and administered there because to do so would be a violation of the Controlled Substances Act.

MANAGEMENT OF SPECIFIC PSYCHIATRIC ISSUES: WHO SHOULD PRESCRIBE?

As mentioned earlier, the decision regarding who should be the prescribing clinician for patients needing psychotropic medication depends on the clinician's level of experience in managing psychiatric disorders. If the clinician is uncomfortable treating co-occurring mental disorders, options include referral to a psychiatrist who can provide all necessary care or a referral to a psychiatrist who can treat the non–substance use mental disorders in conjunction with the clinician prescribing BUP/NX. Alternatively, the patient can be referred to a program that specializes in the treatment of co-occurring disorders.

WHEN TO REFER OR HOSPITALIZE

Acute Suicidal Ideation

Any patient receiving treatment for OUD from an office-based practice must have a way to contact the treating clinician (or covering clinician) 24 hours a day, 7 days a week. Patients should be informed that acute suicidal ideation is a reason to call the treating clinician. Critical elements in the evaluation of suicidal ideation are outlined in Table 10–1. Patients with suicidal ideation who have intent and a plan should be admitted to an inpatient facility that can provide constant care and observation. Such a referral generally begins with an evaluation either in the treating clinician's office or in the local hospital emergency department. If the patient is being interviewed on the telephone, it is important to get information from the patient as to his or her current location and whether any supportive individuals are present. If the patient refuses an evaluation that the clinician believes to be indicated, significant others can be enlisted to assist the patient, or the police can be asked to intervene to assist the individual to the emergency department, where the safety of the patient can be addressed. Patients without intent or plan may need more frequent visits to provide support and structure while working through the difficulties contributing to the suicidal thoughts. Such episodes require an updated treatment plan and possible reevaluation to determine if the patient continues to be a good candidate for office-based treatment of OUD.

Acute Homicidal Ideation

As with suicidal ideation, the occurrence of acute homicidal ideation requires immediate attention from the clinician. The assessment is similar to that described for acute suicidal ideation. Patients experiencing homicidal ideation may require an inpatient level of care for their safety and for the safety of others. If there is an identified victim and the clinician believes the threat to be serious and imminent, there is a duty to warn the intended victim. It is important that a patient with homicidal ideation be admitted to the hospital for a more thorough evaluation and consultation with the treatment team and legal experts to determine the most appropriate course of action. Such patients will require reevaluation to determine whether they are appropriate candidates for continued office-based treatment of OUD.

ADHERENCE TO PRESCRIBED MEDICATIONS

It is difficult to successfully treat a patient who does not take medications as prescribed. There are two immediate issues that can arise in office-based treatment of OUD with BUP/NX. The first is that of prescribing more medication than is needed, resulting in misuse or diversion. Dosage of BUP/NX 12 mg/3 mg to 16 mg/4 mg daily is typically recommended for the treatment of OUD. It is worth emphasizing that 16 mg of buprenorphine daily has been shown to bind to 79%–95% of μ opioid receptors (Greenwald et al. 2003, 2007), so higher doses should not be needed to provide a therapeutic response. Further, the long half-life of buprenorphine and its active metabolite, norbuprenorphine (Zhang et al. 2003), requires at least 12 days to reach steady-state. Therefore, dose changes in close succession are not indicated.

The second issue is deliberate nonadherence on particular days so that opioid use will provide the euphoria being sought. In cases in which the patient reduces or stops his or her medication for a day or two to abuse opioids (BUP/NX can blunt the effect of other abused opioids), it may be helpful to ask the patient to periodically bring in his or her prescription bottles so that a pill count can be done. This will provide additional evidence as to whether the medication is being taken as prescribed. Urine toxicology screens can detect the buprenorphine metabolite, but these screens are not sufficient because this information does not tell the clinician how much of the dose is being taken.

It is also important to ascertain that the patient is taking prescribed psychotropic medication as well. For patients whose psychiatric conditions do not improve, the clinician should consider whether the prescribed medication is not being taken or is not being taken as prescribed. It is necessary to address these issues directly with the patient. For example, patients may be experiencing side effects that they find intolerable, but they may not share this information unless asked. Patients also may lack insight into their psychiatric condition and may not wish to take psychotropic medication. It may be helpful to ask the patient to bring in prescribed psychotropic medications so that a pill count can be completed to help to determine whether the patient is adherent. It is also important to determine whether other substances are being used by the patient who is nonadherent to prescribed medications. Undetected substance use can lead to nonadherence and poor treatment outcomes.

COMPLIANCE WITH PSYCHOTHERAPEUTIC INTERVENTIONS

SUDs are disorders of behavior, but some patients with SUDs are resistant to attending psychosocial therapies that support the pharmacotherapy being provided by the clinician. OUD produces physical dependence that can be effectively managed with long-acting opioids. However, for most individuals, medication alone is not enough to treat the OUD. Although physical dependence (and the associated withdrawal) may be top on the list of problems that the patient wants addressed, the bottom line is that addiction is characterized by aberrant behaviors that spill over into many facets of life. These problems can be addressed best in some form of psychotherapy, counseling, and/or participation in mutual-support groups such as Alcoholics Anonymous or Narcotics Anonymous. If the patient requires counseling or psychotherapy but the treating clinician is not able to provide it, the clinician should refer the patient to another clinician who can provide that intervention (see Chapters 6 and 7). Noncompliance with psychotherapeutic referrals may be discussed with the patient to identify potential barriers and to propose solutions.

Continued Substance Use

When patients with OUD enter any treatment setting—but particularly less structured office-based treatment—one question that always arises is what to do if use of illicit substances continues. The first thing to understand is that in persons with OUD, it is commonplace for substance use to occur at least sporadically, particularly in the initial phases of treatment. Most patients will "test" BUP/NX to determine what occurs when they use opioids again, and most of them find that they do not get the effect that they are accustomed to. Furthermore, most patients with SUD need time to stabilize in treatment before they are able to stop misuse of other drugs and/or alcohol. This fact underscores the importance of several components of treatment: psychotherapy, psychoeducation, urine toxicology screening, and individual evaluation and referral.

Psychosocial therapies are important for helping patients discontinue the behaviors that place them at risk for relapse and helping them develop more adaptive coping mechanisms. Psychoeducation is important for informing patients about the possibility of adverse drug interactions and the side effects of BUP/NX. Once the patient stabilizes on BUP/NX and is established in the recommended psychotherapeutic environment, it will be easier for him or her to stop drug and alcohol use. It is also important to undertake regular but random urine drug screening so that ongoing substance use can be monitored. (For patients with a history of alcohol use, testing for ethyl glucuronide in hair or nails can provide information about recent alcohol use, but this test is not currently available as a point-of-service test.) Each person will need to be individually evaluated; any patient with chronic, unremitting substance use likely will need to be referred to a higher level of care. This might include hospitalization to carry out medical withdrawal from other substances or to stabilize co-occurring psychiatric disorders. In the patient with less severe problems but ongoing substance use, referral to a more structured program, such as methadone maintenance or an intensive outpatient treatment program, may be indicated.

Pharmacotherapy for Co-occurring Psychiatric Disorders

A frequently asked question regarding the treatment of patients with co-occurring OUD and mental disorders is whether they can be treated with the standard psychiatric medications that have an evidence base but that obviously were not developed for patients with OUD or those in BUP/NX treatment. The simple answer to this question is that there is a limited evidence base for treatment of mental disorders in this population. However, the rate of depression in the population with OUD is substantial, ranging from 44% to 54%, as compared with the general population, in which the depression rate is estimated at 16%. Further, estimates ranging from 10% to 30% of those receiving MAT for OUD have co-occurring depression (Pani et al. 2010). Pani et al. reviewed the available studies that focused on pharmacotherapy treatment for depression in patients with OUD and found that antidepressant treatment had no effect on retention in treatment or drug use. Two of three studies showed some benefit of antidepressant treatment in patients with more severe depression. However, it is important to note that the latter finding was based on a small combined sample size of 183 participants from two studies. Antidepressant medication therapy was also associated with higher rates of adverse events than placebo treatment of depression. This review showed little evidence for use of antidepressants to treat depression in patients with OUD being treated with OAT (Pani et al. 2010). Longer-term, well-designed studies are necessary to further illuminate this topic.

In addition to the efficacy of antidepressant pharmacotherapy for treatment of depression in OUD, reviews are also available on the effectiveness of psychosocial therapy combined with MAT for OUD. Amato et al. (2011) reviewed 35 studies with 4,319 participants and found no benefit for 13 different psychosocial interventions, including contingency management, on treatment episode parameters, including retention in treatment, abstinence from opioids, treatment adherence, benefit for psychiatric symptoms, and benefit for depression. However, an earlier review did show an overall significant effect on abstinence at follow up after treatment discontinuation (Amato et al. 2008).

The question, then, is whether antidepressant treatment should be implemented in patients reporting symptoms of depression. Given the currently available literature, it appears that antidepressants may be helpful, but they must be considered carefully. Patients with mild to moderate depression might benefit from MAT for OUD with clinical monitoring. Those with more severe depression are more likely to benefit from treatment with antidepressant pharmacotherapy. Consideration of the risks of untreated depressive symptoms versus the risks and benefits of pharmacotherapy, as well as the risk of adverse events related to concurrent use of opioid therapy and antidepressant pharmacotherapy, will need to guide the decision regarding which patients should be offered pharmacotherapy. Keeping in mind the above considerations, clinicians should consider standard pharmacotherapy and psychotherapy interventions specific to the treatment of the mental disorder in question for patients with OUD who receive BUP/NX pharmacotherapy.

For major depression and anxiety disorders, the first-line treatments are selective serotonin reuptake inhibitors (SSRIs). For anxiety disorders, these medications are especially good choices relative to benzodiazepines, which, if misused by injection, have resulted in deaths and also can be used to enhance the effect of BUP/NX or methadone. Although adverse events with SSRIs have not been reported, several SSRIs may result in drug-drug interactions, at least hypothetically (see section "Drug Interactions With Buprenorphine" below). Therefore, when possible, SSRIs that do not interact with buprenorphine or non-SSRI medications for depression and anxiety should be considered. If the

SSRIs are found to be ineffective, then the serotonin-norepinephrine reuptake inhibitors or bupropion may be tried. The tricyclic antidepressants may also be effective in some patients but will require greater monitoring for side effects.

Pharmacotherapy for ADHD requires careful consideration in any individual with a substance use history. ADHD medications generally should be started after the patient has had a period of abstinence from illicit drugs and the diagnosis of ADHD has been reconfirmed. There are concerns about diversion and misuse because some stimulants produce a "speedball" effect when combined with opioids (Foltin and Fischman 1994). Therefore, unless the patient has a well-documented history of childhood-onset ADHD that has responded positively to treatment with stimulants, it is recommended that nonstimulants such as atomoxetine or bupropion be considered for patients receiving BUP/NX. Extended-release stimulants can be considered in well-stabilized buprenorphine patients, but such patients should be observed carefully for the emergence of euphoria or other behaviors suggestive of medication abuse.

Another common complaint in patients with SUD, including those with OUD, is disrupted sleep. Many will ask for sleep medication. It has become commonplace for physicians to prescribe some atypical antipsychotics for this purpose. In general, the antipsychotics have enough risk of major adverse side effects that they should be avoided except for their approved indication. It is especially important to avoid the use of quetiapine with BUP/NX because of the possibility of an adverse drug interaction (see next section). Sleep hygiene techniques should be taught to all opioid-dependent patients, and avoidance of sleep medications should be the standard. If the problem is so severe that prescribed medication is needed, small amounts of diphenhydramine, trazodone, or ramelteon can be tried for brief periods. However, it is important not to prescribe medication for every complaint because doing so can feed into the pathology of persons with SUD.

Drug Interactions With Buprenorphine

Remarkably little information is available on pharmacokinetic and pharmacodynamic interactions between buprenorphine and other drugs. Most of the studies to date have examined the interaction of buprenorphine with HIV medications (McCance-Katz et al. 2006a, 2006b, 2007) or have compared the extent of interactions between HIV medications and methadone or buprenorphine (McCance-Katz 2005). Buprenorphine is predominantly a substrate of cytochrome P450 (CYP) 3A4. Therefore, as with methadone, drugs that alter CYP3A4 function might alter buprenorphine exposure and its effectiveness in the treatment of OUD. However, buprenorphine has an advantage in its clinical pharmacology that methadone does not: methadone is metabolized to an inactive metabolite, whereas buprenorphine is metabolized to norbuprenorphine, which is also a μ opioid agonist. In the presence of drugs that can induce buprenorphine metabolism, this can help to prevent the onset of withdrawal that has been observed with methadone and some drugs that induce CYP3A4. However, this remains to be demonstrated adequately.

With some HIV medications that induce CYP3A4 enzymes, buprenorphine-treated study participants did not experience withdrawal symptoms, although it is worth noting that these studies were short in duration. With clinical treatment, results may differ and patients taking such drugs need to be monitored for adverse effects. The anticonvulsant medication carbamazepine, which is often used as a mood stabilizer, can induce CYP3A4 (McCance-Katz 2005, McCance-Katz et al. 2007). Whenever possible, another mood-stabilizing drug, such as valproate, might be a better option in patients being treated with BUP/NX.

Some drugs have the potential to inhibit buprenorphine metabolism by inhibiting the action of CYP3A4. There has been a case report of cognitive impairment in patients with HIV treated with atazanavir/ritonavir (Bruce and Altice 2006), and buprenorphine/norbuprenorphine levels were significantly increased in those receiving this drug combination, although in otherwise healthy individuals with OUD sedation was the only adverse event noted with administration of this medication combination (McCance-Katz et al. 2007). Again, patients receiving treatment with medications that might inhibit buprenorphine metabolism should be observed and monitored for adverse opioid effects. Psychotropic medications known to inhibit CYP3A4 include fluoxetine and nefazodone.

There also may be drugs that do not have a direct effect on buprenorphine metabolism but that may have a pharmacodynamic interaction with buprenorphine. For example, the benzodiazepine diazepam has been shown to be associated with increased sedation and memory deficits when given in combination with buprenorphine (Nielsen et al. 2007). Sedating drugs, such as benzodiazepines, nonbenzodiazepines, and antihistamines, should be avoided when possible in the patient being treated with BUP/NX or other opioid therapies. Finally, buprenorphine is not known to alter drug metabolism itself and to date has not been found to substantially alter exposure to other drugs taken concomitantly. Because of the clinical pharmacology of buprenorphine, it may be a better choice for OAT therapy for patients who must also take other medications for co-occurring conditions.

Conclusion

Mental illness occurs frequently in persons with OUD. The safe and effective treatment of these individuals requires thorough evaluation, differentiation of substance-induced from independent mental disorders, and institution of the most appropriate treatment for all current mental disorders in the most appropriate clinical setting. BUP/NX treatment can be undertaken in persons with co-occurring mental disorders, but for some severely ill patients, the best care for OUD and other co-occurring psychiatric disorders will be that delivered in a setting other than an office-based practice. The considerations and practices outlined in this chapter will help clinicians assist patients in finding the most effective treatment interventions for these complex illnesses.

Clinical Pearls

- It is relatively rare to evaluate a patient with opioid use disorder (OUD) who has no other substance problems. The clinician should evaluate and provide treatment for all substance use disorders (SUDs) present in the patient. Failure to treat all the substance problems places the patient at high risk for relapse.

- It is important to differentiate substance-induced from independent mental disorders. The former will resolve with treatment of OUD, whereas the latter will require a specific treatment plan that often will include use of psychotropic medications.

- The currently available literature does not provide evidence that patients with OUD and depression of low severity receiving treatment with opioid agonist therapies benefit from antidepressant pharmacotherapy.

- Psychosocial interventions used concurrently in the treatment of OUD do not address psychiatric symptoms. Patients with mental disorders will need assessment and treatment specific to the diagnosed mental disorder on the basis of severity at presentation.

- Standard first-line treatments should be considered for individuals with OUD and co-occurring mental disorders that are determined to be of a severity requiring pharmacotherapy.

- Medications with abuse liability (e.g., quetiapine, benzodiazepines) should be avoided in patients with OUD. There are other medication choices for the treatment of anxiety disorders that do not have abuse liability. Patients resistant to such medications and/or insistent on prescription of controlled substances should be evaluated carefully to determine whether their behaviors are drug-seeking rather than symptoms of a co-occurring mental disorder.

- Clinicians should be familiar with the referral sources in their community before starting office-based treatment of OUD.

CASE 5 (CONTINUED)

Henrietta, the 43-year-old automobile mechanic who said "drinking has never been a problem," has not paid her bill for a month. She has cut back on her drinking and has been attending group psychotherapy meetings weekly while maintaining negative urine toxicology screens. Today, when she arrives at the office, she is belligerent, and it is very clear that she is intoxicated with alcohol. She refuses to be admitted for alcohol withdrawal treatment and insists on driving herself home.

1. How would you expect your staff to treat Henrietta?

2. How would you respond?

3. How do you address the nonpayment issue?

CASE 8

Maria is a 31-year-old single woman who is referred to your office with the chief complaint "My work Employee Assistance Program wants me to get an evaluation." She is a talented graphics design artist but has been reported as "erratic" and "hotheaded" at work.

The Employee Assistance Program office reports that two urine tests have been positive for opioids. Maria admits to using heroin from time to time but refuses to go into detail—"I'm not hurting anybody." She insists that her only problem is controlling her temper. After you obtain another positive urine test result, Maria admits that her heroin use is out of control and agrees to buprenorphine treatment and weekly group therapy. Her buprenorphine induction goes smoothly, but during her first group session, she engages in a heated argument with several group members and then reveals that she was molested repeatedly as a child.

1. Should this patient have a psychiatric evaluation?

2. What are some psychiatric diagnoses that may help explain Maria's symptoms?

3. Would a more specialized type of therapy group or individual counseling be useful?

4. In this case, would you consider motivation enhancement therapy?

5. Is the Seeking Safety program a better option for this patient?

CASE 9

Karen is a 28-year-old woman who has been gainfully employed as a receptionist for the past year. She started using opioids in her teens and eventually became addicted to intravenous heroin. She has been taking BUP/NX for 2 years. Karen had a few problems with opioids and benzodiazepines during the first year of treatment, but sustained sobriety has been the trend for the past 12 months. She calls, very upset: "They closed our office and fired everyone!" She has been living in a drug- and alcohol-free residential facility in the community but now has to leave because she can no longer afford the rent. Fortunately, she is able to move in with a sober woman friend from Narcotics Anonymous, but she is feeling anxious and discouraged. She says, "I'm scared of becoming homeless, and I think I'm depressed again." She carries the diagnoses of major depressive disorder and generalized anxiety disorder, for which she takes citalopram and trazodone.

1. What helps determine whether Karen's psychiatric symptoms are secondary to her opioid use or represent independent psychiatric disorders?

2. What elements of her history would clarify this diagnostic question?

3. Would you change her psychiatric medications at this time?

4. Given her dual diagnosis, would she be manageable in your office setting?

5. Does it matter which antidepressant is used?

6. If Karen reports clear evidence of a panic attack, would you consider adding a benzodiazepine?

7. In what ways might benzodiazepines be a problem in this case?

Case 10

You cover the psychiatric service for a community hospital on some weekends. When you get to the emergency department, you are asked to evaluate a 28-year-old Iraq War combat veteran for suicidal ideation. He says that he "can't live like this" any longer. He has been taking 3–4 OxyContin 80-mg pills daily for the last 4 months, has been unable to stop, and now realizes that he is addicted. You determine that he meets the threshold for active risk of self-harm, and you admit him to the hospital. During your evaluation, you find that he also meets all of the DSM-5 criteria for PTSD. He also says that he has anger issues about his war experience and sometimes "wants to take everybody out...."

1. How do you determine whether the suicidal ideation is secondary to the patient's drug problem or related to his PTSD? How should this be handled?

2. Would you recommend inpatient opioid withdrawal treatment, or would you consider him a candidate for opioid agonist therapy?

3. How do you address his homicidal language?

4. Is buprenorphine a reasonable choice?

5. How will you incorporate treatment for PTSD into his treatment plan?

References

Amato L, Minozzi S, Davoli M, et al: Psychosocial combined with agonist maintenance treatments versus agonist maintenance treatments alone for treatment of opioid dependence. Cochrane Database of Systematic Reviews 2008, Issue 4, Art. No.: CD004147. DOI: 10.1002/14651858.CD004147.pub3

Amato L, Minozzi S, Davoli M, Vecchi S: Psychosocial combined with agonist maintenance treatments versus agonist maintenance treatments alone for treatment of opioid dependence. Cochrane Database of Systematic Reviews 2011, Issue 10. Art. No.: CD004147. DOI: 10.1002/14651858.CD004147.pub4

American Psychiatric Association: Diagnostic and Statistical Manual of Mental Disorders, 5th Edition. Arlington, VA, American Psychiatric Association, 2013

Bruce RD, Altice FL: Three case reports of a clinical pharmacokinetic interaction with buprenorphine and atazanavir plus ritonavir. AIDS 20(5):783–784, 2006 16514314

Carpentier PJ, Knapen LJM, van Gogh MT, et al: Addiction in developmental perspective: influence of conduct disorder severity, subtype, and attention-deficit hyperactivity disorder on problem severity and comorbidity in adults with opioid dependence. J Addict Dis 31(1):45–59, 2012 22356668

Chen KW, Banducci AN, Guller L, et al: An examination of psychiatric comorbidities as a function of gender and substance type within an inpatient substance use treatment program. Drug Alcohol Depend 118(2–3):92–99, 2011 21514751

Foltin RW, Fischman MW: Effects of buprenorphine on the self-administration of cocaine by humans. Behav Pharmacol 5(1):79–89, 1994 11224254

Ginsberg Y, Quintero J, Anand E, et al: Underdiagnosis of attention-deficit/hyperactivity disorder in adult patients: a review of the literature. Prim Care Companion CNS Disord 16(3), 2014 25317367 Epub before print

Greenwald MK, Johanson CE, Moody DE, et al: Effects of buprenorphine maintenance dose on mu-opioid receptor availability, plasma concentrations, and antagonist blockade in heroin-dependent volunteers. Neuropsychopharmacology 28(11):2000–2009, 2003 12902992

Greenwald M, Johanson CE, Bueller J, et al: Buprenorphine duration of action: mu-opioid receptor availability and pharmacokinetic and behavioral indices. Biol Psychiatry 61(1):101–110, 2007 16950210

McCabe SE, Dickinson K, West BT, Wilens TE: Age of onset, duration, and type of medication therapy for attention-deficit/hyperactivity disorder and substance use during adolescence: A multi-cohort national study. J Am Acad Child Adolesc Psychiatry 55(6):479–486, 2016 27238066

McCance-Katz EF: Treatment of opioid dependence and coinfection with HIV and hepatitis C virus in opioid-dependent patients: the importance of drug interactions between opioids and antiretroviral agents. Clin Infect Dis 41 (suppl 1):S89–S95, 2005 16265622

McCance-Katz EF, Moody DE, Morse GD, et al: Interactions between buprenorphine and antiretrovirals. I. The nonnucleoside reverse-transcriptase inhibitors efavirenz and delavirdine. Clin Infect Dis 43 (suppl 4):S224–S234, 2006a 17109309

McCance-Katz EF, Moody DE, Smith PF, et al: Interactions between buprenorphine and antiretrovirals. II. The protease inhibitors nelfinavir, lopinavir/ritonavir, and ritonavir. Clin Infect Dis 43 (suppl 4):S235–S246, 2006b 17109310

McCance-Katz EF, Moody DE, Morse GD, et al: Interaction between buprenorphine and atazanavir or atazanavir/ritonavir. Drug Alcohol Depend 91(2–3):269–278, 2007 17643869

McCance-Katz EF, Moody DE, Rainey PM: Effect of cocaine use on buprenorphine pharmacokinetics in humans. Am J Addict 19(1):38–46, 2010 20132120

Nielsen S, Dietze P, Lee N, et al: Concurrent buprenorphine and benzodiazepines use and self-reported opioid toxicity in opioid substitution treatment. Addiction 102(4):616–622, 2007 17286641

Pani PP, Vacca R, Trogu E, et al: Pharmacological treatment for depression during opioid agonist treatment for opioid dependence. Cochrane Database of Systematic Reviews 2010, Issue 9. Art. No.: CD008373. DOI: 10.1021/14651858.CD008373.pub2

Ross J, Teesson M, Darke S, et al: The characteristics of heroin users entering treatment: findings from the Australian treatment outcome study (ATOS). Drug Alcohol Rev 24(5):411–418, 2005 16298835

Schottenfeld RS, Pakes J, O'Connor P, et al: Thrice-weekly versus daily buprenorphine maintenance. Biol Psychiatry 47(12):1072–1079, 2000 10862807

Substance Abuse and Mental Health Services Administration: 2014 National Survey on Drug Use and Health: National Findings, Washington, DC, Substance Abuse and Mental Health Services Administration, 2015

Weiss RD, Potter JS, Fiellin DA, et al: Adjunctive counseling during brief and extended buprenorphine-naloxone treatment for prescription opioid dependence: a 2-phase randomized controlled trial. Arch Gen Psychiatry 68(12):1238–1246, 2011 22065255

Zhang W, Ramamoorthy Y, Tyndale RF, et al: Interaction of buprenorphine and its metabolite norbuprenorphine with cytochromes p450 in vitro. Drug Metab Dispos 31(6):768–772, 2003 12756210

11

Medical Comorbidity

Joseph H. Donroe, M.D.
Lynn E. Fiellin, M.D.
David A. Fiellin, M.D.
Jeanette M. Tetrault, M.D.

PATIENTS with opioid use disorder (OUD) who present for treatment often have other medical problems. These medical conditions can result from both past and current risk behaviors. For instance, both injection and non-injection drug use are associated with increased prevalence of infectious complications. It is important for clinicians who treat patients with OUD to screen for and treat (or refer for treatment) common comorbid medical conditions.

Office-based buprenorphine treatment provides an opportunity to integrate the delivery of treatment for substance disorders with screening for and management of comorbid medical conditions. In addition, this setting allows the clinician to discuss relevant preventive measures.

The purpose of this chapter is to review common comorbid medical conditions found in patients with OUD and to review some features of preventive health care for these patients. Topics covered here include admission procedures and referral to primary care; routine preventive care; comorbid hepatitis B, hepatitis C, HIV/AIDS, tuberculosis, and injection drug use–related acute infections; and buprenorphine treatment in the geriatric population. The importance of these topics cannot be overstated because the integration of screening and treatment of comorbid medical disorders with office-based buprenorphine can improve the health of patients being treated with buprenorphine.

Admission Procedures and Referral to Primary Care

All patients with OUD should have a complete medical history taken prior to treatment initiation. At this visit, the clinician should review the following with the patient:

- Medical, surgical, psychiatric, and substance use history
- Medication list and allergies
- Prior history of treatment for substance use disorders
- Social determinants of health such as support systems, employment, level of education, and housing situation

Clinicians should have the ability to perform, or refer for, physical examination, with attention to potential stigmata of drug use, including careful inspection of skin and soft tissue (especially at sites of injection), lymph node examination, liver size and contour, cardiac examination with auscultation for murmurs, and focused neurological exam. Liver function tests should be evaluated at baseline and monitored periodically throughout the course of treatment, particularly in patients with chronic viral illnesses or if baseline testing is abnormal (Saxon et al. 2013; Vergara-Rodriguez et al. 2011). Although prior studies raised concern for potential buprenorphine-related hepatotoxicity, more recent data suggested that buprenorphine infrequently causes significant liver damage (Saxon et al. 2013; Tetrault et al. 2016). However, patients with chronic viral illnesses (e.g., HIV, hepatitis C and heapatitis B) are more likely to develop alterations in measures of liver health during buprenorphine treatment (Kraus et al. 2011; Saxon and Bisaga 2014; Tetrault et al. 2016).

Any patient with chronic underlying medical conditions or a new diagnosis of acute or chronic infectious etiologies should be referred for ongoing primary care. Patients with chronic pain and OUD present unique challenges and may require a primary care or more specialized referral (see Chapter 12, "Acute and Chronic Pain"). Because of buprenorphine's high binding affinity, managing patients treated with buprenorphine who have acute moderate to severe pain can be particularly challenging; however, guidance is available (Alford et al. 2006; Donroe et al. 2016).

Routine Preventive Care

Patients with illicit substance use have higher rates of transmittable infectious diseases, and on the basis of published recommendations and guidelines (Bibbins-Domingo et al. 2016; Branson et al. 2006; Cantor et al. 2016; Centers for Disease Control and Prevention 2012; LeFevre and U.S. Preventive Services Task Force 2014a, 2014b; Moyer and U.S. Preventive Services Task Force 2013), clinicians should consider screening asymptomatic patients for the following:

- Hepatitis B virus (HBV) and hepatitis C virus (HCV) infection
- Latent tuberculosis infection (LTBI)
- Other sexually transmitted infections, including chlamydia, gonorrhea, syphilis, and HIV

Current guidelines recommend opt-out screening for HIV in all patients between the ages of 13 and 64 years, meaning testing should be performed routinely unless the patient explicitly refuses (Branson et al. 2006).

Patients with OUD should be vaccinated against hepatitis A and hepatitis B if they have not been exposed or immunized previously. Immunization against hepatitis B is described further in the next section. Immunization against hepatitis A involves a two-dose vaccine series separated by at least 6 months (for single-antigen formulations). All patients also should be vaccinated against influenza yearly and receive a tetanus-diphtheria booster every 10 years, with at least one dose being a tetanus-diphtheria-pertussis vaccine. The following individuals should receive the pneumococcal vaccine: all adults with certain immunocompromising conditions; immunocompetent adults age 65 years and older; and adults younger than 65 years who are smokers or have alcohol use disorder, diabetes, or chronic heart, lung, or liver disease. Providers should refer to the Centers for Disease Control and Prevention (CDC) guidelines for recommendations on which pneumococcal vaccine or vaccine combination to administer (D. K. Kim et al. 2016).

Hepatitis B

Epidemiology

HBV is an important cause of chronic hepatitis, cirrhosis, and hepatocellular carcinoma (HCC) worldwide. The United States is considered a low prevalence region, with an estimated 850,000 to 2.2 million individuals infected with chronic HBV—many of whom are unaware of their HBV status—and a yearly rate of acute infection declining to approximately 19,200 according to recent CDC estimates (Centers for Disease Control and Prevention 2016b; LeFevre and U.S. Preventive Services Task Force 2014b). Less than 1% of adults with acute HBV infection will progress to fulminant hepatitis, and less than 5% will develop chronic infection (Trépo et al. 2014).

HBV is contracted primarily via blood or other bodily fluids. Although vertical transmission from mother to child is a significant risk factor worldwide, it plays a less important role in non-endemic regions. High prevalence groups in the United States include the following:

- HIV-positive individuals
- Persons with past or present injection drug use (IDU)
- Household contacts with or sexual partners of persons with HBV infection
- Men who have sex with men

In addition to these groups, screening is also recommended for persons born in high-prevalence (≥2%) HBV countries, unvaccinated U.S.-born adults whose parents were born in regions with a very high prevalence (≥8%) of HBV, persons with elevated liver enzymes of unknown etiology, and all pregnant women, among others (LeFevre and U.S. Preventive Services Task Force 2014b; Weinbaum et al. 2008).

Among persons with active IDU, it is estimated that 50% have serological evidence of prior exposure to HBV, and in the majority of these cases there is evidence of active viral infection. In addition, approximately 70% of patients who inject drugs are infected with HBV within 5 years (Garfein et al. 1996).

LABORATORY DIAGNOSIS

Testing for acute HBV infection is typically prompted by the constellation of symptoms of hepatitis plus elevated liver transaminases, the levels of which can be quite high, with alanine transaminase (ALT) values typically being greater than aspartate transaminase (AST) values. Chronic HBV infection is usually asymptomatic, and cases are detected through screening of asymptomatic individuals with risk factors as described above or patients with newly diagnosed cirrhosis.

As shown in Figure 11–1, screening tests for HBV includes serologies for the following:

- Hepatitis B surface antigen (HBsAg)
- Hepatitis B surface antibody (anti-HBs)
- Antibody (IgM and IgG) to hepatitis B core antigen (anti-HBc)

The presence of HBsAg in the serum, detected as early as 1 week to as late as 12 weeks after exposure to the virus, is the hallmark of active infection and will be present in both acute or chronic states (Younossi 2000). *Acute HBV infection* is further characterized by the appearance of anti-HBc (both IgM and IgG), which occurs 1–2 weeks after the appearance of HBsAg and at the time of transaminase increase. *Chronic HBV infection* is characterized by persistent HBsAg and anti-HBc IgG. For individuals whose acute infection does not

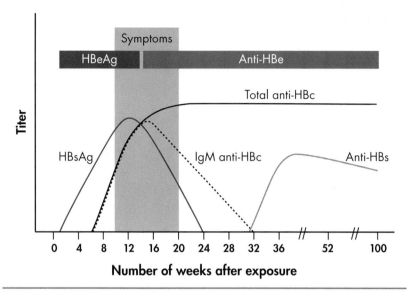

FIGURE 11–1.   **Hepatitis B serology.**
Anti-HBc=antibody to hepatitis B core antigen (HBcAg); anti-HBe=antibody to hepatitis B envelope antigen (HBeAg); anti-HBs=antibody to hepatitis B surface antigen (HBsAg); IgM anti-HBc=immunoglobulin M antibody to HBcAg.
Source.   Courtesy of Centers for Disease Control and Prevention, Division of Viral Hepatitis.

progress to chronic infection, HBsAg typically clears within 3–6 months. The loss of HBsAg and the appearance of anti-HBs signals recovery and protective immunity from re-infection (LeFevre and U.S. Preventive Services Task Force 2014b; Trépo et al. 2014). Patients with immunity through natural infection will therefore be positive for anti-HBs and anti-HBc IgG antibodies. Individuals with immunity by vaccination will be positive for anti-HBs antibody alone.

Further HBV-specific testing recommended for individuals with chronic HBV infection includes the following:

- HBV e antigen (HBeAg)
- HBV e antibody (anti-HBe)
- HBV DNA by PCR assay

HBV DNA appears soon after infection, and levels vary during the course of chronic infection. HBeAg also appears early in the disease and is usually associated with high HBV DNA levels (Trépo et al. 2014). Seroconversion to anti-HBe positivity with loss of HBeAg occurs in most cases of adult acquired HBV and usually indicates decreased viral replication and decreased infectivity.

ACUTE HBV INFECTION

Following exposure to HBV in a susceptible host, the virus enters hepatocytes and remains dormant for 1 to several months before liver enzymes first become elevated. The clinical presentation of acute HBV infection can vary widely depending on age and immune status and can range from asymptomatic to (rarely) fulminant hepatitis. Most commonly, there is a mild nonspecific and short-lived prodrome of nausea, vomiting, anorexia, malaise, and abdominal pain. Jaundice occurs in approximately 30% of all patients with acute HBV infection and is often the symptom that prompts medical care and further workup (Shiffman 2010).

CHRONIC HBV INFECTION

The risk of progression of acute HBV to chronic HBV indirectly correlates with age. Acute infection progresses to chronic infection, characterized by the persistence of HBsAg for at least 6 months, in less than 5% of newly infected adults (Trépo et al. 2014). Among untreated adults with chronic HBV, the cumulative 5-year incidence of cirrhosis is 5%–20%. Of patients with HBV cirrhosis, the 5-year cumulative risk of hepatic decompensation is 20%, and the risk of HCC is 2%–5% (Terrault et al. 2016). In contrast to patients with acute HBV infection, patients with chronic HBV are typically asymptomatic unless exhibiting signs of cirrhosis.

Initial evaluation of all patients with chronic HBV infection should include the following:

- HBV DNA viral load
- Testing for HBeAg and anti-HBe
- Liver panel, including albumin
- Coagulation studies
- Complete blood count (CBC) with platelets
- Testing for HAV, HCV, hepatitis D virus (HDV), and HIV

Patients without immunity should receive the HAV vaccine, and close contacts without immunity should receive the HBV vaccine. An evaluation of the degree of liver fibrosis is helpful for guiding therapy and is needed for HCC surveillance. Liver biopsy is the gold standard, but noninvasive methods, such as vibration-controlled transient elastography and serum tests including aspartate aminotransferase (AST)–to–platelet ratio index (APRI), Fibro Test, FibroSure, and FIB-4 index, are available (Terrault et al. 2016).

Persons with chronic HBV infection should be counseled about maintaining liver health (e.g., avoidance of alcohol and herbal products) and risk of transmission through sexual contact and sharing of needles, toothbrushes, razors, and so forth. Patients with chronic HBV infection who are at high risk of HCC should undergo HCC surveillance with ultrasound every 6 months. High risk groups include the following:

- Asian men ages > 40 years and Asian women ages > 50 years
- Persons with cirrhosis
- Persons with a family history of HCC
- People of African descent ages > 20 years

Surveillance should continue for these groups even if treatment is undertaken, because the risk of HCC likely persists (Bruix et al. 2011).

PREVENTION AND TREATMENT

Vaccination against hepatitis B is highly effective and is recommended universally for children and susceptible adults with specific indications, including OUD. The recommended vaccination schedule is a series of three shots administered at 0, 1, and 6 months, although an accelerated schedule of 0, 1, and 4 months is acceptable and may improve adherence (Hwang et al. 2010; D. K. Kim et al. 2016). If there is a longer than recommended time between doses, the vaccine series can be simply continued and does not need to be restarted. When patient follow-up is uncertain, the first dose of hepatitis B vaccine can be given once blood work for HBV screening is drawn (Centers for Disease Control and Prevention 2012).

No guidelines currently exist for the pharmacological treatment of acute HBV infection. Thus, the clinical management of acute HBV infection is primarily one of supportive measures, though lamivudine may play a role in some presentations (Shiffman 2010; Wiegand et al. 2014). Patients should be counseled with regard to risk of transmission to household and sexual contacts until anti-HBs is evident.

The objective of treatment of chronic HBV infection is to eradicate active replication, thereby decreasing hepatic injury and improving morbidity and mortality. *Virological cure*, defined as eradication of HBV, is not yet attainable, although improved outcomes through suppression of HBV replication is achievable (Terrault et al. 2016). Pharmacological treatment options include interferon alfa; pegylated interferon; the nucleoside analogues lamivudine, telbivudine, and entecavir; and the nucleotide analogues adefovir and tenofovir (Table 11–1). The most recent treatment guidelines from the American Association for the Study of Liver Diseases recommend considering HBV DNA viral load, HBeAg, ALT value, and presence of cirrhosis when making decisions to treat patients with chronic HBV infection. Duration of treatment is not well

TABLE 11–1.   **Pharmacological options available for the treatment of chronic hepatitis B virus infection**

Medication Class		Dosage	Advantages	Side Effects
Pegylated interferon alfa-2a	Immuno-suppressant	180 μg weekly im	Resistance unlikely	Flu-like symptoms, autoimmune disorders, depression, cytopenias
Lamivudine	Nucleoside analogue	100 mg daily po	Well tolerated	High rate of resistance, pancreatitis
Entecavir	Nucleoside analogue	0.5 or 1.0 mg daily po	Potent viral suppression; low rate of resistance; well tolerated	
Telbivudine	Nucleoside analogue	600 mg daily po	Well tolerated; pregnancy category B	Cross-resistance with lamivudine; rhabdomyolysis and peripheral neuropathy rare but may occur
Adefovir	Nucleotide analogue	10 mg daily po	Activity against lamivudine-resistant virus	Nephrotoxicity; nephrogenic diabetes insipidus, slow viral suppression
Tenofovir	Nucleotide analogue	300 mg daily po	Well tolerated	Potential nephrotoxicity; osteomalacia

Note.   im = intramuscularly; po = orally.

established but should be thought of as long term when discussing decisions to treat with patients. Treatment endpoints depend on such factors as the presence of cirrhosis, HBeAg seroconversion, HBV detectability, persistent ALT elevation, and loss of HBsAg (Terrault et al. 2016).

HBV AND OPIOID AGONIST TREATMENT

There appear to be few unique precautions that need to be adhered to in patients receiving buprenorphine who are infected with HBV. There are no known interactions between buprenorphine and any of the antiviral medications used to treat hepatitis B. However, if interferon treatment is used, patients should be monitored closely for relapse to drug use because the flu-like syndrome that often accompanies interferon treatment may mimic symptoms of opioid withdrawal.

Hepatitis C

EPIDEMIOLOGY

At least 4.6 million persons in the United States are HCV-antibody positive, and nearly 3.5 million persons are infected with HCV, although roughly half are unaware of their infection. Upward of 85% of incident cases of HCV go on to develop chronic infection, and HCV is the leading cause of liver transplantation in the United States (American Association for the Study of Liver Diseases–Infectious Diseases Society of America 2016b; Centers for Disease Control and Prevention 2016a; Kohli et al. 2014).

IDU remains the most common cause of HCV seroconversion in the United States, responsible for more than 60% of all new infections (American Association for the Study of Liver Diseases–Infectious Diseases Society of America 2016b). It is important to remember that HCV is transmitted not only through sharing needles but also through sharing works (e.g., tubing, syringe, wastewater) with an infected individual. There is evidence to suggest that opioid agonist therapy with methadone or buprenorphine can be effective in reducing transmission of HCV among persons who inject drugs (Alavian et al. 2013; Perlman et al. 2015; Tsui et al. 2014). Sexual transmission of HCV is inefficient, but patients practicing high-risk sexual behavior or those with multiple sexual partners should use barrier methods of contraception. Other causes of HCV transmission include needle stick injuries, receipt of a blood transfusion prior to 1992, and, infrequently, mother-to-child transmission.

NATURAL HISTORY

Although acute HCV infection can cause severe hepatic injury, this is rare, and infection is most often asymptomatic or associated with mild nonspecific symptoms, such as myalgias and malaise. HCV RNA appears in the blood weeks before increases in ALT or the development of HCV antibodies (anti-HCV). Because the syndrome is so benign, patients usually do not present for medical care, and the infection goes undetected (A. Kim 2016).

Exposure to HCV generally results in development of an anti-HCV antibody roughly 10–12 weeks after exposure; however, this antibody does not confer protection. After acute infection, approximately 15%–25% of those infected will spontaneously clear the infection, usually within 1 year, with clearance defined as repeated undetectable HCV RNA levels (Centers for Disease Control and Prevention 2016a; A. Kim 2016).

Of those going on to develop chronic infection, 15%–20% develop liver cirrhosis within 25 years, and up to 5% will die from HCV-related liver cancer or complications of end-stage liver disease (Centers for Disease Control and Prevention 2016a). Factors known to influence the progression of liver fibrosis include male gender, older age at onset of disease, co-infection with HIV, and presence of other liver insults, including hepatitis B, fatty liver, and alcohol consumption (Fattovich et al. 1997). Chronic HCV infection is usually asymptomatic, but extrahepatic manifestations do occur and include the following manifestations:

- Hematological: cryoglobulinemic vasculitis, non-Hodgkin lymphoma
- Endocrine: thyroid disease, diabetes
- Rheumatological: arthralgias and arthritis, chronic fatigue
- Dermatological: porphyria cutanea tarda
- Renal: glomerular disease

LABORATORY DIAGNOSIS

Screening for HCV is recommended (Moyer and U.S. Preventive Services Task Force 2013) for adult patients

- With past or current IDU or intranasal drug use
- Born between 1945 and 1965
- Who received a blood transfusion before 1992
- Receiving long-term hemodialysis treatment
- With a history of incarceration
- With percutaneous exposure, such as in an occupational setting or in an unregulated tattoo parlor

Individuals with ongoing risk factors, such as IDU, should be screened periodically.

Screening for HCV infection rests with measurement of serum anti-HCV. Once a detectable antibody is noted, quantitative or qualitative HCV RNA testing should be performed to confirm viremia. Quantitative testing is recommended prior to initiation of pharmacological therapy. HCV RNA testing is also indicated for persons in whom re-infection is detected and for persons with negative anti-HCV who are immunocompromised, on chronic hemodialysis, or presumed to have been exposed to HCV within the prior 6 months (American Association for the Study of Liver Diseases–Infectious Diseases Society of America 2016b). Transaminase levels are nonspecific and should not be used for screening. ALT values may be elevated, may be normal, or may fluctuate throughout the course of disease (A. Kim 2016). For patients considering treatment, an HCV genotype should be obtained because results will influence treatment regimens. There are six different genotypes of HCV with multiple subtypes. Genotype 1 (specifically 1a) is the most common type in the United States, with genotypes 2, 3, and 4 being less common.

Additional workup of patients diagnosed with HCV infection includes the following tests:

- CBC with platelets
- Coagulation studies
- Liver panel with albumin for evidence of cirrhosis
- HIV and HBV testing
- Assessment of liver fibrosis, performed invasively or noninvasively as described for HBV (see subsection "Chronic HBV Infection" earlier in this chapter)

NONPHARMACOLOGICAL MANAGEMENT OF CHRONIC HCV INFECTION

All patients with active HCV infection should be linked to care with a provider experienced in managing chronic liver disease and HCV treatment. Important elements of care beyond pharmacological treatment include counseling to minimize alcohol use, with a goal of abstinence, and avoidance of other hepatotoxic agents, such as herbal products. Additional counseling should address ongoing risk factors for HCV exposure and risk of new genotype acquisition, as well as strategies to minimize transmission of the virus to others and to reduce the risk of acquisition of new viral genotypes. Vaccination against HAV and HBV is recommended for susceptible hosts. It is further recommended that patients with cirrhosis receive the pneumococcal vaccine, screening for esophageal varices, and close monitoring for signs of decompensation. Screening for HCC with ultrasound every 6 months should be performed indefinitely, even after curative treatment.

PHARMACOLOGICAL TREATMENT OF CHRONIC HCV

The near-term goal of treatment of HCV infection is *sustained virological response* (SVR), defined as the continued absence of detectable HCV RNA for 12 or more weeks after cessation of therapy. It is recognized that all patients with active HCV infection will benefit from, and should be considered for, treatment, with the exception of cases involving patients with life expectancies less than 12 months in which treatment of HCV would not influence mortality

(American Association for the Study of Liver Diseases–Infectious Diseases Society of America 2016b; A. Kim 2016).

According to current recommendations, treatment should not be withheld from patients with OUD, and treatment of active users of drugs and alcohol should be considered on a case-by-case basis (American Association for the Study of Liver Diseases–Infectious Diseases Society of America 2016b; National Institutes of Health 2002). There is mounting evidence supporting good adherence to treatment and low re-infection rates among patients who inject drugs who are treated for chronic HCV (American Association for the Study of Liver Diseases–Infectious Diseases Society of America 2016b; Hellard et al. 2009; A. Kim 2016). In fact, evidence supporting the exclusion of this population from chronic HCV treatment is lacking. Given that IDU is the most important risk factor for HCV infection in the United States, treatment of HCV in this population coupled with opioid agonist therapy and harm reduction strategies (e.g., needle exchange programs) may considerably impact overall incidence and prevalence of HCV disease. Models of HCV treatment programs on site in opioid agonist treatment settings have been shown to be feasible and effective (Bruggmann and Litwin 2013; Butner et al. 2017; Litwin et al. 2009).

The traditional management of HCV infection with pegylated interferon alfa and ribavirin has fallen out of favor in light of the introduction in 2011 of direct-acting antiviral (DAA) agents, which have excellent efficacy and safety profiles. This is an evolving area, and as seen in Table 11–2, there are currently three classes of DAAs: protease inhibitors, NS5A inhibitors, and NS5B polymerase inhibitors. Combination therapy is recommended because of the decreased efficacy of monotherapy, and suggested regimens depend on HCV genotype, prior treatment failure, and presence of cirrhosis. Efficacy of therapy is influenced by viral factors (genotype, resistant variants) and host factors (favorable features include persons who are treatment naïve and without cirrhosis). In hosts with favorable features and genotype 1, SVR is expected in >95% of cases. For genotype 2, SVR is as high as 99%, and for genotype 3, SVR can be as high as 95%. Less data are available for other genotypes (A. Kim 2016). At minimum, treatment monitoring should be performed at baseline and week 4 and include the following:

- CBC
- Creatinine
- Liver panel
- Quantitative HCV RNA

TABLE 11–2.   Direct-acting antiviral therapies for initial treatment of hepatitis C infection[a]

Therapy	Dose, mg	Brand name	Genotype	Comments
Protease inhibitors				
Grazoprevir	100	Zepatier (in combo)	1, 4, 6	Avoid in decompensated cirrhosis
Paritaprevir	150	Technivie, Viekira (in combo)	vc1, 4	Avoid in decompensated cirrhosis; use caution in HIV co-infection
Simeprevir	150	Olysio	1, 4	Avoid in decompensated cirrhosis; associated phototoxicity
NS5A inhibitors				
Daclatasvir	60	Daklinza	All	Drug interactions
Elbasvir	50	Zepatier (combo)	1, 4, 6	RAV
Ledipasvir	90	Harvoni (combo)	1, 4, 5, 6	Absorption decreased with acid suppression
Ombitasvir	25	Technivie, Viekira XR (combo)	1, 4	
Velpatasvir	100	Epclusa (combo)	All	
NS5B polymerase inhibitors				
Dasabuvir	250	Viekira XR (combo)	1	
Sofosbuvir	400	Solvaldi	All	

TABLE 11–2.   Direct-acting antiviral therapies for initial treatment of hepatitis C infection[a] (*continued*)

Therapy	Dose, mg	Brand name	Genotype	Comments
Combination therapies[b]				
Daclatasvir+Sofosbuvir	—	Daklinza+Solvaldi	1a, 1b, 3[c]	Genotype 3 cirrhosis—consider NS5A RAV testing; add ribavirin; 24-week therapy
Elbasvir–grazoprevir	—	Zepatier	1a,[c] 1b,[c] 4[c]	Consider NS5A RAV testing
Ledipasvir–sofosbuvir	—	Harvoni	**1a, 1b**,[c] 4, [c] 5, [c] 6[c]	
Ombitasvir–paritaprevir–ritonavir	—	Technivie	4[c]	Add ribavirin; requires close hepatic monitoring
Simeprevir+sofosbuvir	—	Olysio+Solvaldi	1a, 1b	
Sofosbuvir–velpatasvir	—	Epclusa	1a,[c] 1b, **2**, **3**,[c] **4**,[c] **5**,[c] **6**[c]	Genotype 3 cirrhosis—consider NS5A RAV testing; add ribavirin

Note.   combo=part of fixed combination product; RAV=resistance-associated variants.
[a]Does not include second-line regimens or regimens for treating patients with decompensated cirrhosis or prior treatment failure. Review medication interactions prior to initiating therapy.
[b]All treatment regimens are 12 weeks unless noted in comments. Recommended first-line therapies in bold.
[c]Indicates that recommendation applies for patients with and without compensated cirrhosis (Child-Turcotte-Pugh Class A).

Quantitative HCV RNA testing should be repeated at 12 weeks following completion of therapy if levels at week 4 are undetectable. For detectable levels at week 4, testing should be repeated at week 6. If HCV RNA levels increase more than tenfold, therapy should be stopped (American Association for the Study of Liver Diseases–Infectious Diseases Society of America 2016a). Some specific DAA combinations require further monitoring and can be reviewed on a case-by-case basis.

DAAS AND BUPRENORPHINE

Although data remain limited, coadministration of DAAs with buprenorphine, combination buprenorphine-naloxone, or methadone appears safe, and no dose adjustments are recommended. Daclatasvir may increase buprenorphine levels, without any major clinical impact (Meemken et al. 2015; Ogbuagu et al. 2016).

HIV/AIDS

EPIDEMIOLOGY

HIV is a blood-borne retroviral infection. Transmission occurs through sexual contact, parenteral exposure, perinatal exposure, and breastfeeding. It is estimated that there are roughly 1.2 million individuals living with HIV/AIDS in the United States, and 12.5% are unaware of their infection. AIDS is defined as a CD4 count below 200 cells/mm^3 or the presence of an opportunistic infection known to be associated with HIV (Centers for Disease Control and Prevention 2006). By recent estimates, 8% of the nearly 40,000 new infections each year occur through IDU (Broz et al. 2014). In addition to direct transmission through IDU, patients with OUD are at risk for HIV transmission through high-risk sexual contact (Sullivan et al. 2008).

LABORATORY DIAGNOSIS

HIV screening is recommended for everyone ages 13–65 unless the individual explicitly opts out (Branson et al. 2006). Unfortunately, many office-based providers of buprenorphine do not routinely test according to these guidelines (Edelman et al. 2012). Testing for established or acute infection begins with a fourth-generation HIV-1/2 antigen/antibody combination immunoassay that detects HIV-1 and HIV-2 antibodies as well as HIV-1 p24 antigen. The sensitivity of this test is 99%–100%. If positive, the specimen is tested with an HIV-1/HIV-2 antibody differentiation immunoassay. A positive test result indicates infection. Negative specimens at this step are further tested with an HIV-1 nucleic acid test (NAT). A positive test at this stage indicates acute

HIV-1 infection. A negative NAT indicates a false positive result from the original immunoassay (Centers for Disease Control and Prevention 2014a).

Once a patient is diagnosed with HIV, the patient should undergo further testing, including CD4 count, HIV viral load, and HIV resistance testing (Aberg et al. 2014). Patients should also be referred for treatment with an HIV specialist.

Natural History

The course of HIV disease can be followed clinically by monitoring the CD4 lymphocyte count and viral load. Low CD4 count is the strongest predictor of the development of opportunistic infections. Most opportunistic infections occur at a CD4 count below 50 cells/mm^3. High viral load remains an independent predictor of disease progression, and the goal of treatment is to suppress the viral load to undetectable levels. In the setting of untreated disease, patients become increasingly immunocompromised and ultimately succumb to overwhelming infection.

Treatment

Treatment is currently recommended for all HIV-infected individuals regardless of CD4 count (Panel on Antiretroviral Guidelines for Adults and Adolescents 2016). Prior to initiation of treatment, the following testing should be performed:

- CBC
- Chemistries
- Liver panel
- Urinalysis
- Fasting blood glucose and lipids
- Screening for HAV, HBV, HCV, sexually transmitted diseases, and opportunistic infections

The mainstay of treatment is combination antiretroviral therapy. For treatment-naïve individuals, an antiretroviral regimen consists of two nucleoside reverse transcriptase inhibitors (NRTIs) in combination with a third active antiretroviral drug from one of four drug classes: an integrase strand transfer inhibitor (INSTI), a non-nucleoside reverse transcriptase inhibitor (NNRTI), a fusion inhibitor, or a protease inhibitor (PI) with a pharmacokinetic booster (cobicistat or ritonavir). The treatment of HIV is an ever-changing landscape of possible combinations, and Table 11–3 shows the medications currently used.

HIV and Opioid Agonist Treatment

The only notable interactions between buprenorphine and antiretroviral drugs is with the protease inhibitors atazanavir and ritonavir. Both may increase buprenorphine concentrations and cause sedation; however, the clinical impact may be insignificant (Ogbuagu et al. 2016; Vergara-Rodriguez et al. 2011). None-

TABLE 11–3.   Medications and trade names used for treatment of HIV

Medication	Trade names
Non-nucleoside reverse transcriptase inhibitors	
Delavirdine (DLV)	Rescriptor
Efavirenz (EFV)[a]	Sustiva
Etravirine (ETR)	Intelence
Nevirapine (NVP)[a]	Viramune
Rilpivirine (RPV)[a]	Edurant
Nucleoside reverse transcriptase inhibitors	
Abacavir (ABC)	Ziagen
Abacavir + lamivudine + zidovudine (ABC/ZDV/3TC)	Trizivir
Abacavir + lamivudine (ABC/3TC)	Epzicom
Didanosine (ddl)	Videx, Videx EC
Emtricitabine (FTC)	Emtriva, Coviracil
Emtricitabine + tenofovir alafenamide (FTC/TAF)	Descovy
Emtricitabine + tenofovir disoproxil fumarate (FTC/TDF)	Truvada
Lamivudine (3TC)	Epivir
Lamivudine + zidovudine (3TC/ZDV)	Combivir
Stavudine (d4T)	Zerit
Tenofovir disoproxil fumarate (TDF)	Viread
Tenofovir alafenamide (TAF)	
Zidovudine[a] (ZDV)	Retrovir
Protease inhibitors	
Atazanavir (ATV)[b]	Reyataz
Atazanavir + cobicistat (ATV/c)	Evotaz
Darunavir (DRV)[a]	Prezista
Darunavir + cobicistat (DRV/c)	Prezcobix
Fosamprenavir (FPV)[a]	Lexiva
Indinavir (IDV)	Crixivan
Lopinavir + ritonavir (LPV/r)[a]	Kaletra
Nelfinavir (NFV)	Viracept
Ritonavir (RTV)[b]	Norvir
Saquinavir (SQV)[a]	Invirase
Tipranavir (TPV)[a]	Aptivus

TABLE 11–3.   **Medications and trade names used for treatment of HIV** *(continued)*

Medication	Trade names
Fusion inhibitor	
Enfuvirtide (T20)	Fuzeon
CCR5 antagonist	
Maraviroc (MVC)	Selzentry
Integrase inhibitors	
Dolutegravir (DTG)	Tivicay
Elvitegravir (EVG)	Vitekta
Raltegravir (RAL)	Isentress
Class combinations	
Abacavir+dolutegravir+lamivudine (ABC/DTG/3TC)	Triumeq
Efavirenz+emtricitabine+tenofovir DF (EFV/FTC/TDF)	Atripla
Elvitegravir+cobicistat+emtricitabine+tenofovir A (EVG/c/FTC/TAF)	Genvoya
Elvitegravir+cobicistat+emtricitabine+tenofovir DF (EVG/c/FTC/TDF)	Stribild
Emtricitabine+rilpivirine+tenofovir A (FTC/RPV/TAF)	Odefsey
Emtricitabine+rilpivirine+tenofovir DF (FTC/RPV/TDF)	Complera

[a]May cause clinically significant interaction with methadone, requiring dose adjustment or increased monitoring.
[b]May cause clinically significant interaction with buprenorphine, requiring dose adjustment or increased monitoring.

theless, clinicians should remain vigilant and consider starting patients at a lower buprenorphine dose. Potential drug interactions between HIV medications and buprenorphine and methadone are noted in the subscripts in Table 11–3.

It is established that methadone maintenance reduces risk of HIV transmission and improves HIV medication adherence and outcomes (Gowing et al. 2006; MacArthur et al. 2012; Sullivan et al. 2005). Recent work also has suggested that buprenorphine has a similar impact on HIV transmission, medication adherence, and outcomes (Altice et al. 2011; Edelman et al. 2014a; Sullivan and Fiellin 2005; Sullivan et al. 2006, 2008; Tetrault et al. 2012). Additionally, pre-exposure prophylaxis (PrEP) has been demonstrated to significantly reduce HIV transmission for persons who inject drugs (Choopanya et al. 2013). It is currently recommended that persons with substantial risk of acquiring HIV who inject drugs be offered PrEP with daily fixed dose combination oral tenofovir disoproxil fumarate 300 mg and emtricitabine 200 mg. The cost-effectiveness of

PrEP coupled with frequent HIV testing and treatment depends on medication adherence, individual risk, and the community HIV prevalence (Bernard et al. 2016). Patients considered to be at high risk of acquiring HIV in whom PrEP should be considered include those with any illicit IDU in the past 6 months and at least one of the following:

- Any sharing of injection or drug preparation equipment in the past 6 months
- Involvement with a methadone or buprenorphine treatment program in the past 6 months
- Any high-risk sexual activity

For patients who initiate PrEP, renal function should be monitored at least every 6 months, and HIV screening should be done at least every 3 months (Centers for Disease Control and Prevention 2014b).

Tuberculosis

Current guidelines recommend screening for latent tuberculosis infection in asymptomatic adults at increased risk of infection (Bibbins-Domingo et al. 2016; Centers for Disease Control and Prevention 2013). Those groups include the following:

- Persons who were born or resided in countries with increased tuberculosis (TB) prevalence
- Persons who live in or have lived in high-risk congregate settings such as homeless shelters or correctional facilities
- Persons who inject drugs
- Individuals with HIV

Screening for exposure to TB can be performed with either the tuberculin skin test (TST) or interferon gamma release assays (IGRAs), both of which are moderately sensitive and highly specific in countries with low prevalence of infection (Bibbins-Domingo et al. 2016). IGRAs are preferred in patients who have received the TB vaccine and in those who will have difficulty making the 48- to 72-hour follow-up appointment for interpretation of the TST. A positive TST is defined as follows:

- Reaction of ≥5 mm of induration in patients with HIV who are otherwise immunosuppressed and those with recent close TB contact
- Reaction of ≥10 mm of induration in patients who inject drugs, have exposure to high-risk congregate settings, and/or are recent immigrants from a high-prevalence country
- A reaction of ≥15 mm of induration in persons with no known risk factors for TB

Positive testing by either TST or IGRAs indicates the person was infected with *Mycobacterium tuberculosis* but does not distinguish active TB disease from LTBI. Further testing for active pulmonary (including chest X-ray) or extrapulmonary infection is required, and if findings from this testing are negative, treatment for LTBI should be considered. If active TB disease is suspected, specialty referral to a pulmonologist and possible hospitalization needs to be made as soon as possible for management.

The goal of treatment of LTBI is to prevent development or reactivation of active infection. Treatment regimens for LTBI include the following:

- Isoniazid (INH) daily or twice weekly for nine months (preferred regimen)
- INH daily or twice weekly for 6 months (alternative, based on treatment adherence)
- INH plus rifapentine once weekly for 3 months
- Rifampin daily for 4 months

Baseline AST, ALT, and bilirubin testing are recommended for individuals at risk for liver disease. Periodic testing during treatment is considered on a case-to-case basis, though it should be done for individuals with abnormal baseline testing or if symptoms suggestive of hepatitis develop. If a patient's liver function test values increase to three times the upper limit of normal, therapy should be withheld (Centers for Disease Control and Prevention 2013). Adherence to treatment is a common concern, and directly observed therapy can be instituted as a means to increase treatment adherence.

LTBI TREATMENT AND OPIOID AGONIST THERAPY

Methadone programs have been effective for linking opioid agonist treatment to INH chemoprophylaxis and increasing medication adherence (Batki et al. 2002; O'Connor et al. 1999). Similar data are not available for buprenorphine-maintained patients. Rifampin has been reported to significantly reduce serum buprenorphine levels and precipitate withdrawal in patients taking maintenance buprenorphine (McCance-Katz et al. 2011). All patients should be counseled to abstain from alcohol use during treatment for LTBI with INH.

Complication of Injection Drug Use

IDU is a risk factor for acute infections, particularly in patients with little IDU experience or those who inject more frequently (Brown and Ebright 2002; Gordon and Lowy 2005; Schoener et al. 2002). The severity of infection is influenced by underlying co-occurring chronic infections such as HIV and HCV and timing of presentation because patients with OUD may present late in the course of illness (Lloyd-Smith et al. 2010; Palepu et al. 2001). The most common infections are skin and soft tissue infections and their complications, including osteomyelitis, bacteremia and sepsis, endocarditis, septic arthritis, ulcers, thrombophlebitis, discitis, and myositis. Responsible pathogens are commonly skin and mouth flora, including *Staphylococcus aureus*, streptococcal species, gram-negative bacteria, and anaerobic bacteria. Methicillin-resistant *S. aureus* and polymicrobial infections, including mixed aerobic and anaerobic infections, are prevalent in injection drug users (Brown and Ebright 2002; Gordon and Lowy 2005).

Treatment principles include obtaining culture data when possible, incision and drainage of abscesses, appropriate antibiotic selection, and triage to the hospital based on assessment of illness severity. Comprehensive management also should include education around injection practices as a harm reduction strategy. Factors increasing the risk of infectious complications of IDU can be encountered at each step of the injection process. The drug itself may increase risk, with more skin and soft tissue infections seen with injecting "speedballs" (heroin plus cocaine) and black tar heroin. Nonsterile injection technique, including touching or licking the needle, failure to clean the skin prior to injecting, and reusing or sharing needles, predisposes the user to acute and chronic infection. Finally, injection practices such as "booting" (repeatedly flushing and pulling back during injection), "groin hits" (injecting into inguinal vessels), "skin popping" (subcutaneous injection), "pocket shots" (injecting in the neck veins), and intramuscular injection can all increase the risk of infection (Gordon and Lowy 2005; Roszler et al. 1989; Schoener et al. 2002; Tamir et al. 2015). Utilization of needle exchange programs and supervised injection facilities should be encouraged when available. Safe injection practices can be taught and include the following:

- Using boiled or sterile water
- Cleaning the skin with alcohol
- Cleaning drug paraphernalia with bleach
- Avoiding needle sharing and reusing needles
- Rotating injection sites to minimize vein sclerosis
- Avoiding the groin, neck, and arteries as injection sites
- Limiting injections in the hands and feet

Buprenorphine Treatment in Geriatric Patients

To date, there are few published data on the use of buprenorphine for the treatment of OUD in patients older than 65 years. In fact, there is little known about the use of illicit substances in this population (Edelman et al. 2014b). If buprenorphine treatment is considered, gradual dose escalation and monitoring for medication interactions and fall risk should be undertaken (Center for Substance Abuse Treatment 2004).

Conclusion

Patients with OUD frequently have comorbid medical conditions, especially infectious diseases. Screening for and treatment or referral to treatment of these comorbid conditions is paramount to provision of the best possible care for this patient population. Knowledge of these potential comorbid conditions is important for any clinician treating patients with opioid agonist therapy. Office-based buprenorphine allows for linkage of treatment of substance use with comprehensive medical care.

Clinical Pearls

- Patients admitted to buprenorphine treatment should have a comprehensive history and access to a physical examination as well as evaluation of baseline liver function tests.

- Clinicians treating patients with opioid agonist treatment should consider screening patients for HIV, hepatitis B, hepatitis C, tuberculosis, and sexually transmitted diseases, including HIV, syphilis, gonorrhea, and chlamydia, as well as offering immunizations for hepatitis A, hepatitis B, influenza, pneumococcal disease, and tetanus, if appropriate.

- Treatment modalities for hepatitis B, hepatitis C, and HIV are complex and continue to emerge. Physicians caring for patients with these comorbid conditions should have an understanding of treatment options and their potential interactions with buprenorphine.

- Hepatitis B, hepatitis C, HIV, and latent tuberculosis infections and their management are not contraindications to office-based treatment with buprenorphine.

- OUD in the geriatric population may require an individualized treatment approach, and further guidance identifying proper strategies for the care of this special population will likely emerge over time.

CASE 11

Rosie is a 56-year-old woman with chronic homeless who has been receiving buprenorphine therapy in your clinic for the past 2 years. She had a "hard life on the streets" and was diagnosed with HCV infection 10 years ago. She has not considered doing anything about it because she has not felt sick and did not think anyone would treat her. Her AST and ALT levels have been running at 1.5 times the high-normal values. She says that she has one drink a day most days of the week and smokes one pack of cigarettes a day. She calls and says, "My eyes look kind of yellow, and I don't feel so great...." You obtain laboratory test results that reveal AST and ALT levels five times the upper limit of normal and a total bilirubin level of 3 mg/dL (normal range, 0.3–1.9 mg/dL).

1. What are the possible causes of Rosie's jaundice? Is this likely to be related to her buprenorphine treatment?

2. Should you stop the buprenorphine treatment?

3. Would she be an appropriate candidate for treatment of her HCV?

4. What is your mechanism for referral to a gastroenterologist?

References

Aberg JA, Gallant JE, Ghanem KG, et al: Primary care guidelines for the management of persons infected with HIV: 2013 update by the HIV medicine association of the Infectious Diseases Society of America. Clin Infect Dis 58(1):e1–e34, 2014 24235263

Alavian SM, Mirahmadizadeh A, Javanbakht M, et al: Effectiveness of methadone maintenance treatment in prevention of hepatitis C virus transmission among injecting drug users. Hepat Mon 13(8):e12411, 2013 24069039

Alford DP, Compton P, Samet JH: Acute pain management for patients receiving maintenance methadone or buprenorphine therapy. Ann Intern Med 144(2):127–134, 2006 16418412

Altice FL, Bruce RD, Lucas GM, et al: HIV treatment outcomes among HIV-infected, opioid-dependent patients receiving buprenorphine/naloxone treatment within HIV clinical care settings: results from a multisite study. J Acquir Immune Defic Syndr 56 (suppl 1):S22–S32, 2011 21317590

American Association for the Study of Liver Diseases–Infectious Diseases Society of America: Monitoring patients who are starting hepatitis C treatment, are on treatment, or who have completed therapy. Alexandria, VA, American Association for the Study of Liver Diseases, 2016a. Available at: http://www.hcvguidelines.org/full-report/monitoring-patients-who-are-starting-hepatitis-c-treatment-are-treatment-or-have. Accessed January 7, 2017.

American Association for the Study of Liver Diseases–Infectious Diseases Society of America: Recommendations for testing, managing, and treating hepatitis C. Alexandria, VA, American Association for the Study of Liver Diseases, 2016b. Available at: http://www.hcvguidelines.org. Accessed January 7, 2017.

Batki SL, Gruber VA, Bradley JM, et al: A controlled trial of methadone treatment combined with directly observed isoniazid for tuberculosis prevention in injection drug users. Drug Alcohol Depend 66(3):283–293, 2002 12062463

Bernard CL, Brandeau ML, Humphreys K, et al: Cost-effectiveness of HIV preexposure prophylaxis for people who inject drugs in the United States. Ann Intern Med 2016 27110953 [Epub ahead of print]

Bibbins-Domingo K, Grossman DC, Curry SJ, et al: Screening for latent tuberculosis infection in adults: US preventive services task force recommendation statement. JAMA 316(9):962–969, 2016 27599331

Branson BM, Handsfield HH, Lampe MA, et al: Revised recommendations for HIV testing of adults, adolescents, and pregnant women in health-care settings. MMWR Recomm Rep 55(RR-14):1–17; quiz CE11–CE14, 2006 16988643

Brown PD, Ebright JR: Skin and soft tissue infections in injection drug users. Curr Infect Dis Rep 4(5):415–419 2002 12228028

Broz D, Wejnert C, Pham HT, et al: HIV infection and risk, prevention, and testing behaviors among injecting drug users—National HIV Behavioral Surveillance System 20 U.S. cities 2009. MMWR Surveill Summ 63(6):1–51 2014 24990587

Bruggmann P, Litwin AH: Models of care for the management of hepatitis C virus among people who inject drugs: one size does not fit all. Clin Infect Dis 57 (suppl 2):S56–S61, 2013 23884067

Bruix J, Sherman M; American Association for the Study of Liver Diseases: Management of hepatocellular carcinoma: an update. Hepatology 53(3):1020–1022, 2011 21374666

Butner JL, Gupta N, Fabian C, et al: Onsite treatment of HCV infection with direct acting antivirals within an opioid treatment program. J Subst Abuse Treat 75:49–53 2017 28237054

Cantor AG, Pappas M, Daeges M, et al: Screening for syphilis: updated evidence report and systematic review for the US Preventive Services Task Force. JAMA 315(21):2328–2337, 2016 27272584

Center for Substance Abuse Treatment: Clinical Guidelines for the Use of Buprenorphine in the Treatment of Opioid Addiction. Treatment Improvement Protocol (TIP) Series 40. DHHS Publ No (SMA) 04-3939. Rockville, MD, Substance Abuse and Mental Health Services Administration, 2004

Centers for Disease Control and Prevention: HIV/AIDS Surveillance Report: Cases of HIV Infection and AIDS in the United States and Dependent Areas. Atlanta, GA, Centers for Disease Control and Prevention, 2006. Available at: http://www.cdc.gov/hiv/topics/surveillance/basic.htm#hivest. Accessed January 8, 2009.

Centers for Disease Control and Prevention: Integrated prevention services for HIV infection, viral hepatitis, sexually transmitted diseases, and tuberculosis for persons who use drugs illicitly: summary guidance from CDC and the U.S. Department of Health and Human Services. MMWR Recomm Rep 61(RR-5):1–40, 2012 23135062

Centers for Disease Control and Prevention: Latent Tuberculosis Infection: A Guide for Primary Health Care Providers. Atlanta, GA, Centers for Disease Control and Prevention, 2013. Available at: https://www.cdc.gov/tb/publications/ltbi/targetedtesting.htm. Accessed January 5, 2017.

Centers for Disease Control and Prevention: Laboratory Testing for the Diagnosis of HIV Infection: Updated Recommendations. Atlanta, GA, Centers for Disease Control and Prevention, 2014a. Available at: https://stacks.cdc.gov/view/cdc/23447. Accessed January 5, 2016.

Centers for Disease Control and Prevention: Preexposure Prophylaxis for the Prevention of HIV Infection in the United States—2014 Clinical Practice Guideline. Atlanta, GA, Centers for Disease Control and Prevention, 2014b. Available at: https://www.cdc.gov/hiv/pdf/prepguidelines2014.pdf. Accessed January 8, 2017.

Centers for Disease Control and Prevention: Hepatitis C FAQs for Health Professionals. Atlanta, GA, Centers for Disease Control and Prevention, 2016a. Available at: https://www.cdc.gov/hepatitis/hcv/hcvfaq.htm. Accessed January 5, 2017.

Centers for Disease Control and Prevention: Viral Hepatitis—Hepatitis B Information. Atlanta, GA, Centers for Disease Control and Prevention, 2016b. Available at: https://www.cdc.gov/hepatitis/hbv/hbvfaq.htm#overview. Accessed January 4, 2017.

Choopanya K, Martin M, Suntharasamai P, et al: Antiretroviral prophylaxis for HIV infection in injecting drug users in Bangkok, Thailand (the Bangkok Tenofovir Study): a randomised, double-blind, placebo-controlled phase 3 trial. Lancet 381(9883):2083–2090, 2013 23769234

Donroe JH, Holt SR, Tetrault JM: Caring for patients with opioid use disorder in the hospital. CMAJ 188(17–18):1232–1239, 2016 27647616

Edelman EJ, Dinh AT, Moore BA, et al: Human immunodeficiency virus testing practices among buprenorphine-prescribing physicians. J Addict Med 6(2):159–165, 2012 22367499

Edelman EJ, Chantarat T, Caffrey S, et al: The impact of buprenorphine/naloxone treatment on HIV risk behaviors among HIV-infected, opioid-dependent patients. Drug Alcohol Depend 139:79–85, 2014a 24726429

Edelman EJ, Tetrault JM, Fiellin DA: Substance use in older HIV-infected patients. Curr Opin HIV AIDS 9(4):317–324, 2014b 24824888

Fattovich G, Giustina G, Degos F, et al: Morbidity and mortality in compensated cirrhosis type C: a retrospective follow-up study of 384 patients (see comment). Gastroenterology 112(2):463–472, 1997 9024300

Garfein RS, Vlahov D, Galai N, et al: Viral infections in short-term injection drug users: the prevalence of the hepatitis C, hepatitis B, human immunodeficiency, and human T-lymphotropic viruses. Am J Public Health 86(5):655–661, 1996 8629715

Gordon RJ, Lowy FD: Bacterial infections in drug users. N Engl J Med 353(18):1945–1954, 2005 16267325

Gowing LR, Farrell M, Bornemann R, et al: Brief report: Methadone treatment of injecting opioid users for prevention of HIV infection. J Gen Intern Med 21(2):193–195, 2006 16336624

Hellard M, Sacks-Davis R, Gold J: Hepatitis C treatment for injection drug users: a review of the available evidence. Clin Infect Dis 49(4):561–573, 2009 19589081

Hwang L-Y, Grimes CZ, Tran TQ, et al: Accelerated hepatitis B vaccination schedule among drug users: a randomized controlled trial. J Infect Dis 202(10):1500–1509, 2010 20936979

Kim A: Hepatitis C virus. Ann Intern Med 165(5):ITC33–ITC48, 2016 27595226

Kim DK, Bridges CB, Harriman KH: Advisory Committee on Immunization Practices recommended immunization schedule for adults aged 19 years or older: United States 2016. Ann Intern Med 164(3):184–194, 2016 26829913

Kohli A, Shaffer A, Sherman A, et al: Treatment of hepatitis C: a systematic review. JAMA 312(6):631–640, 2014 25117132

Kraus ML, Alford DP, Kotz MM, et al: Statement of the American Society of Addiction Medicine Consensus Panel on the use of buprenorphine in office-based treatment of opioid addiction. J Addict Med 5(4):254–263, 2011 22042215

LeFevre ML; U.S. Preventive Services Task Force: Screening for chlamydia and gonorrhea: U.S. Preventive Services Task Force recommendation statement. Ann Intern
Med 161(12):902–910, 2014a 25243785

LeFevre ML; U.S. Preventive Services Task Force: Screening for hepatitis B virus infection in nonpregnant adolescents and adults: U.S. Preventive Services Task Force
recommendation statement. Ann Intern Med 161(1):58–66, 2014b 24863637

Litwin AH, Harris KA Jr, Nahvi S, et al: Successful treatment of chronic hepatitis C
with pegylated interferon in combination with ribavirin in a methadone maintenance treatment program. J Subst Abuse Treat 37(1):32–40, 2009 DOI: 10.1016/
j.jsat.2008.09.009 19038524

Lloyd-Smith E, Wood E, Zhang R, et al: Determinants of hospitalization for a cutane-
ous injection-related infection among injection drug users: a cohort study. BMC
Public Health 10:327, 2010 20534148

MacArthur GJ, Minozzi S, Martin N, et al: Opiate substitution treatment and HIV
transmission in people who inject drugs: systematic review and meta-analysis. BMJ
345:e5945, 2012 23038795

McCance-Katz EF, Moody DE, Prathikanti S, et al: Rifampin, but not rifabutin, may
produce opiate withdrawal in buprenorphine-maintained patients. Drug Alcohol
Depend 118(2–3):326–334, 2011 21596492

Meemken L, Hanhoff N, Tseng A, et al: Drug-drug interactions with antiviral agents
in people who inject drugs requiring substitution therapy. Ann Pharmacother
49(7):796–807, 2015 25902733

Moyer VA; U.S. Preventive Services Task Force: Screening for hepatitis C virus infection in adults: U.S. Preventive Services Task Force recommendation statement.
Ann Intern Med 159(5):349–357, 2013 23798026

National Institutes of Health: Management of Hepatitis C: Consensus Conference
Statement June 10–12, 2002. Bethesda, MD, National Institutes of Health, 2002

O'Connor PG, Shi JM, Henry S, et al: Tuberculosis chemoprophylaxis using a liquid
isoniazid-methadone admixture for drug users in methadone maintenance. Addiction 94(7):1071–1075, 1999 10707445

Ogbuagu O, Friedland G, Bruce RD: Drug interactions between buprenorphine, methadone and hepatitis C therapeutics. Expert Opin Drug Metab Toxicol 12(7):721–
731, 2016 27140427

Palepu A, Tyndall MW, Leon H, et al: Hospital utilization and costs in a cohort of injection drug users. CMAJ 165(4):415–420 2001 11531049

Panel on Antiretroviral Guidelines for Adults and Adolescents: Guidelines for the Use of
Antiretroviral Agents in HIV-1-Infected Adults and Adolescents. Washington,
D.C., U.S. Department of Health and Human Services, 2016. Available at: https://
aidsinfo.nih.gov/contentfiles/lvguidelines/adultandadolescentgl.pdf. Accessed
January 5, 2017.

Perlman DC, Jordan AE, Uuskula A, et al: An international perspective on using opioid
substitution treatment to improve hepatitis C prevention and care for people who
inject drugs: Structural barriers and public health potential. Int J Drug Policy
26(11):1056–1063, 2015 26050614

Roszler MH, McCarroll KA, Donovan KR, et al: The groin hit: complications of intravenous drug abuse. Radiographics 9(3):487–508, 1989 2727357

Saxon AJ, Bisaga A: Monitoring of Liver Function Tests and Hepatitis in Patients Receiving Buprenorphine (With or Without Naloxone). Providence, RI, Providers' Clinical Support System, 2014. Available at http://pcssmat.org/wp-content/uploads/2014/03/PCSS-MATGuidanceMonitoringLiverFunctionTests-and-HepatitisIn BupPatients.Saxon_.pdf. Accessed January 3, 2017.

Saxon AJ, Ling W, Hillhouse M, et al: Buprenorphine/naloxone and methadone effects on laboratory indices of liver health: a randomized trial. Drug Alcohol Depend 128(1–2):71–76, 2013 22921476

Schoener EP, Hopper JA, Pierre JD: Injection drug use in North America. Infect Dis Clin North Am 16(3):535–551, vii, 2002 12371114

Shiffman ML: Management of acute hepatitis B. Clin Liver Dis 14(1):75–91, viii–ix, 2010 20123442

Sullivan LE, Fiellin DA: Buprenorphine: its role in preventing HIV transmission and improving the care of HIV-infected patients with opioid dependence. Clin Infect Dis 41(6):891–896, 2005 16107991

Sullivan LE, Metzger DS, Fudala PJ, et al: Decreasing international HIV transmission: the role of expanding access to opioid agonist therapies for injection drug users. Addiction 100(2):150–158, 2005 15679744

Sullivan LE, Barry D, Moore BA, et al: A trial of integrated buprenorphine/naloxone and HIV clinical care. Clin Infect Dis 43(suppl 4):S184–S190, 2006 17109305

Sullivan LE, Moore BA, Chawarski MC, et al: Buprenorphine/naloxone treatment in primary care is associated with decreased human immunodeficiency virus risk behaviors. J Subst Abuse Treat 35(1):87–92, 2008 17933486

Tamir SO, Marom T, Len A, et al: Deep neck infections in cervical injection drug users. Laryngoscope 125(6):1336–1339, 2015 25387948

Terrault NA, Bzowej NH, Chang KM, et al: AASLD guidelines for treatment of chronic hepatitis B. Hepatology 63(1):261–283, 2016 26566064

Tetrault JM, Moore BA, Barry DT, et al: Brief versus extended counseling along with buprenorphine/naloxone for HIV-infected opioid dependent patients. J Subst Abuse Treat 43(4):433–439, 2012 22938914

Tetrault JM, Tate JP, Edelman EJ, et al: Hepatic safety of buprenorphine in HIV-infected and uninfected patients with opioid use disorder: the role of HCV-infection. J Subst Abuse Treat 68:62–67, 2016 27431048

Trépo C, Chan HL, Lok A: Hepatitis B virus infection. Lancet 384(9959):2053–2063, 2014 24954675

Tsui JI, Evans JL, Lum PJ, et al: Association of opioid agonist therapy with lower incidence of hepatitis C virus infection in young adult injection drug users. JAMA Intern Med 174(12):1974–1981, 2014 25347412

Vergara-Rodriguez P, Tozzi MJ, Botsko M, et al: Hepatic safety and lack of antiretroviral interactions with buprenorphine/naloxone in HIV-infected opioid-dependent patients. J Acquir Immune Defic Syndr 56 (suppl 1):S62–S67, 2011 21317596

Weinbaum CM, Williams I, Mast EE, et a: Recommendations for identification and public health management of persons with chronic hepatitis B virus infection. MMWR Recomm Rep 57(RR-8):1–20, 2008 18802412

Wiegand J, Wedemeyer H, Franke A, et al: Treatment of severe, nonfulminant acute hepatitis B with lamivudine vs placebo: a prospective randomized double-blinded multicentre trial. J Viral Hepat 21(10):744–750, 2014 24329913

Younossi ZM; Cleveland Clinic of Medicine: Viral hepatitis guide for practicing physicians. Cleve Clin J Med 67 (suppl 1):SI6–SI45, 2000 11068358

12

Acute and Chronic Pain

Daniel P. Alford, M.D., M.P.H., FACP, DFASAM

ADEQUATE treatment of pain is recognized as an essential dimension of quality medical care. Managing pain is complex when patients also have a history of a substance use disorder (SUD). Treatment of pain can be particularly challenging in a patient with an opioid use disorder (OUD) who is receiving opioid agonist therapy (OAT) (i.e., methadone or buprenorphine) (Alford et al. 2006). Although non-opioid analgesics (e.g., nonsteroidal anti-inflammatory drugs [NSAIDs]) are recommended as first-line therapy for treating most pain, severe pain may require the use of opioid analgesics. Some of the most often cited reasons for clinicians not prescribing opioid analgesics are fear of causing iatrogenic drug addiction, concerns about prescription drug diversion (e.g., patients selling their prescription), and concerns about regulatory (e.g., Drug Enforcement Administration [DEA]) scrutiny (Upshur et al. 2006).

A common concern by clinicians is that the use of opioid analgesics in patients receiving OAT may result in relapse to active drug use. However, there is no evidence that exposure to opioid analgesics in the presence of pain increases relapse in patients maintained on OAT. A small retrospective study of methadone-maintained postsurgical patients who received opioid analgesics found no difference in relapse indicators when compared with matched methadone-maintained patients (Kantor et al. 1980). Similarly, no evidence of relapse was noted in six methadone-maintained patients treated with opioid analgesics for cancer pain (Manfredi et al. 2001). In fact, relapse prevention theories would suggest that the stress associated with unrelieved pain is more likely to be a trigger for relapse than adequate analgesia. This is supported by studies in which patients maintained on OAT stated that unrelieved pain played a substantial role in their initiating and continuing illicit opioid use (Karasz et al. 2004; Potter et al. 2010).

There is also concern that opioid analgesics might cause severe respiratory or central nervous system (CNS) depression in patients maintained on OAT. Tolerance to the respiratory and CNS depressant effects of opioids occurs rapidly and reliably (Gutstein and Akil 2006). Patients with cancer with worsening pain who require opioid analgesic dose escalations typically do not exhibit respiratory and CNS depressant effects with the administration of additional opioids (Manfredi et al. 2001). It has been suggested that acute pain serves as a natural antagonist to opioid-associated respiratory and CNS depression (Eriator 1998). Therefore, the concern about severe drug toxicity with opioid analgesics in patients maintained with OAT is not supported by clinical or empirical experience.

Not uncommonly, patients with a history of an OUD are perceived by health care providers to be demanding when hospitalized with acute pain. This scenario develops in part because of the patients' distrust of the medical community, concern about being stigmatized, and fears that their pain will be undertreated or that their OAT may be altered or discontinued (Merrill et al. 2002; St Marie 2014). Patients' anxiety related to these concerns, which can be profound and well founded, can complicate provision of adequate pain relief. Clinicians' concern that they are being manipulated by "drug-seeking" patients is difficult to quantify and is emotion laden. Pain is always subjective, even when validated pain scales are used, making assessment of its presence and severity difficult. During an initial assessment it is difficult, if not impossible, to differentiate between inappropriate drug-seeking (e.g., SUD) and appropriate pain relief–seeking behaviors. A careful clinical assessment for objective evidence of acute pain (e.g., tachycardia) will help support the clinically appropriate use of opioid analgesics in patients with a history of an OUD. It is important to remember that patients maintained on OAT are typically receiving opioid maintenance doses that block the euphoric effects of coadministered opioids, theoretically decreasing the likelihood of opioid analgesic misuse.

Complicating the use of opioids in managing pain is the confusing and often misunderstood terminology used in pain management and addiction medicine. *Physical dependence* and *tolerance* are typical and predictable physiological adaptations of opioid exposure. These manifestations, in and of themselves, do not indicate maladaptive behaviors and do not meet the diagnostic criteria of an OUD in DSM-5 (American Psychiatric Association 2013) without, for example, loss of control or continued use despite harm.

Pain medicine specialists and addiction treatment providers commonly operate in separate spheres without much communication or collaboration. However, the well-described interplay between addiction and pain calls into question this artificial separation. This chapter covers the epidemiology and neurobiology of pain in patients with OUD, buprenorphine analgesic pharmacology, and acute and chronic pain management in patients receiving buprenorphine maintenance therapy.

Epidemiology and Neurobiology

Pain is common in patients with OUD, including those maintained on OAT (i.e., methadone or buprenorphine). One survey found that 52% of 228 treatment-seeking veterans with OUDs complained of moderate to very severe pain lasting more than 30 days (Trafton et al. 2004). Cross-sectional surveys among patients with OUDs treated with OAT report a prevalence of chronic pain ranging from 36% to 61% (Barry et al. 2013; Jamison et al. 2000; Rosenblum et al. 2003).

The clinical conditions of pain and addiction are not unrelated phenomena. Martin and Inglis (1965, p. 224), observed more than 50 years ago that patients with opioid addiction had "an abnormally low tolerance for painful stimuli." In a recent cross-sectional study, severe chronic pain and pain-related dysfunction were common in primary care patients with heroin use or prescription opioid misuse, with many reporting that their drug use was to self-medicate their pain (Alford et al. 2016). Opioids, whether administered with analgesic or addictive intent, activate opioid receptors, which provide both analgesia and reward. The presence of one condition appears to influence the expression of the other. Clinical examples of this include 1) how the presence of acute pain appears to decrease the euphoric response to an opioid and 2) how the presence of addictive disease appears to worsen the experience of pain (Zacny et al. 1996). Pain experience is worsened by subtle opioid withdrawal syndromes, sleep disturbances, and affective changes, all consequences of SUDs. Supporting a negative effect of addiction on pain tolerance, both stimulant and opioid abusers have been shown to be less pain tolerant than peers in remission (Compton 1994).

Buprenorphine Pharmacology

Buprenorphine is available worldwide as a parenteral, sublingual, buccal, and transdermal analgesic. Buprenorphine is a partial opioid agonist at the μ opioid receptor, resulting in supraspinal analgesia, euphoria, respiratory depression, and decreased gastrointestinal motility. Whereas full opioid agonists (e.g., morphine, oxycodone, methadone) have no analgesic or respiratory depressant ceiling effect, buprenorphine has a ceiling effect on respiratory depression but likely not on analgesia (Khanna and Pillarisetti 2015). This lack of analgesic ceiling effect is based on animal (Cowan 2007) and human experimental studies (Dahan et al. 2006).

Buprenorphine's high affinity at the μ opioid receptor makes buprenorphine difficult to displace. Initially, there was concern that this high affinity would effectively block the analgesic properties of coadministered opioid analgesics; however, both preclinical (Englberger et al. 2006; Kögel et al. 2005) and clinical studies (Hansen et al. 2016; Jones et al. 2009; Kornfeld and Manfredi 2010; Macintyre et al. 2013) do not support this fear. Full agonist opioids coadministered with buprenorphine result in additive analgesic effects (van Niel et al. 2016).

Pharmacological explanations account for why patients with OUD do not receive adequate analgesia from maintenance buprenorphine therapy prescribed for OUD treatment. Not only do the analgesic and OUD treatment profiles of buprenorphine differ, the neuroplastic changes associated with chronic opioid exposure (i.e., tolerance) may effectively diminish buprenorphine's analgesic effectiveness (White 2004). Buprenorphine's duration of action for analgesia (6–8 hours) is substantially shorter than its suppression of opioid withdrawal and craving and maintenance of opioid blockade (24–48 hours) (Johnson et al. 2005). Because buprenorphine is usually dosed every 24 hours for OUD, the period of even partial pain relief with this medication is small. Tolerance is another factor why these patients derive little analgesia from maintenance buprenorphine therapy. Analgesic tolerance develops for different medications within the opioid class, a phenomenon referred to as *cross-tolerance* (Collett 1998). Doverty et al. (2001) found patients receiving methadone maintenance therapy to be cross-tolerant to the analgesic effects of morphine, and when analgesia was obtained, its duration was shorter than expected. Therefore, cross-tolerance between the opioids used for maintenance therapy and other opioids used for analgesia may explain why patients maintained with OAT often require higher and more frequent doses of opioid analgesics to achieve adequate pain control.

Pain Assessment

Because of the complex interplay between pain and OUD, a comprehensive clinical approach is needed. As with all patients, self-reporting remains the gold standard for assessing pain. Although a number of clinical pain assessment measures exist (Breivik et al. 2008), none have been validated specifically in patients with OUD, in whom anxiety, fear, past experiences, and other psychological elements may impact pain ratings. Simple scales provide cross-sectional estimates of an individual's pain intensity and can be used longitudinally to measure the impact of interventions targeting pain. On a 10-point scale, mild pain is typically considered equivalent to a self-reported level of 1–3, moderate pain is in the range of 4–6, and severe pain is anything greater than that (Breivik et al. 2008).

To understand the impact of chronic pain on function, measures such as the Brief Pain Inventory (Tan et al. 2004) or the Graded Chronic Pain Scale (Von Korff et al. 1992) can be used. In addition, physicians should obtain information and results from prior pain evaluations, including imaging and other testing, treatments tried, past psychiatric therapy, and the impact of these prior interventions on pain and functional abilities.

Acute Pain Management

The appropriate treatment of acute pain in patients receiving OAT (i.e., methadone or buprenorphine) includes uninterrupted OAT equivalence to address the patient's baseline opioid requirement for addiction treatment plus aggressive pain management. Continuing the patient's baseline opioid requirements avoids worsening pain symptoms due to the increased pain sensitivity associated with opioid withdrawal. Thus, daily opioid treatment requirements, or the patient's "opioid debt," must be met before attempting to achieve analgesia (Peng et al. 2005). As with all patients with pain, nonpharmacological and non-opioid pain treatments should be implemented aggressively. However, severe acute pain often requires a short course of opioid analgesics. Literature suggests that undertreating acute pain may lead to decreased responsiveness to subsequent opioid analgesics, thus making pain control more difficult (Mao et al. 1995). To decrease the total amount of opioids given to these patients, multimodal analgesia (e.g., NSAIDs, acetaminophen), including adjuvant analgesics (e.g., antidepressants, anticonvulsants) that enhance opioid effects, may be coadministered (Kehlet and Dahl 1993).

To decrease their anxiety, clinicians should reassure patients that treatment of their OUD will continue and that their pain will be aggressively and safely managed. Considering the increased pain sensitivity and cross-tolerance with OAT, adequate pain control generally necessitates higher opioid doses at shorter dosing intervals. Initially, analgesic dosing should be continuous or scheduled rather than on an as-needed basis. Allowing pain to reemerge before requesting the next dose causes unnecessary suffering and anxiety and increases tension between the patient and treatment team.

Empirical data on the use of patient-controlled analgesia in patients with SUD and acute pain are limited. Paige et al. (1994) reported that although women receiving methadone maintenance therapy had higher pain scores after cesarean section surgery, there was no statistically significant difference in opioid analgesic usage compared with control subjects. Clinical experience supports consideration of using patient-controlled analgesia in patients receiving OAT; increased patient control over analgesia minimizes patient anxiety over pain management.

The pharmacological properties of opioids must be considered when selecting an opioid analgesic for a patient receiving OAT. Mixed agonist-antagonist opioid analgesics such as pentazocine (Talwin), nalbuphine (Nubain), and butorphanol (Stadol) must be avoided because they may displace the maintenance buprenorphine from the μ opioid receptor, thus precipitating acute opioid withdrawal (Scimeca et al. 2000). Opioid analgesic combination products containing fixed doses of acetaminophen and an opioid (e.g., Percocet, Vicodin) should be limited to situations not requiring high doses to avoid acetaminophen-induced hepatic toxicity. Alternatively, each medication could be prescribed individually at appropriate doses to achieve the desired analgesic effect and to avoid hepatic damage.

Clinical experience treating acute pain in patients maintained with buprenorphine is increasing. Preclinical and clinical studies now suggest that concurrent use of opioid analgesics in patients maintained on buprenorphine is effective (van Niel et al. 2016). When a high-dose parenteral opioid analgesic is being used, the highly variable rates of buprenorphine dissociation from the μ opioid receptor necessitate 1) close monitoring of the patient's level of consciousness and respiratory status and 2) the availability of the opioid antagonist naloxone. On the basis of the most current evidence, several possible approaches exist for treating acute pain requiring opioid analgesia in patients maintained on buprenorphine therapy.

1. Continue buprenorphine maintenance therapy but divide the dose (every 6–8 hours) to take advantage of the drug's analgesic properties. For example, for buprenorphine 16 mg daily, the split dose could be 4 mg every 6 hours. Then, titrate a short-acting opioid analgesic (e.g., morphine, hydromorphone) to analgesic effect. Higher doses of full opioid agonist analgesics may be required because of cross-tolerance.
2. Continue buprenorphine maintenance therapy but divide the dose (every 6–8 hours) to take advantage of the drug's analgesic properties and add additional buprenorphine to treat acute pain. Because of the apparent lack of analgesic ceiling effect and the presence of a respiratory depression ceiling effect, it is possible to safely administer additional buprenorphine (parenteral, sublingual, or buccal) to the patient's maintenance dose. For example, if the patient is prescribed 16 mg sublingual per day, split the daily dose to 4 mg sublingual every 6 hours with an additional 0.3 mg intramuscular (or 2 mg sublingual) every 6–8 hours for breakthrough pain.
3. If the patient is hospitalized in acute pain, the patient's baseline opioid requirement can be managed, and thus opioid withdrawal can be prevented

by converting buprenorphine therapy to a long-acting opioid (e.g., methadone 30–40 mg daily, extended-release morphine 15 mg twice daily). Titrate a short-acting opioid analgesic to effect. Higher doses of full opioid agonist analgesics may be required because of cross-tolerance. When the acute pain resolves, discontinue the opioid agonist analgesics and long-acting opioid and resume buprenorphine maintenance using an induction protocol. It is important to remember that buprenorphine induction can precipitate opioid withdrawal. Therefore, patients regularly receiving a full opioid agonist analgesic should be in mild opioid withdrawal before restarting buprenorphine therapy. Extended-release morphine (typically dosed every 12 hours) has a shorter half-life than methadone, so it may be easier to convert morphine back to buprenorphine because methadone has a very long half-life (greater than 24 hours).

Chronic Pain Management

The management of chronic pain in patients receiving OAT is complex. Outcomes in chronic pain management frequently are expressed in terms of improved quality of life and function rather than complete remission of pain. Improvements in physical capabilities, social interactions, and health care utilization have been used variously as indicators of good chronic pain management. It is therefore important to set realistic expectations with patients regarding goals of care, with an emphasis on functional outcomes. Similarly, management of chronic pain in patients receiving OAT should be reflected by improved functionality in these domains. It is in the context of well-treated SUDs that good pain management outcomes can be expected. Of note, interventions known to improve chronic pain (e.g., cognitive therapy, behavior modification, involvement of family, treatment of concurrent psychological or psychiatric problems, stress management, group support) are similar to those effective in managing SUDs. The positive effects of various types of interventions on both chronic pain and SUDs suggest that exposure to these types of interventions in either context would yield improvements in the other.

Patients maintained on buprenorphine also can be managed using nonpharmacological interventions (e.g., acupuncture, cognitive-behavioral therapy, massage, relaxation, physical therapy) and/or non-opioid medications (e.g., acetaminophen, NSAIDs, antidepressants, anticonvulsants). Because of its inherent analgesic properties, sublingual buprenorphine could be dosed every 6–8 hours to treat both OUD (an on-label indication—that is, one that is within U.S. Food and Drug Administration–approved drug labeling) and pain (an off-label indication). Malinoff et al. (2005) reported that 86% of patients treated with divided doses of sublingual buprenorphine (mean dosage 8 mg/day) had moderate to substantial pain relief along with improved mood and function. Effectiveness of sublingual buprenorphine in treating chronic pain was summarized in a systematic review of 10 trials involving 1,190 patients (Cote and Montgomery 2014). However, because of the heterogeneity of studies, pooling results and meta-analysis were not possible. Moreover, the majority of studies were observational and low quality, resulting in the authors' concluding that current evidence remains insufficient to determine the effectiveness of sublingual buprenorphine for treatment of chronic pain.

If a patient receiving buprenorphine maintenance therapy requires a full opioid agonist for adequate treatment of chronic pain, it is reasonable to divide the buprenorphine dose to every 6–8 hours to take advantage of its analgesic properties. This will allow the patient to have both the OUD and the chronic pain treated simultaneously with sublingual buprenorphine. Currently, there are no studies examining the efficacy of chronic use of a full opioid agonist analgesic for chronic pain management in a patient maintained on buprenorphine for an OUD. Alternatively, the patient could be transferred to an opioid treatment program for methadone maintenance treatment of his or her OUD, which would allow the patient to receive concurrent opioid analgesic treatment by his or her primary care provider or pain specialist for chronic pain management.

Conclusion

SUDs elicit neurophysiological, behavioral, and social responses that worsen the pain experience and complicate the provision of adequate analgesia. Treating acute and chronic pain in patients receiving OAT (i.e., methadone or buprenorphine) is clinically challenging but can be achieved. Patients with a history of OUD may have an increased sensitivity to painful stimuli and therefore may experience acute and chronic pain differently from other patients. Moreover, OAT with the medication taken once a day does not provide analgesia to patients in acute or chronic pain. Because of opioid cross-tolerance and increased pain sensitivity in these patients, opioid analgesics often need to be administered in higher doses and at shortened intervals.

In treating acute pain in patients receiving buprenorphine maintenance therapy, the clinician should provide 1) reassurance regarding uninterrupted OAT equivalence in order to avoid opioid withdrawal and 2) reassurance regarding aggressive pain management, including patient-controlled analgesia to mitigate patient anxiety and facilitate successful treatment of pain. For patients maintained on buprenorphine who have chronic pain, non-opioid analgesics and nonpharmacological approaches should be tried. If chronic opioid use is required for treatment of pain, it may be necessary to split the buprenorphine dose or to transfer the patient to an opioid treatment program for methadone maintenance therapy with concurrent opioid analgesics prescribed by the clinician managing the patient's pain.

Clinical Pearls

Strategies for treatment of acute or chronic pain in patients with opioid use disorder include the following:

- Acute Pain Management

  - Reassure the patient that his or her opioid use disorder history will not prevent adequate pain management.
  - Relieve patient anxiety by discussing, in a nonjudgmental manner, the plan for pain management.
  - Continue the usual or equivalent dose of opioid agonist therapy to avoid opioid withdrawal.
  - Try non-opioids and nonpharmacological strategies.
  - If opioid analgesics are required, the following strategies should be used:

    - Prescribe higher doses at shorter intervals to account for cross-tolerance.
    - Initially prescribe (or order) continuous scheduled dosing rather than writing "prn" orders and include an order to "hold opioid dose if patient is sedated."
    - Avoid using mixed agonist-antagonist opioids because they will precipitate an acute withdrawal syndrome.
    - Administer according to one of the following options:

      Option 1

      Continue buprenorphine maintenance therapy but divide the dose to every 6–8 hours to take advantage of buprenorphine's analgesic properties.

      Use concurrent short-acting opioid analgesics to achieve analgesia.

      Option 2

      Continue buprenorphine maintenance therapy but divide the dose to every 6–8 hours to take advantage of buprenorphine's analgesic properties.

      Give supplemental doses of buprenorphine to achieve analgesia.

Return to the usual daily maintenance dosage when pain resolves.

Option 3 (if patient is hospitalized)

Convert therapy from buprenorphine to long-acting full opioid agonist (e.g., methadone 30–40 mg/day, extended-release morphine 15 mg bid) to manage opioid daily requirement.

Use concurrent short-acting opioid analgesics to achieve analgesia.

Order naloxone (Narcan) to the bedside.

Convert therapy back to buprenorphine before discharge.

- Chronic Pain Management

  — Try non-opioids and nonpharmacological strategies.

  — If opioid analgesics are required, administer according to one of the following options:

    Option 1

    Divide the daily buprenorphine dose to use every 6- to 8-hour dosing.

    Option 2

    Refer the patient to an opioid treatment program for methadone maintenance therapy to treat opioid use disorder and to a primary care provider or pain specialist to treat chronic pain with opioid analgesics.

CASE 6 (CONTINUED)

Martha, the 35-year-old woman who had trouble reconciling her 12-step program and taking buprenorphine, eventually found them mutually inclusive; she has continued as an active member of AA and is taking 16 mg buprenorphine/naloxone per day. She now needs her gallbladder removed; her surgeon calls asking for help managing her medication during the perioperative period. He expects her to be hospitalized for 2 days and to have pain for a week to 10 days.

1. What are the recommendations for the perioperative pain management of a patient taking buprenorphine?

2. Do you have to taper doses until the buprenorphine is completely discontinued?

3. If you taper down to completely discontinue buprenorphine, how do you cross over to another opioid?

4. How do you use methadone in the perioperative period?

CASE 12

Fred is a 44-year-old senior noncommissioned officer who was injured 4 years ago in Iraq by an improvised explosive device and has residual chronic lower extremity and low back pain. He was treated through pain management services at a Veterans Health Administration medical center with a complicated course that included trials of opioids, non-opioid medication, regional block, and physical treatments. During the course of treatment, he became addicted to opioids and was eventually referred for buprenorphine treatment. He has achieved excellent control of his opioid use disorder and "tolerable" control of his pain with sublingual buprenorphine 8 mg/naloxone 2 mg three times a day. He is now successfully pursuing a master of business administration degree. He calls from the emergency department (ED) and tells you that he fell and reinjured his leg. The ED physician wants to prescribe some additional pain medication.

1. What would be the strategies for addressing acute pain in this patient?

2. What are the available non-opioid therapies?

3. What are the available nonpharmacological therapies?

4. When do you seek collaboration with other specialists?

5. Does buprenorphine provide adequate pain relief?

6. Compare and contrast strategies for treating pain in the context of agonist maintenance treatment.

References

Alford DP, Compton P, Samet JH: Acute pain management for patients receiving maintenance methadone or buprenorphine therapy. Ann Intern Med 144(2):127–134, 2006 16418412

Alford DP, German JS, Samet JH, et al: Primary care patients with drug use report chronic pain and self-medicate with alcohol and other drugs. J Gen Intern Med 31(5):486–491, 2016 26809204

American Psychiatric Association: Diagnostic and Statistical Manual of Mental Disorders, 5th Edition. Arlington, VA, American Psychiatric Association, 2013

Barry DT, Savant JD, Beitel M, et al: Pain and associated substance use among opioid dependent individuals seeking office-based treatment with buprenorphine-naloxone: a needs assessment study. Am J Addict 22(3):212–217, 2013 23617861

Breivik H, Borchgrevink PC, Allen SM, et al: Assessment of pain. Br J Anaesth 101(1):17–24, 2008 18487245

Collett BJ: Opioid tolerance: the clinical perspective. Br J Anaesth 81(1):58–68, 1998 9771273

Compton MA: Cold-pressor pain tolerance in opiate and cocaine abusers: correlates of drug type and use status. J Pain Symptom Manage 9(7):462–473, 1994 7822886

Cote J, Montgomery L: Sublingual buprenorphine as an analgesic in chronic pain: a systematic review. Pain Med 15(7):1171–1178, 2014 24995716

Cowan A: Buprenorphine: the basic pharmacology revisited. J Addict Med 1(2):68–72, 2007 21768937

Dahan A, Yassen A, Romberg R, et al: Buprenorphine induces ceiling in respiratory depression but not in analgesia. Br J Anaesth 96(5):627–632, 2006 16547090

Doverty M, White JM, Somogyi AA, et al: Hyperalgesic responses in methadone maintenance patients. Pain 90(1–2):91–96, 2001 11166974

Englberger W, Kögel B, Friderichs E, et al: Reversibility of opioid receptor occupancy of buprenorphine in vivo. Eur J Pharmacol 534(1–3):95–102, 2006 16490191

Eriator I: Narcotic analgesics for chronic pain management. Curr Rev Pain 2(4):193–200, 1998

Gutstein HB, Akil H: Opioid analgesics, in Goodman and Gilman's The Pharmacological Basis of Therapeutics, 11th Edition. Edited by Brunton LL, Lazo JS, Parker KL. New York, McGraw-Hill, 2006, pp 547–590

Hansen LE, Stone GL, Matson CA, et al: Total joint arthroplasty in patients taking methadone or buprenorphine/naloxone preoperatively for prior heroin addiction: a prospective matched cohort study. J Arthroplasty 31(8):1698–1701, 2016 26899477

Jamison RN, Kauffman J, Katz NP: Characteristics of methadone maintenance patients with chronic pain. J Pain Symptom Manage 19(1):53–62, 2000 10687327

Johnson RE, Fudala PJ, Payne R: Buprenorphine: considerations for pain management. J Pain Symptom Manage 29(3):297–326, 2005 15781180

Jones HE, O'Grady K, Dahne J, et al: Management of acute postpartum pain in patients maintained on methadone or buprenorphine during pregnancy. Am J Drug Alcohol Abuse 35(3):151–156, 2009 19462298

Kantor TG, Cantor R, Tom E: A study of hospitalized surgical patients on methadone maintenance. Drug Alcohol Depend 6(3):163–173, 1980 6107237

Karasz A, Zallman L, Berg K, et al: The experience of chronic severe pain in patients undergoing methadone maintenance treatment. J Pain Symptom Manage 28(5):517–525, 2004 15504628

Kehlet H, Dahl JB: The value of "multimodal" or "balanced analgesia" in postoperative pain treatment. Anesth Analg 77(5):1048–1056, 1993 8105724

Khanna IK, Pillarisetti S: Buprenorphine—an attractive opioid with underutilized potential in treatment of chronic pain. J Pain Res 8:859–870, 2015 26672499

Kögel B, Christoph T, Strassburger W, et al: Interaction of mu-opioid receptor agonists and antagonists with the analgesic effect of buprenorphine in mice. Eur J Pain 9(5):599–611, 2005 16139189

Kornfeld H, Manfredi L: Effectiveness of full agonist opioids in patients stabilized on buprenorphine undergoing major surgery: a case series. Am J Ther 17(5):523–528, 2010 19918165

Macintyre PE, Russell RA, Usher KA, et al: Pain relief and opioid requirements in the first 24 hours after surgery in patients taking buprenorphine and methadone opioid substitution therapy. Anaesth Intensive Care 41(2):222–230, 2013 23530789

Malinoff HL, Barkin RL, Wilson G: Sublingual buprenorphine is effective in the treatment of chronic pain syndrome. Am J Ther 12(5):379–384, 2005 16148422

Manfredi PL, Gonzales GR, Cheville AL, et al: Methadone analgesia in cancer pain patients on chronic methadone maintenance therapy. J Pain Symptom Manage 21(2):169–174, 2001 11226767

Mao J, Price DD, Mayer DJ: Mechanisms of hyperalgesia and morphine tolerance: a current view of their possible interactions. Pain 62(3):259–274, 1995 8657426

Martin JE, Inglis J: Pain tolerance and narcotic addiction. Br J Soc Clin Psychol 4(3):224–229, 1965 5872680

Merrill JO, Rhodes LA, Deyo RA, et al: Mutual mistrust in the medical care of drug users: the keys to the "narc" cabinet. J Gen Intern Med 17(5):327–333, 2002 12047728

Paige D, Proble L, Watrous G, et al: PCA use in cocaine using patients: a pilot study. Am J Pain Manage 4:101–105, 1994

Peng PW, Tumber PS, Gourlay D: Review article: perioperative pain management of patients on methadone therapy. Can J Anaesth 52(5):513–523, 2005 15872131

Potter JS, Chakrabarti A, Domier CP, et al: Pain and continued opioid use in individuals receiving buprenorphine-naloxone for opioid detoxification: secondary analyses from the Clinical Trials Network. J Subst Abuse Treat 38 (suppl 1):S80–S86, 2010 20307799

Rosenblum A, Joseph H, Fong C, et al: Prevalence and characteristics of chronic pain among chemically dependent patients in methadone maintenance and residential treatment facilities. JAMA 289(18):2370–2378, 2003 12746360

Scimeca MM, Savage SR, Portenoy R, et al: Treatment of pain in methadone-maintained patients. Mt Sinai J Med 67(5–6):412–422, 2000 11064492

St Marie B: Health care experiences when pain and substance use disorder coexist: "just because I'm an addict doesn't mean I don't have pain." Pain Med 15(12):2075–2086, 2014 25041442

Tan G, Jensen MP, Thornby JI, et al: Validation of the Brief Pain Inventory for chronic nonmalignant pain. J Pain 5(2):133–137, 2004 15042521

Trafton JA, Oliva EM, Horst DA, et al: Treatment needs associated with pain in substance use disorder patients: implications for concurrent treatment. Drug Alcohol Depend 73(1):23–31, 2004 14687956

Upshur CC, Luckmann RS, Savageau JA: Primary care provider concerns about management of chronic pain in community clinic populations. J Gen Intern Med 21(6):652–655, 2006 16808752

van Niel JC, Schneider J, Tzschentke TM: Drug Res (Stuttg) 66(11):562–570, 2016 27504867

Von Korff M, Ormel J, Keefe FJ, et al: Grading the severity of chronic pain. Pain 50(2):133–149, 1992 1408309

White JM: Pleasure into pain: the consequences of long-term opioid use. Addict Behav 29(7):1311–1324, 2004 15345267

Zacny JP, McKay MA, Toledano AY, et al: The effects of a cold-water immersion stressor on the reinforcing and subjective effects of fentanyl in healthy volunteers. Drug Alcohol Depend 42(2):133–142, 1996 8889412

13

Opioid Use by Adolescents

Ximena Sanchez-Samper, M.D.
Sharon Levy, M.D., M.P.H.

SCREENING for alcohol and illicit drug use is recommended for any practice that cares for adolescents and young adults. In this chapter, we review validated screening tools and management approaches for use in this population. We cover standard treatment options with a focus on the treatment of adolescents with severe opioid use disorder (OUD) and the promising role of buprenorphine in the treatment of this high-risk population.

Epidemiology

OUD among adolescents is a substantial problem in the United States. According to data from the National Institute on Drug Abuse's Monitoring the Future study, use of "narcotics other than heroin" doubled among high school students between the years 1994 (6.6%) and 2002 (13.5%), with marked increases in the use of long-acting oxycodone tablets and hydrocodone-acetaminophen combination tablets (Johnston 2016). In 2009, the annual prevalence for oxycodone and hydrocodone use reached its highest level since these data have been collected, with 2.0%, 5.1%, and 4.9% of 8th, 10th, and 12th graders, respectively, reporting oxycodone use in the past year and 2.5%, 8.1%, and 9.7% of them, respectively, reporting hydrocodone use in the past year (Johnston 2016). In 2015 alone, about 276,000 adolescents ages 12–17 were reported to be misusing pain relieving drugs, 21,000 adolescents had used heroin, and 6,000 are estimated to have had a heroin use disorder (Center for Behavioral Health Statistics and Quality 2016).

Teenagers may not fully appreciate the risks of misusing prescription opioids because these drugs are legal and easily accessible (Boyd et al. 2006). Many adolescents who misuse opioids to get high may become addicted quickly and transition to heroin use when they can no longer afford the street price of opioid medications. A decrease in the price of heroin has increased accessibility to teens, and an increase in purity has allowed for non-intravenous administration, which has made the drug more attractive to adolescents (Hopfer et al. 2003). Approximately 21% of individuals reporting first-time heroin use in the years 2002–2011 were younger than age 18 (Muhuri et al. 2013). Although all adolescents are at risk, heroin use is more common among teens with early-onset substance use or those who have developed polysubstance dependence (Hopfer et al. 2002). In the general adult population, males account for nearly three-quarters of users (Center for Behavioral Health Statistics and Quality 2015), and approximately 90% of individuals seeking treatment for heroin use are white (Cicero et al. 2014). Intravenous use accounts for more than half of all heroin use by adolescents (Center for Behavioral Health Statistics and Quality 2015), which raises a significant public health concern because of an increased risk of contracting and spreading HIV, hepatitis, and other infectious diseases (Marsch 2005).

Risk and Protective Factors

Individual, peer, family, and community factors all impact the likelihood of drug use and the likelihood of an adolescent progressing to substance use disorders (SUDs; Oetting and Beauvais 1987; Weinberg 2001). Healthy parental attitudes and role modeling decrease the likelihood that teens will try drugs or affiliate with peers who use drugs. Conversely, conflicted parent-child relationships, parental ineffectiveness, insufficient parental monitoring, inconsistent discipline, deprived socioeconomic status, and parental alcohol or drug use have all been robustly correlated with adolescent opioid use (Teichman and Kefir 2000). Lower levels of parental education are correlated with heroin use by teens, with rates highest among those whose parents did not complete grade school (Catalano et al. 1992).

Early-onset substance use predicts a rapid progression to SUDs. Early use of nicotine and alcohol increases the risk of developing SUDs later in life, including cannabis, stimulant, opioid, and/or alcohol use disorders (Hopfer et al. 2002). Marijuana use, in particular, has been associated with increased susceptibility to OUD (Lynskey et al. 2003). Teens diagnosed with SUDs are also more likely than their peers to continue substance use into adulthood (Hingson et al. 2006).

Legal problems and co-occurring childhood psychopathology are also risk factors for progression from opioid use to OUDs, especially among adolescent females. The most frequently identified antecedent psychiatric disorders include behavioral disorders (conduct disorder, attention-deficit/hyperactivity disorder [ADHD]), mood disorders, anxiety disorders, and learning disorders (Currie et al. 2005; Goodwin et al. 2002; Wilens et al. 2003).

Substance Use and Co-occurring Disorders

SUDs frequently co-occur with other mental health disorders, and OUD is no exception. The most common co-occurring disorders include mood and anxiety disorders, conduct disorder, oppositional defiant disorder, and ADHD (Currie et al. 2005; Goodwin et al. 2002; Wilens et al. 2004). Adolescents with SUDs are also more likely than their peers to have been victims of physical or sexual abuse (Jaycox et al. 2004).

Use of psychoactive substances can induce, mimic, or exacerbate underlying mental illness. Adolescents with OUD and co-occurring mental health disorders are more likely to require inpatient hospitalization, are less likely to be compliant with medications, are more likely to drop out of treatment, and are at higher risk of relapse. Despite these poor outcomes, simultaneous treatment of the co-occurring mental health disorder helps to alleviate the substance use. Therefore, all adolescents with OUD should be evaluated for co-occurring mental health disorder(s) and should be treated for both disorders simultaneously.

Screening and Assessment

Screening for drug use using a validated instrument is a recommended component of routine health care for all adolescents. The goal of screening is to identify an individual's experience with psychoactive substances—from abstinence through severe SUD—in order to guide an appropriate response, from primary prevention for those who have never used substances to referral to treatment for those with severe SUDs. Use of a validated tool ensures appropriate risk level identification. Clinical impressions, which rely on observable disruptions in behavior and/or functioning, are notably insensitive for identifying substance use problems and even SUDs (Wilson et al. 2004).

Several screens have been validated for use with adolescents. Screens can be divided into two broad categories—problem-based screens, such as the CRAFFT screening tool (Knight et al. 2003), or newer frequency-based screens, such as the Brief Screener for Tobacco, Alcohol, and other Drugs (BSTAD; Kelly et al. 2014) and Screen to Brief Intervention tool (S2BI; Levy et al. 2014). Frequency-based screens may be quicker and more efficient to administer and also can give separate risk levels for individual substances; therefore, these screens are recommended by the American Academy of Pediatrics (Levy and Kokotailo 2011).

Regardless of which screen is chosen, the risk level–based response is identical. For example, the recommended response to a report of no past year substance use is to deliver a prevention message in an effort to delay or prevent initiation of use. The American Academy of Pediatrics has identified four distinct levels of intervention based on results of risk level screening: positive reinforcement (for abstinence), brief health advice (for substance use without a disorder), brief intervention (for mild, moderate, or severe SUD), and referral to treatment (for severe SUD) (S.L. Levy et al. 2016).

Beyond screening, substance use should be considered in the differential diagnosis of any teen who presents with new-onset behavioral, emotional, or school problems or when an adult suspects substance use because a teen has appeared intoxicated or has been in possession of drugs or drug paraphernalia. Recognition of the physical and behavioral manifestations of common psychoactive substances can aid in focusing an assessment, testing, and prompt intervention. Clinician and family understanding of risk and protective factors may be the single most important element for identifying at-risk youth and intervening early.

Adolescents who report any use of opioids (other than as prescribed by a clinician) should receive further assessment to determine the motivation and pattern of use, associated problems, attempts at quitting, and previous treatment to determine the stage of use and whether an SUD is present. Opioid use occurs on a continuum from *misuse* to *severe substance use disorder* as described below. Treatment strategies are most effective when they target the stage of use.

Although not a formal diagnosis, *opioid misuse* is characterized by any use of opioids without a prescription for pain relief or use of more opioid than was prescribed. Because of the highly addictive nature of opioids, teens using these medications without medical supervision may develop opioid addiction.

Mild opioid use disorder is defined as meeting two or three of the SUD symptom criteria specified in DSM-5 (American Psychiatric Association 2013). Adolescents with mild OUD typically use for reasons other than relief of pain (e.g., to become intoxicated) and may have begun to experience adverse consequences as a result of use. Substance-related problems may include decreased school performance, suspensions, relationship problems with parents or peers, motor vehicle accidents, injuries, emergency department visits, physical or sexual assaults, and legal problems. These may be accompanied by significant changes in dress, behavior, and peer group.

Moderate opioid use disorder is defined as meeting four or five of the symptom criteria for OUD in DSM-5. Typically, adolescents with moderate OUD have continued to use opioids in the context of significant problems or impairment in functioning.

Severe opioid use disorder, or addiction, is defined as meeting six or more symptom criteria for OUD in DSM-5 and refers to loss of control over drug use. Severe OUD is characterized by a maladaptive pattern of compulsive opioid use, preoccupation, and associated negative consequences. Tolerance and withdrawal are nearly universal. Clinical manifestations typically include continual use of substances when available, solitary use, disrupted family relationships, and loss of outside supports. Intravenous use, nasal insufflation, and smoking are common. Formal diagnostic criteria are specified in DSM-5 (see Chapter 4, "Patient Assessment").

If a teen denies drug use in the context of substantial evidence to the contrary, a confidential interview is recommended. The clinician can ask for an explanation of the reported observations (e.g., "Why is your mother so worried that you are using drugs?" or "Why were you carrying pills in your purse?"). Urine drug testing for opioids also may be a useful part of an assessment, but the procedure has significant limitations. A drug test may be negative in the context of drug use if the window of detection (< 72 hours for most opioid preparations) is missed or if a specimen is adulterated or substituted. Although most standard urine drug screens include an opiate panel that detects morphine and codeine, synthetic opioids are not always detected by these screens, and tests for those substances may need to be ordered separately (Levy et al. 2006; see also Chapter 6, "Buprenorphine Treatment in Office-Based Settings"). Conversely, false-positive screening results may occur because of medications or foods cross-reacting with an opiate screening panel; thus, all positive results should be confirmed with a definitive test such as gas chromatography–mass spectrometry. Drug testing cannot differentiate use of a medication as prescribed from misuse. Furthermore, a single positive confirmed test result is neither necessary nor sufficient for making the diagnosis of an OUD. Despite these limitations, a positive test result for opioids in the context of clinical suspicion of drug use may be a useful way to start an honest conversation with an adolescent.

A physical examination including assessment of a full set of vital signs should be performed as part of a complete assessment for an OUD. Signs of acute intoxication or chronic opioid use are rare in adolescents but should be noted if present. Patients who present in opioid withdrawal may benefit from inpatient medical withdrawal for symptomatic relief.

Prevention and Pharmacotherapy

TEENS WITHOUT OPIOID USE DISORDER

Primary Prevention

Anticipatory guidance from the provider is recommended when prescribing opioid medications. Although pain medications are highly effective and safe when used as prescribed, they are also highly addictive and can be dangerous when misused. Parental monitoring to ensure that medications are always used as directed is advised whenever possible. Any leftover medication can be discarded by returning it to the pharmacy. Medications should never be shared or given to anyone other than the patient for whom the prescription was written.

Pain medication can be safe for use even in patients with SUDs, and pain should not be left untreated because of a history of SUD. However, in these situations, increased supervision and monitoring to avoid misuse is advisable. Parents can be asked to hold, dispense, and observe all medication doses. When treating chronic pain, the clinician can request that all prescriptions initiate from a single prescriber and use state prescription drug monitoring programs to prevent patients from obtaining duplicates. Patients and parents may be asked to sign consent to maintain open communication among all treating clinicians. Parents can bring in medication bottles for pill counts. Early refills should generally be avoided (Hertz and Knight 2006).

Brief Advice

Adolescents who misuse opioids but do not have an SUD may respond to brief counseling and advice. In these cases, the clinician can recommend that the adolescent discontinue use of prescription opioid medications entirely and briefly discuss the risk of progressing to OUD with continued use because of the addictive potential of opioids. An assessment for pain can be conducted if appropriate, and the adolescent should be seen again for a follow-up health visit.

Brief Intervention

Adolescents with a diagnosis of mild or moderate OUD but not addiction (severe OUD) may benefit from a relatively brief intervention. Motivational techniques that 1) encourage teens to consider any negative consequences they have already experienced or are concerned about related to their drug use and 2) explore their ambivalence regarding continued use may be particularly helpful (Knight et al. 2005; Marsch et al. 2005). We recommend that these teens be followed closely to ensure that they are able to achieve and maintain abstinence or to refer them for more intensive treatment if they progress to severe OUD.

TEENS WITH SEVERE OPIOID USE DISORDER

Adolescents with a diagnosis of severe OUD require long-term treatment to keep them in stable recovery. Treatment should be comprehensive and tailored to the adolescent's particular needs; no single approach is suitable for all individuals. Brief medically supervised opioid withdrawal, unless followed by a long-term treatment plan, is associated with very high rates of relapse. Similarly, standard drug-free outpatient counseling has minimal efficacy in both adolescents and adults. Few teens with opioid addiction will be able to remain drug free without ongoing treatment, and providing treatment to young patients may present an opportunity to prevent commonly associated biopsychosocial and secondary medical problems. In most cases, effective treatment for adolescents with severe OUD should be medication—either opioid agonist or opioid antagonist therapy in conjunction with evidence-based behavioral therapies. Buprenorphine has added an important option for the treatment of these high-risk patients.

Role of Pharmacotherapy

A large body of evidence has demonstrated that pharmacotherapy is effective in treating adults with OUDs, both for withdrawal and for long-term maintenance (see Chapter 3, "Efficacy and Safety of Buprenorphine"). Few medication studies have included adolescents, but accumulating evidence suggests that opioid agonist therapy can be effective in reducing relapse rates in adolescent populations by stabilizing neurochemistry, ameliorating withdrawal, and curbing cravings (Fiellin 2008; Woody et al. 2008). However, there is little guidance regarding the optimal length of buprenorphine treatment for adolescents. Before describing the use of buprenorphine in adolescents, we review other pharmacotherapy options.

Short-Term Pharmacotherapy (Withdrawal Treatment)

Withdrawal treatment refers to the medical management of symptoms of withdrawal (see Chapter 5, "Clinical Use of Buprenorphine"). Because of the pharmacological properties of opioids, recurrent use results in upregulation of the μ opioid receptor, intercellular and intracellular dysregulation, activation of the dopamine-based reward system, and development of dependence. If opioid use is discontinued abruptly, adolescents with OUD may experience unpleasant withdrawal symptoms, which is often the precipitating event that brings them into treatment (Rowan et al. 2000). Otherwise-healthy adolescents can tolerate withdrawal without serious medical consequences, although the unpleasant symptoms may lead to relapse to opioid use for symptomatic relief. Inpatient withdrawal treatment is a reasonable option for patients who meet criteria for severe OUD. For adolescents in opioid withdrawal with underlying medical conditions, such as diabetes or cystic fibrosis, or with significant psychiatric co-morbidity, inpatient detoxification is the standard of care.

Medication withdrawal treatment protocols for adults are well established, and similar protocols can be used for teens. Medication options include brief inpatient treatment with clonidine, methadone, or buprenorphine or a more gradual outpatient buprenorphine taper. Clonidine is a centrally active α_2-adrenergic blocker that decreases sympathetic outflow. It has been used to decrease symptoms associated with opioid withdrawal; it does not bind to the opioid receptor, and its abuse potential is limited. A randomized controlled trial conducted among 13- to 18-year-olds with severe OUD compared clonidine with buprenorphine withdrawal treatment. The buprenorphine group had significantly greater retention in treatment (72% vs. 39%), significantly less opioid use (64% vs. 32% of urine samples tested negative for opioids), and significantly greater retention in care after withdrawal treatment (61% vs. 5%) (Marsch et al. 2005). These findings, which are comparable to findings of similar trials in adults, suggest that buprenorphine is clinically more effective than clonidine for the treatment of opioid withdrawal symptoms. There are no published studies comparing methadone to buprenorphine for withdrawal treatment of adolescents. Adolescents should be discharged from a medical withdrawal treatment program only when a plan for continued care is in place (Chang and Kosten 2005).

Long-Term Pharmacotherapy

The American Academy of Pediatrics recommends medication-assisted treatment for adolescents with OUD (Committee on Substance Use and Prevention 2016) and has endorsed a buprenorphine waiver course specifically designed for professionals who treat this age group (http://www.aap.org). Treatment options include methadone, buprenorphine, and naltrexone. In 2000, Congress passed the Drug Addiction Treatment Act (DATA), which permits office-based buprenorphine treatment, thus expanding options and access to opioid agonist therapy (see Chapter 1, "Opioid Use Disorder in America"). Buprenorphine presents several advantages over methadone for the treatment of adolescents, including an improved safety profile and reduced potential for misuse. However, the treatment of adolescents with severe OUD presents specific challenges to providers because limited evidence-based research for treatment exists (Institute of Medicine Committee on Federal Regulation of Methadone Treatment 1995; Sees et al. 2000).

Methadone maintenance.   Patients with OUD may be treated with long-term agonist therapy with the goal of reducing cravings, decreasing relapse rates, and improving overall functioning. Methadone and buprenorphine are currently the only two opioid agonist therapies available in the United States. Methadone maintenance has long been a mainstay of treatment for adults with OUD, although access to treatment, especially for youth, is limited (Fiellin et al. 2001).

Methadone is a full agonist of the μ opioid receptor. It has a long half-life, which allows for steady-state dosing without the peaks and troughs associated with euphoria and withdrawal. Methadone maintenance therapy improves functioning, decreases heroin use as evidenced by urine drug testing, leads to reductions in criminal activity, increases treatment retention and employment status, decreases the risk of spreading highly transmissible diseases, and reduces mortality associated with severe OUD by approximately two-thirds in adult cohorts (Mattick et al. 2003).

Under certain conditions, methadone has been approved for use in adolescents younger than 18 years for treatment of withdrawal symptoms; however, it can be prescribed for maintenance therapy only through specially licensed clinics, which limits its availability. Federal regulations limit methadone maintenance treatment to individuals with at least 1 year of severe OUD, making methadone less accessible to younger users with shorter histories of OUD. Furthermore, U.S. Department of Health and Human Services guidelines specify that methadone clinics cannot accept patients younger than 18 years for maintenance treatment unless they have undergone two unsuccessful attempts at short-term withdrawal treatment or drug-free treatment within a 12-month period and have obtained parental consent (Fudala et al. 2003; Jasinski et al. 1978).

Buprenorphine.   An overview of buprenorphine is provided in this section, and specifics of initiating buprenorphine treatment are discussed later in this chapter (see section "Buprenorphine Treatment in Adolescents"). Buprenorphine is a Schedule III, synthetic partial μ opioid receptor agonist and an antagonist at the μ opioid receptor. Because of its mixed partial agonist-antagonist profile, it has several advantages, including a greater margin of safety than full μ opioid agonists, a less intense abstinence syndrome with fewer autonomic symptoms, lower abuse potential, and an improved safety profile with limited potential for overdose. The agonist activity of buprenorphine has a ceiling effect and therefore causes less respiratory depression than full agonists (although deaths due to respiratory suppression have been reported when buprenorphine is used in combination with alcohol, benzodiazepines, or other central nervous system–depressant drugs) (Mattick et al. 2014; see also Chapter 2, "General Opioid Pharmacology," and Chapter 3). Buprenorphine has a higher affinity for opioid receptors than full agonists and displaces full agonists, causing rapid and severe withdrawal symptoms if given to a patient without sufficient receptor availability. When used as maintenance therapy, buprenorphine provides a μ opioid blockade that diminishes a patient's ability to become intoxicated with other opioids while the μ opioid receptors are saturated (Colson et al. 2012).

Because buprenorphine has a long half-life (24–60 hours), most adolescent patients can be maintained with 8–16 mg daily, which can be given in single or divided doses. Physicians who have received a special waiver from the U.S.

Food and Drug Administration (FDA) can prescribe buprenorphine in an office-based setting, which reduces stigma and expands treatment access for adolescents (Woody et al. 2008). In an effort to increase access to buprenorphine, changes to DATA allow physicians who have been prescribing buprenorphine for at least 1 year to apply for an expanded cap, allowing them to prescribe buprenorphine for a panel of up to 100 patients. After an additional year, physicians can apply to increase their panel to 275 patients. Nonetheless, shortages of buprenorphine providers exist. The problem of access is exacerbated for adolescents; currently less than 1% of buprenorphine prescribers are pediatricians.

Buprenorphine is as efficacious as methadone in adults with OUDs when equi-effective doses of these medications are provided. It has been approved for use as opioid agonist therapy in adults whose use meets DSM-IV-TR (American Psychiatric Association 2000) criteria for opioid dependence. Safety and efficacy of buprenorphine for patients under age 16 years and older has not been well established. Unlike the federal regulations for methadone maintenance treatment, there is no requirement to document a 1-year history of severe opioid use disorder. This permits the treatment of younger individuals with shorter histories of OUD, a major benefit when treating adolescents.

Although evidence suggests that teens can benefit from buprenorphine maintenance therapy, the optimal length of treatment is unknown. Woody et al. (2008) published a randomized cohort study of 152 treatment-seeking adolescents ages 15–21 years whose use met DSM-IV-TR criteria for opioid dependence. Participants were randomly assigned to receive either 14-day opioid withdrawal treatment or 12 weeks of opioid agonist therapy. Patients who received 12 weeks of buprenorphine treatment reported less use of opioids and other illicit substances, had fewer opioid-positive urine test results, and were retained in the study longer. These differences disappeared after medications were discontinued (Woody et al. 2008).

Naltrexone.   Naltrexone is a μ opioid receptor antagonist with high affinity for the receptor (see Chapter 9, "Methadone, Naltrexone, and Naloxone"). Oral naltrexone has been approved by the FDA for the treatment of both alcohol use disorder and OUD. A sustained-release depot formulation of naltrexone has received FDA approval for the treatment of alcohol use disorder and OUD. Naltrexone, particularly in the sustained-release formulation, may be a good option for adolescents with relatively short histories of opioid use; for teens with active alcohol or sedative use disorders for whom buprenorphine may be relatively contraindicated; and for teens who are homeless or unstably housed or living in dormitories with minimal supervision, for whom the misuse and diversion potential of buprenorphine may make it riskier. There is no published research on the efficacy of naltrexone for OUD in adolescent patients.

Buprenorphine Treatment in Adolescents

PRELIMINARY EVALUATION

Before opioid agonist therapy is initiated, a complete evaluation is recommended, including a thorough substance use history assessment; medical, mental health, vocational, and psychosocial history assessments; and a physical examination. This gives the treating clinician the opportunity to address any active problems that would interfere with long-term recovery or refer the patient for treatment. Testing for HIV, hepatitis B, hepatitis C, and other infectious diseases as indicated is recommended. Symptoms of mild depression or inattention may improve with abstinence and can be monitored if they are not debilitating. However, all patients should be screened for more significant co-occurring psychiatric symptoms, and simultaneous treatment of comorbidities is recommended. Homelessness or living with a parent or guardian with active SUD poses special challenges; patients without a stable home and guardian can be referred to social services for support. School dropout and unemployment rates are high among adolescents with severe OUD; addressing educational and vocational difficulties as soon as the patient is stable may improve long-term outcomes.

SETTING TREATMENT GOALS

The optimal length of medication treatment has not been scientifically determined, and the risks of long-term exposure to buprenorphine or naltrexone on the still-developing adolescent brain are unknown. We recommend, therefore, that the clinician discuss the length of treatment with patients and, when appropriate, parents or guardians. Although there is little published evidence, in our clinical practice we recommend that adolescents continue to take buprenorphine until they have been abstinent from illicit opioid use for at least 1 year before considering discontinuation. This approach is consistent with DSM-5 criteria for "severe opioid use disorder in sustained remission, on maintenance therapy," given that relapse rates for other addictions tend to fall sharply over the course of the first year of abstinence and then begin to level off. Buprenorphine should be tapered slowly to avoid withdrawal symptoms and/or resurgence of cravings. Close follow-up and ongoing drug testing to monitor for relapse are recommended even after medications are discontinued. Naltrexone can be considered for patients who have successfully tapered off buprenorphine and do not have withdrawal symptoms.

THE TREATMENT CONTRACT

Establishing a set of expectations for adolescents beginning buprenorphine treatment is recommended. A written contract may be helpful (Table 13–1). We recommend that adolescents be encouraged to abstain from all substances, including alcohol, which can be dangerous in combination with buprenorphine as they enter treatment. However, ongoing substance use is an indication of a need for more treatment and/or a higher level of care and not a reason to terminate treatment or discharge an adolescent from care. Random drug tests to monitor for use of alcohol, opioid, or other drug use and to assess medication adherence with buprenorphine are an important component of treatment. Patients who are unable to achieve abstinence from substances other than opioids can be referred for complementary treatment. Because of the risk of accidental oversedation or overdose, office-based buprenorphine treatment may need to be stopped if a patient is unable to stop using alcohol or sedatives. We recommend that adolescents with severe OUD enter counseling to help them identify and avoid triggers for drug use, to learn healthy mechanisms for relieving stress, and to learn other life skills. Some individuals also will need specific counseling to address other issues such as depression, anxiety, and anger.

Adolescents can benefit from the availability of parents or guardians who participate in treatment and provide structure whenever possible. As with treatment-seeking adults who benefit from family involvement, parental participation may improve adolescent treatment adherence, allow for prompt intervention when a relapse occurs, and minimize diversion risk (Dasinger et al. 2004).

GETTING STARTED: THE INITIAL BUPRENORPHINE DOSE

Adolescents should be advised not to use opioids before buprenorphine induction—about 12–24 hours or longer depending on the half-life of their drug of choice (see Chapter 5). Buprenorphine therapy may be started at home if a patient (along with a parent or guardian) can be taught to reliably monitor signs of withdrawal and wait until withdrawal has progressed enough to avoid inducing precipitated withdrawal. However, we recommend observed induction for all adolescent patients to give the clinician the opportunity to assess and quantify signs of withdrawal, to teach the teenager to take medications sublingually, to teach the parent or guardian how to observe a medication dose, and to answer questions.

Close monitoring for side effects and continued cravings is important until patients are taking a stable dose of buprenorphine. Because of the long half-life of buprenorphine, a single daily dose is effective, although many adolescents prefer divided doses to mimic previous drug use patterns. Patients should be

---

TABLE 13–1. **Sample agreement for medication treatment**

❑ Yes   1. I agree to stop using all drugs, including opiates, alcohol, marijuana, and other street drugs. I will request additional support if I am unable to remain drug free.

❑ Yes   2. I understand that it is dangerous to mix buprenorphine with alcohol or other sedatives (such as Valium, Ativan, Xanax, Klonopin)—so dangerous that it could result in **accidental overdose, oversedation, coma, or death**. I will not use **ALCOHOL** or **SEDATIVES** while I am being treated with buprenorphine. My doctor will discontinue my buprenorphine treatment if I violate this agreement.

❑ Yes   3. I agree to cooperate with urine drug testing whenever requested to detect whether I have used alcohol, prescription drugs, or street drugs.

❑ Yes   4. If I slip and use opiates, alcohol, or an illicit drug, I will discuss this honestly with staff.

❑ Yes   5. I agree that my home medication supplies will be kept in the care of my parent or guardian. My parents will provide me one dose at a time and observe me take my medication. I will never sell, share, or otherwise distribute my medication. If my medication is taken accidentally by a child or a pet, I will call 911 or Poison Control at 1-800-222-1222.

❑ Yes   6. I will always take my medication by placing it under my tongue to dissolve and be absorbed. I will never inject buprenorphine because IV use can lead to sudden and severe opiate withdrawal. I will not skip or alter doses without speaking to my doctor.

❑ Yes   7. I will schedule and keep all recommended appointments. My parent or guardian will accompany me to all of my appointments until I have been cleared to come by myself. If I or my parent must reschedule an appointment because of an emergency, I will call the office as soon as I am aware of the need to change.

❑ Yes   8. My parent or guardian will bring my medication bottle in to every visit for a pill count. Once I have been cleared to come by myself, I will give my refill prescriptions directly to my parent or guardian. My parent or guardian will report a pill count by phone whenever requested.

❑ Yes   9. I will report my history and symptoms, including reports of side effects and cravings, honestly.

❑ Yes   10. I will not drive a car or use dangerous machinery while taking buprenorphine until I have been cleared to do so. I will request medical clearance prior to resuming any dangerous activities.

---

warned to avoid driving for the first few weeks of taking the medication because drowsiness has been reported as a side effect of buprenorphine.

BEHAVIORAL TREATMENTS

OUD is a complex illness that can impact every aspect of an adolescent's functioning. Because of the pervasive consequences of OUD, comprehensive treatment involves behavioral therapy in addition to medication. Options for behavioral therapy range from office-based management to hospitalization. The clinician performing an assessment can explore the patient's readiness for treatment (Miller 1998; "Treating Teens: A Guide to Adolescent Drug Programs" 2002), withdrawal risk, medical complications, psychiatric comorbidities, and home environment in an attempt to determine the least restrictive treatment setting.

Manual-driven protocols for psychotherapeutic treatment exist in the form of individual, group, and family therapy. These protocols often implement skills-based approaches via cognitive-behavioral therapy, which can be delivered at various levels of care (in outpatient settings, inpatient settings, or residential treatment programs) (Dasinger et al. 2004; Deas 2006; Kaminer et al. 2002). Long-term treatments may be provided in outpatient settings, but some patients require greater supervision in such settings as long-term residential facilities to achieve and maintain abstinence.

The American Academy of Child and Adolescent Psychiatry has developed a list of principles for adolescent treatment (Bukstein et al. 2005). Typically, treatment can be rendered at outpatient or inpatient/residential levels. These treatment levels are described in the following subsections.

In 2001, the American Society of Addiction Medicine (ASAM) revised its comprehensive national guidelines for placement, continued stay, and discharge of patients with alcohol and other drug problems. The separate guidelines devised for adults and adolescents detail five broad levels of care that range from early intervention to medically managed intensive inpatient treatment and correspond to addiction severity, related problems, and potential for behavior change and recovery (Mee-Lee 2013). Adolescents should be treated in the least restrictive environment (i.e., level of care) that supports their clinical needs. Adolescents who voluntarily accept therapeutic placement will usually engage more readily in their care, which is a key factor influencing SUD treatment success.

OUTPATIENT CARE

Outpatient care is the mainstay of substance abuse treatment for adolescents who are medically and behaviorally stable and may consist of individual, group, or family therapy alone or in combination. A variety of psychosocial therapies have been demonstrated to be effective in the treatment of SUDs (Table 13–2). Outpatient care varies in intensity. *Day treatment* or *intensive outpatient programs* and *partial hospitalization programs* are highly structured programs that meet for several hours each day for several weeks and generally combine both individual and group treatment. These programs usually are recommended for adolescents who are transitioning from inpatient care back into the community or for those who are in the early stages of the recovery process. *Office-based management* refers to less intensive treatment, with patients receiving individual and/or group therapy in sessions ranging from several times per week to several times per month (Bukstein et al. 2005; Dasinger et al. 2004; "Treating Teens: A Guide to Adolescent Drug Programs" 2002).

Psychiatric Hospitalization

Psychiatric hospitalization may be warranted for adolescents with unstable co-occurring mental illness. A full range of services, including assessment and consultation, psychopharmacology, family therapy, and recommendations or referrals for aftercare in an inpatient psychiatric treatment facility, can help to stabilize these patients (Deas 2006). Once medically stable, an adolescent may be a candidate for a less restrictive acute residential treatment (ART) program as an alternative to prolonged inpatient hospitalization. On the basis of a multimodal approach and therapeutic milieu model, ART programs work closely with parents and teens to build and strengthen interpersonal relationships, learn more about themselves through group therapy and classroom experience, and reinforce emerging healthy alternative behaviors for managing feelings and impulsive behaviors and avoiding substance use. Further evaluation to address specific concerns such as childhood trauma, eating disorders, learning disorders, and school conflict can be coordinated as necessary. The goal of an ART program is to promote transition from the therapeutic milieu back to the community (Hawthorne et al. 1999; Stevens and Morral 2013).

Long-Term Residential Programs

Long-term residential programs provide services over an average period of 3–12 months and offer a variety of daily therapeutic sessions, including individual, group, and family therapy as well as psychoeducation and psychopharmacology. They can accommodate adolescents with both psychiatric disorders and SUDs who have been unable to stop using opioids and/or who have other self-injurious behaviors. Locked facilities are available for youth at risk of running away (Bukstein et al. 2005).

TABLE 13–2. **Description of various psychosocial therapies**

Therapy	Description	Mechanisms
Psychoeducation	Helps patient access and learn strategies to deal with substance abuse and mental illness and their effects	Used in conjunction with other forms of treatment as a tool for understanding a patient's illness Helps patients gain self-awareness, identify community resources, and develop a better understanding of the steps of recovery
Cognitive-behavioral therapy[a]	Designed to teach skills for maintaining abstinence by identifying and modifying thoughts and feelings that precede substance use and trying new ways of behaving	Manual-based, structured therapy Teaches patients to use refusal skills or avoid risky situations Patients record events, feelings, thoughts, behaviors Identifies and helps changes unrealistic assumptions and habits
Motivation enhancement therapy[a]	Patient-centered approach aimed at resolving ambivalence about engaging in treatment or stopping drugs	Stimulates discussion about personal substance use Evokes internally motivated change statements Embraces a dynamic and fluctuating view of willingness or readiness to change Encourages small steps toward larger goals
Group therapy	Provides a cost-effective, "safe" environment in which to examine issues related to peer pressure and relationships	Offers the feeling of "safety in numbers" for adolescents Facilitates interpersonal and intrapersonal growth through the use of the group dynamic Developmentally normal preference among adolescents Member must be screened to determine group appropriateness
12-step fellowships (AA, NA, Alateen)	Peer-based support that uses the 12-step model	Allows members to share their experiences, strengths, and hopes Adolescents should have an appropriate sponsor Adult meetings may not be appropriate for certain adolescents

TABLE 13–2. **Description of various psychosocial therapies** *(continued)*

Therapy	Description	Mechanisms
Multidimensional family therapy[a]	Form of family therapy specifically designed to treat adolescents with substance abuse and behavioral problems	Manual-based therapy with up to four individual and family sessions per week Utilizes intensive advocacy and phone contact with the adolescent's school and the court system
Brief strategic family therapy[a]	Designed to prevent, reduce, and/or treat adolescent drug use, high-risk sexual behaviors, conduct problems, delinquency, violence, and other problems	Aims to improve family functioning (effective, positive parenting) and improve adolescent prosocial behaviors (school attendance and performance)
Multisystemic therapy[a]	Intensive 4-month program addressing needs of youth at high risk of incarceration or foster care	Integrates comprehensive psychiatric and substance abuse services with in-home family sessions
Contingency management	Based on the behavioral principle that good behaviors, when rewarded (in a positive and supportive manner), are likely to be repeated	Requires that patients be called weekly, at random, to provide urine specimens and rewards them for each negative specimen Adolescent-appropriate rewards can include gift certificates, clothing, music, sports equipment, or movie theater tickets
Therapeutic communities	Therapeutic community model enhanced to meet the developmental needs of teenagers ages 13–17 with substance use, mental health, and behavioral disorders	Integrates residential treatment with on-site public school education at the junior high and senior high school level Some programs may include trade or technical training sponsored by local community colleges

Note.   AA = Alcoholics Anonymous; NA = Narcotics Anonymous.
[a]Indicates evidence-based practices (EBPs). See www.uncg.edu/csr/asatp/ebpmatrix.pdf for the complete matrix of EBPs with links to more information.

THERAPEUTIC COMMUNITIES

Therapeutic communities are drug-free residential settings that provide treatment for adolescents with addictions and behavioral disorders who have failed to respond to less intensive treatments and are unable to live at home. Adolescents treated in therapeutic community programs are more likely than those in outpatient programs to have prior addiction treatment experience and criminal justice histories and are likely to have experienced more severe consequences. These closely supervised programs are typically longer than residential programs (12–24 months) and use a hierarchical model that reflects increased levels of personal and social responsibility that are acquired as progress is made through the various levels of treatment (Morral et al. 2004). Therapeutic communities differ from other treatment approaches mainly through their use of community and peer interactions as a means of learning and assimilating new attitudes, perceptions, and behaviors previously associated with drug use. However, modifications may be required to accommodate adolescent developmental differences, such as including on-site schooling and family support services.

Conclusion

Adolescence is a time of physical, emotional, and psychological maturation, and experimentation with risky behaviors is common. Screening for substance use, including opioids, is a recommended component of routine medical care for adolescents. Adolescents who have used opioids but whose use does not meet criteria for severe opioid use disorder (OUD) may benefit from relatively brief office-based interventions. Adolescents whose use does meet criteria for severe OUD should have a thorough assessment before beginning treatment. Although promising treatment interventions are emerging, additional research is needed to evaluate behavioral and pharmacological treatment options. This research will help identify how to best minimize opioid withdrawal symptoms and promote treatment retention and long-term opioid abstinence in the context of the maturing adolescent brain. Few medication studies have included adolescents, but accumulating evidence suggests that buprenorphine can be effective in reducing relapse rates with adolescent populations by stabilizing neurochemistry, ameliorating withdrawal, and curbing cravings.

Clinical Pearls

- Opioid use, addiction, and overdose continue to be a problem for adolescents and young adults.

- Several validated screening tools for adolescent substance use are available. Newer, frequency-based screens are efficient at determining risk level of individual substances and guiding intervention.

- Pain medication can be safe for use even in adolescents with substance use disorders (SUDs), and pain should not be left untreated because of a history of SUD. However, increased supervision and monitoring to avoid misuse is recommended for all patients with SUDs.

- No single approach is suitable for all individuals; treatment should be comprehensive and tailored to the particular needs of the individual. In most cases, treatment should include medication in conjunction with evidence-based behavioral therapies. Screening for psychiatric and medical comorbidities is recommended.

- Few medication studies have included adolescents, but accumulating evidence suggests that buprenorphine can be effective in reducing relapse rates with adolescent populations by stabilizing neurochemistry, ameliorating withdrawal, and curbing cravings.

- A combination of behavioral therapy and medication is recommended and can be delivered in settings ranging from office-based management to the hospital level of care.

- Psychoactive substances can induce, mimic, co-occur with, and/or exacerbate underlying mental illness; therefore, evaluation for co-occurring mental health disorders and appropriate treatment is recommended.

CASE 13

Tommy is a 16-year-old male who started intravenous heroin use when he was 13. He now uses up to 15 bags of heroin a day, has previously undergone two failed treatments for opioid withdrawal, and has some very serious legal jeopardy hinged on his remaining sober. Both of his parents are in AA and oppose "using drugs to treat an addiction." He smokes marijuana from time to time but does not drink or use other drugs. He was referred to your clinic by the drug court.

1. How does the approach to OUD differ in an adolescent?

2. Can you legally prescribe buprenorphine to a 16-year-old?

3. Is parental consent a requirement?

4. What is a reasonable treatment goal in this case?

References

American Psychiatric Association: Diagnostic and Statistical Manual of Mental Disorders, 4th Edition, Text Revision. Arlington, VA, American Psychiatric Association, 2000

American Psychiatric Association: Diagnostic and Statistical Manual of Mental Disorders, 5th Edition. Arlington, VA, American Psychiatric Association, 2013

Boyd CJ, McCabe SE, Cranford JA, Young A: Adolescents' motivations to abuse prescription medications. Pediatrics 118(6):2472–2480, 2006 17142533

Bukstein OG, Bernet W, Arnold V, et al: Practice parameter for the assessment and treatment of children and adolescents with substance use disorders. J Am Acad Child Adolesc Psychiatry 44(6):609–621, 2005 15908844

Catalano RF, Morrison DM, Wells EA, et al: Ethnic differences in family factors related to early drug initiation. J Stud Alcohol 53(3):208–217, 1992 1285743

Center for Behavioral Health Statistics and Quality: 2014 National Survey on Drug Use and Health: Detailed Tables. Rockville, MD, Substance Abuse and Mental Health Services Administration, 2015

Center for Behavioral Health Statistics and Quality: Key Substance Use and Mental Health Indicators in the United States: Results From the 2015 National Survey on Drug Use and Health. Rockville, MD, Substance Abuse and Mental Health Services Administration, 2016

Center for Substance Abuse Treatment: Triage and placement in treatment services, in SAMHSA/CSAT Treatment Improvement Protocols. Rockville, MD, Substance Abuse and Mental Health Services Administration, 1999a

Center for Substance Abuse Treatment: Therapeutic communities, in SAMHSA/CSAT Treatment Improvement Protocols. Rockville, MD, Substance Abuse and Mental Health Services Administration, 1999b

Center for Substance Abuse Treatment: Services in Intensive Outpatient Treatment Programs. Rockville, MD, Substance Abuse and Mental Health Services Administration, 2006

Chang G, Kosten T: Treatment approaches, in Substance Abuse: A Comprehensive Textbook. Edited by Lowinson J, Ruiz P, Millman R, et al. New York, Lippincott Williams and Wilkins, 2005, pp 579–586

Cicero TJ, Ellis MS, Surratt HL, et al: The changing face of heroin use in the United States: a retrospective analysis of the past 50 years. JAMA Psychiatry 71(7):821–826, 2014 24871348

Colson J, Helm S, Silverman SM: Office-based opioid dependence treatment. Pain Physician 15(3 suppl):ES231–ES236, 2012 22786460

Committee on Substance Use and Prevention: Medication-assisted treatment of adolescents with opioid use disorders. Pediatrics Sept 138(3), August 22, 2016 27550978 [Epub ahead of print]

Currie SR, Patten SB, Williams JV, et al: Comorbidity of major depression with substance use disorders. Can J Psychiatry 50(10):660–666, 2005 16276858

Dasinger LK, Shane PA, Martinovich Z: Assessing the effectiveness of community-based substance abuse treatment for adolescents. J Psychoactive Drugs 36(1):27–33, 2004 15152707

Deas D: Adolescent substance abuse and psychiatric comorbidities. J Clin Psychiatry 67 (suppl 7):18–23, 2006 16961420

Fiellin DA: Treatment of adolescent opioid dependence: no quick fix. JAMA 300(17):2057–2059, 2008 18984896

Fiellin DA, O'Connor PG, Chawarski M, et al: Methadone maintenance in primary care: a randomized controlled trial. JAMA 286(14):1724–1731, 2001 11594897

Fournier ME, Levy S: Recent trends in adolescent substance use, primary care screening, and updates in treatment options. Curr Opin Pediatr 18(4):352–358, 2006 16914986

Fudala PJ, Bridge TP, Herbert S, et al: Office-based treatment of opiate addiction with a sublingual-tablet formulation of buprenorphine and naloxone. N Engl J Med 349(10):949–958, 2003 12954743

Goodwin RD, Stayner DA, Chinman MJ, et al: The relationship between anxiety and substance use disorders among individuals with severe affective disorders. Compr Psychiatry 43(4):245–252, 2002 12107861

Hawthorne WB, Green EE, Lohr JB, et al: Comparison of outcomes of acute care in short-term residential treatment and psychiatric hospital settings. Psychiatr Serv 50(3):401–406, 1999 10096647

Hertz JA, Knight JR: Prescription drug misuse: a growing national problem. Adolesc Med Clin 17(3):751–769, abstract xiii, 2006 17030290

Hingson RW, Heeren T, Winter MR: Age at drinking onset and alcohol dependence: age at onset, duration, and severity. Arch Pediatr Adolesc Med 160(7):739–746, 2006 16818840

Hopfer CJ, Khuri E, Crowley TJ, et al: Adolescent heroin use: a review of the descriptive and treatment literature. J Subst Abuse Treat 23(3):231–237, 2002 12392810

Hopfer CJ, Khuri E, Crowley TJ: Treating adolescent heroin use. J Am Acad Child Adolesc Psychiatry 42(5):609–611, 2003 12707565

Institute of Medicine Committee on Federal Regulation of Methadone Treatment: Who are the recipients of treatment?, in Federal Regulation of Methadone Treatment. Edited by Rettig RA, Yarmolinksy A. Washington, DC, National Academies Press, 1995

Jasinski DR, Pevnick JS, Griffith JD: Human pharmacology and abuse potential of the analgesic buprenorphine: a potential agent for treating narcotic addiction. Arch Gen Psychiatry 35(4):501–516, 1978 215096

Jaycox LH, Ebener P, Damesek L, et al: Trauma exposure and retention in adolescent substance abuse treatment. J Trauma Stress 17(2):113–121, 2004 15141784

Johnston LD: Monitoring the Future National Survey Results on Drug Use, 1975–2015: Overview, Key Findings on Adolescent Drug Use. Ann Arbor, MI, University of Michigan Institute for Social Research, 2016

Kaminer Y, Burleson JA, Goldberger R: Cognitive-behavioral coping skills and psychoeducation therapies for adolescent substance abuse. J Nerv Ment Dis 190(11):737–745, 2002 12436013

Kelly SM, Gryczynski J, Mitchell SG, et al: Validity of brief screening instrument for adolescent tobacco, alcohol, and drug use. Pediatrics 133(5):819–826, 2014 24753528

Knight JR, Sherritt L, Harris SK, et al: Validity of brief alcohol screening tests among adolescents: a comparison of the AUDIT, POSIT, CAGE, and CRAFFT. Alcohol Clin Exp Res 27(1):67–73, 2003 12544008

Knight JR, Sherritt L, Van Hook S, et al: Motivational interviewing for adolescent substance use: a pilot study. J Adolesc Health 37(2):167–169, 2005 16026730

Levy SJ, Kokotailo PK; Committee on Substance Abuse: Substance use screening, brief intervention, and referral to treatment for pediatricians. Pediatrics 128(5):e1330–e1340, 2011 22042818

Levy S, Weiss R, Sherritt L, et al: An electronic screen for triaging adolescent substance use by risk levels. JAMA Pediatr 168(9):822–828, 2014 25070067

Levy SL, Williams JF, Committee on Substance Use and Prevention: Substance use screening, brief intervention, and referral to treatment. Pediatrics 138(1), 2016 27325634 [Epub ahead of print]

Levy S, Harris SK, Sherritt L, et al: Drug testing of adolescents in ambulatory medicine: physician practices and knowledge. Arch Pediatr Adolesc Med 160(2):146–150, 2006 16461869

Lynskey MT, Heath AC, Bucholz KK, et al: Escalation of drug use in early onset cannabis users vs co-twin controls. JAMA 289(4):427–433, 2003 12533121

Marsch LA: Treatment of adolescents, in Treatment of Opioid Dependence. Edited by Marsch LA, Strain E, Stitzer M. Baltimore, MD, Johns Hopkins University Press, 2005, pp 497–507

Marsch LA, Bickel WK, Badger GJ, et al: Comparison of pharmacological treatments for opioid-dependent adolescents: a randomized controlled trial. Arch Gen Psychiatry 62(10):1157–1164, 2005 16203961

Mattick RP, Ali R, White JM, et al: Buprenorphine versus methadone maintenance therapy: a randomized double-blind trial with 405 opioid-dependent patients. Addiction 98(4):441–452, 2003 12653814

Mattick RP, Breen C, Kimber J, Davoli M: Buprenorphine maintenance versus placebo or methadone maintenance for opioid dependence. Cochrane Database of Systematic Reviews 2014, Issue 2, Art. No.: CD002207, DOI: 10.1002/14651858.CD002207.pub4

Mee-Lee D (ed): The ASAM Criteria: Treatment Criteria for Addictive, Substance-Related, and Co-occurring Conditions. Carson City, NV, The Change Companies, 2013

Miller WR: Why do people change addictive behavior? The 1996 H. David Archibald Lecture. Addiction 93(2):163–172, 1998 9624719

Morral AR, McCaffrey DF, Ridgeway G: Effectiveness of community-based treatment for substance-abusing adolescents: 12-month outcomes of youths entering phoenix academy or alternative probation dispositions. Psychol Addict Behav 18(3):257–268, 2004 15482081

Muhuri PK, Gfroerer JC, Davies CM: Associations of Nonmedical Pain Reliever Use and Initiation of Heroin Use in the United States. Rockville, MD, CBHSQ Data Review, 2013

Nemecek D, Lopez WM, Blank AR: CIGNA Standards and Guidelines/Medical Necessity Criteria: For Treatment of Behavioral Health and Ssubstance Use Disorders. Eden Prairie, MN, CIGNA Behavioral Health, 2015

Oetting ER, Beauvais F: Peer cluster theory, socialization characteristics, and adolescent drug use: a path analysis. J Couns Psychol 34(2):205–213, 1987

Rowan AB, Fudala PJ, Mulligan J: The medical management of adolescent heroin dependence. Curr Psychiatry Rep 2(6):527–530, 2000 11123006

Sees KL, Delucchi KL, Masson C, et al: Methadone maintenance vs 180-day psychosocially enriched detoxification for treatment of opioid dependence: a randomized controlled trial. JAMA 283(10):1303–1310, 2000 10714729

Stevens S, Morral A: Adolescent Substance Abuse Treatment in the United States: Exemplary Models from a National Evaluation Study. New York, Routledge, 2013

Teichman M, Kefir E: The effects of perceived parental behaviors, attitudes, and substance-use on adolescent attitudes toward and intent to use psychoactive substances. J Drug Educ 30(2):193–204, 2000 10920598

Treating Teens: A Guide to Adolescent Drug Programs. San Francisco, CA, Drug Strategies, 2002

Vaughan BL, Knight JR: Intensive drug treatment, in Adolescent Healthcare: A Practical Guide, 5th Edition. Edited by Neinstein LS, Gordon C, Katzman D. Philadelphia, PA, Lippincott Williams and Wilkins, 2009, pp 671–675

Weinberg NZ: Risk factors for adolescent substance abuse. J Learn Disabil 34(4):343–351, 2001 15503578

Wilens TE, Faraone SV, Biederman J, et al: Does stimulant therapy of attention-deficit/hyperactivity disorder beget later substance abuse? A meta-analytic review of the literature. Pediatrics 111(1):179–185, 2003 12509574

Wilens TE, Biederman J, Kwon A, et al: Risk of substance use disorders in adolescents with bipolar disorder. J Am Acad Child Adolesc Psychiatry 43(11):1380–1386, 2004 15502597

Wilson CR, Sherritt L, Gates E, et al: Are clinical impressions of adolescent substance use accurate? Pediatrics 114(5):e536–e540, 2004 15520086

Woody GE, Poole SA, Subramaniam G, et al: Extended vs short-term buprenorphine-naloxone for treatment of opioid-addicted youth: a randomized trial. JAMA 300(17):2003–2011, 2008 18984887

14

Women's Health and Pregnancy

Anna T. LaRose, M.D.
Hendrée E. Jones, Ph.D.

THROUGHOUT history and across cultures, women have typically used less alcohol and fewer illicit psychoactive substances than men. This fact may be due to differences in physiology, women's roles as caretakers, and the impact of psychoactive substances on fetal development in pregnancy. However, sedative and opioid use in the United States by women during the 1800s was fairly high compared with men's use, in large part because women were more likely than men to be prescribed such substances by their health care providers. More recently, with the advent of prescription medications, patterns of illicit substance use began to shift.

In the present day, history again repeats itself, with women being vulnerable to the use and consequences of nonmedical use of prescription opioids. For example, although more men than women are likely to die of a prescription narcotic overdose, the percentage increase in deaths between 1999 and 2010 was greater among women than among men. Factors that may contribute to the severity of current prescription medication misuse include 1) large increases in the number of prescriptions written and dispensed, 2) greater social acceptability of medication use for a variety of health and mental health issues, 3) aggressive marketing by pharmaceutical companies, and 4) health care providers lacking adequate training in the overlap between pain and addiction and the risks of opioid use disorder (OUD) and how to treat individuals who have it. In addition to prescription opioid misuse, women also use illicit opioids, and those who do are at higher risk for medical and psychiatric complications. As the use of illicit substances and misuse of prescription medications increase in the female population, it is important to investigate use patterns, treatment, and recovery of women. In this chapter, we primarily discuss opioid use in women, including information about opioid use epidemiology in women; issues important in treating women with OUD; and pharmacotherapy of opioid use in pregnancy, with a focus on key aspects of the use of buprenorphine-naloxone (BUP/NX).

Epidemiology of Opioid Use Disorders

The most recent findings from the National Survey on Drug Use and Health (NSDUH) show that rates of substance use among males were greater than those among females. However, use among females has increased over the years. In addition, adolescent males and females have similar rates of substance use. In the general population, rates for lifetime and past-year nonmedical prescription opioid use were 14% and 5%, respectively. Men were found to be 1.3 times more likely to have past-year use than women, although findings from other studies are conflicting (Back et al. 2010).

According to 2011 data from the Drug Abuse Warning Network (Substance Abuse and Mental Health Services Administration 2013), more than one million emergency department (ED) visits annually involved illicit psychoactive substances, and a similar number of ED visits involved nonmedical use of prescription medications. The long-term trend shows increases in ED visits due to nonmedical use of prescription medications. Almost 40% of ED visits for nonmedical use of prescription medications are due to opioids. Females make up about half of the ED visits for substance use, although data suggest that fewer females present to EDs for heroin overdose than do males.

Deaths due to prescription opioid use have consistently been greater than overdose deaths due to heroin use in part because more people have access to opioid medications. More than 50% of overdose deaths in 2013 were due to prescription medications, and of those, more than 70% were due to opioid medications. Rates for prescription overdose deaths in females exceeded 6,000 in 2010 and increased by 400% from 1999 to 2010, whereas the corresponding increase for men was 263% (Centers for Disease Control and Prevention 2013, 2015). Although there are more overdose deaths due to prescription opioids than to heroin, heroin deaths tripled from 2010 to 2013. These rates of heroin-related overdose deaths increased in both men and women, with a larger increase in men.

When treatment admissions are considered, the Treatment Episode Data Set shows that in 2011 about a third of individuals seeking general substance abuse treatment were women. Slightly more women seek treatment for heroin use than for prescription opioid use, although significantly more women than men seek treatment for prescription medication use. When seeking treatment, women ages 18–24 and ages 25–34 had the highest rates of nonmedical use of prescription analgesics as primary substances of use. Women older than 65 years had three times higher rates of nonmedical prescription analgesics use compared with men in their cohort (Substance Abuse and Mental Health Services Administration 2014b).

Although males have significantly higher rates of substance use and substance use disorders (SUDs), recent data show that relative to men, women are using illicit psychoactive substances in increasing numbers and have equivalent rates of ED visits for psychoactive use. Adolescent females and males have equivalent rates of substance use. Women are more likely to use prescription opioids than to use heroin, yet rates of death from heroin have increased in women in recent years. Women generally seek treatment for OUD less often than do men, and women are more likely than men to seek treatment for nonmedical prescription opioid use. Given these alarming trends, addressing the special needs of women who use opioids is an important concern in clinical practice.

Screening for Opioid Use Disorder in Women

Screening for opioid use in women is an important part of medical assessment (Jones et al. 2014). Generally, substance use screening tools that were developed for the general population are less sensitive in detecting such use in women (Suarez Ordoñez et al. 2015). In addition, there is some evidence that self-administered tools may be more informative and accurate than face-to-face screening in women (Ondersma et al. 2014). One of the screening tools that has been studied in women that includes assessment of substance use is the Texas Christian University Drug Screen II (TCUDS II). Validated screening tools for the general adult population include the National Institute on Drug Abuse (NIDA) Drug Use Screening Tool, the CAGE-AID (CAGE adapted to include drugs), and the Drug Abuse Screening Test (DAST-10). Prenatal substance abuse screening includes use of the 5Ps (peers, partner [with problem], parents, past use, and present use). When the clinician is assessing for OUD, it is important to assess for co-occurring SUDs, medical consequences of use, and psychiatric issues because these problems occur at higher rates in women than in men with SUDs (National Institute on Drug Abuse 2015; Substance Abuse and Mental Health Services Administration 2009).

When women are being screened for substance use, they must be approached in a nonjudgmental way, and questions about substance use need to be normalized and asked at initial patient contact with all women. Furthermore, substance use occurs on a continuum from no use to a severe use disorder. Thus, not all women who use substances need treatment. However, in women who are pregnant, there can be greater maternal and fetal consequences of tobacco, alcohol, and psychoactive substance use, and the levels of such use that becomes a concern are generally lower than for nonpregnant women.

Special Issues in Women With Substance Use Disorders

Women face unique medical, psychological, and psychosocial challenges that can impact substance use and treatment seeking. Unlike their male counterparts, women are less likely to use for purely recreational purposes and are less likely to use intravenously. Women are more likely than men to use psychoactive substances to alleviate depression and anxiety. Women who use substances have been found to have high rates of childhood and adult trauma. They also have higher rates of mood disorders and posttraumatic stress disorder (PTSD) than the general population. Women who use substances are also especially vulnerable to trauma when they use, including assault, rape, and intimate partner violence (Substance Abuse and Mental Health Services Administration 2009).

Although women have lower rates of substance use and SUDs than do men, the phase from initiation to an SUD diagnosis is thought to progress more rapidly in women for a number of substances, including alcohol, marijuana, and opioids. This phenomenon is known as *telescoping*. As use escalates, women are at high risk for medical and psychiatric sequelae of substance use. They have a greater risk of harm from use given the metabolism of substances (due to differences in body weight and composition versus males) and physiological vulnerability to harmful consequences of substance use (Greenfield et al. 2010).

General Considerations When Treating Women With SUDs

When women enter SUD treatment, their medical and/or psychological functioning may be severely compromised. Treatment for SUDs should be offered in conjunction with medical and psychiatric treatment. Awareness of the specific needs of women is crucial. Women with SUDs face more stigma from providers and the general public, especially if they have children. Stigma can lead to guilt, shame, and social isolation and prevent women from seeking treatment for their substance use. Social relationships also can hinge on use, and relationships are very important for women's mental health. Minimizing stigma and creating a strong therapeutic alliance are critical to the effective treatment of women with SUDs. In addition, women often take on the role of primary caretakers in our society. For women to enter into and engage in treatment, securing resources for their children, grandchildren, and/or elderly parents may be necessary. Furthermore, women do not always have financial independence and in general earn less than men. They often depend on partners, who often are not supportive of their recovery. Addressing financial barriers is another important aspect of treating women.

Psychosocial treatments, including psychotherapy, are important to offer to women with SUDs. Women can benefit from both individual and group therapy for SUDs as well as for psychiatric disorders, including PTSD, especially given the quicker progression of SUDs of women seeking treatment and psychiatric comorbidities found in many women with SUDs. Also, certain women, especially women with histories of trauma, may choose to have female providers and may prefer women-only groups; these services should be easily available in clinics treating women. Women-only groups can be helpful because the many topics of interest to women can be addressed, and women may feel more at ease in single-gender groups. Limited data have shown that gender-specific group therapy for women is at least equivalent in efficacy to mixed-gender groups (Greenfield et al. 2014).

Pregnancy is a critical time to address substance use in women. In general, pregnancy is often a time when women with SUDs seek treatment, yet national and state legislation around reporting substance use during pregnancy and plans of safe care reporting and monitoring create barriers to treatment for many women. Discussing these issues with female patients and determining specific state requirements is necessary when providing treatment services for women with SUDs.

BRIEF INTERVENTIONS

A *brief intervention* is a very time limited intervention that can be used for both pregnant and nonpregnant women. The intervention can be a single session of a few minutes aiming to provide education and feedback to the patient about substance use and its dangers. It also can consist of multiple sessions focused on increasing the patient's motivation to change her substance use behaviors. Although brief interventions may be effective with light or moderate substance use, many women using substances regularly may be in need of referral to specialized treatment.

PHARMACOTHERAPY FOR OPIOID USE DISORDERS IN WOMEN

In terms of pharmacotherapy for OUDs, a general approach to first-line treatment for women is similar to first-line treatment for men and includes opioid agonist pharmacotherapy with either methadone or BUP/NX. Given the availability of BUP/NX in the doctor's office, its lower misuse liability, and the ability to transfer to methadone if buprenorphine proves inadequate for treatment, BUP/NX is an excellent choice for many women with OUDs. Every patient's medication decision needs to be an individualized one between patient and provider.

There are limited studies in women and opioid agonist pharmacotherapy; of the studies that include men and women, women typically make up about a fifth of the samples, and few of the studies have examined sex differences. Most studies have found no treatment response difference in men versus women. In a randomized controlled trial (RCT) comparing medications that included methadone and BUP/NX, there were significant decreases in self-reported illicit opioid use for both women and men within both the BUP/NX and methadone medication conditions, indicating that both medications benefit both sexes. However, women receiving BUP/NX had less objective substance use than women receiving methadone, and within the BUP/NX condition, women had significantly fewer opioid-positive urine screening test results than did men (Jones et al. 2005b). This finding may be in part a result of sex differences in buprenorphine's pharmacokinetics, differences in body composition, differences in cytochrome P450–dependent metabolism (Moody et al. 2011), interaction of estrogen and progesterone with buprenorphine, and differences in opioid binding capacity (Zubieta et al. 1999).

For methadone, a literature review concluded that with methadone, reported volume-of-distribution differences are likely related to differences between the body weight and composition of men and women; however, no direct pharmacodynamic parameters were related to sex (Graziani and Nisticò 2015). There is also no specific dosing adjustment in women compared with men with BUP/NX. One small retrospective study found that females given the same doses of BUP/NX as males had a higher concentration of buprenorphine and its metabolites than did the males, but there is no research to date supporting a relationship between BUP/NX dose and treatment response in women (Moody et al. 2011).

Pregnant women provided pharmacotherapy with either methadone or buprenorphine may require dose increases as pregnancy advances because of increasing blood volume and hormonal enzyme induction. In pregnant women taking buprenorphine, the mono formulation is recommended by most experts over the BUP/NX combination product because of the concern regarding limited preclinical data showing fetal and maternal hormone changes. However, there are no clear data supporting this recommendation. A review of seven various trials showed no significant maternal outcomes for women exposed to BUP/NX compared with buprenorphine alone (Lund et al. 2013). In the same review, the only significant neonatal outcomes found were shorter neonates in the BUP/NX group compared with the buprenorphine-alone group and lower 5-minute Apgar scores in the BUP/NX group compared with the buprenorphine-alone group, although both neonatal length and Apgar scores were considered to be within normal ranges in both groups. If a woman becomes pregnant, switching to the buprenorphine mono product is an option if there are concerns about prenatal exposure to naloxone. If only BUP/NX is available, if the patient does not want to switch from BUP/NX to the mono product, or if there are concerns about diversion of the mono product, the risks and benefits should be discussed with the patient, and the provider can consider continuing BUP/NX, especially if the alternative is discontinuation of all pharmacological treatment of the OUD in the pregnant patient.

In general, buprenorphine shows fewer drug interactions than does methadone (Jones et al. 2008b), and when such interactions do occur, they appear to increase the effects of buprenorphine. Of particular concern is the interaction between buprenorphine (and methadone) and benzodiazepines. Concurrent use of both substances can lead to increased risk of medical complications and, in extreme cases, death.

Finally, the only FDA-approved medication alternative to opioid agonist treatment for OUD is naltrexone. Naltrexone also can be used in both men and women and has a small yet important place in the medications offered, but it is usually offered as a second-line treatment (Ayanga et al. 2016). There are no studies to date for use of naltrexone for OUD in pregnant women.

Pregnancy and Opioid Use

EPIDEMIOLOGY

The most recent findings from the NSDUH, from combined 2012–2013 data, show that 5.4% of pregnant women ages 15–44 used illicit substances, with younger women using more frequently than older women (14.6% of pregnant women ages 15–17 vs. 3.2% of pregnant women ages 26–44) (Substance Abuse and Mental Health Services Administration 2014a). Recent data on opioid use in pregnant women are limited because subgroup analysis is not often reported, but pregnant women have not been excluded from the most recent opioid use epidemic. Maternal use of heroin or nonmedical use of opioid analgesics led to prenatal exposure of approximately 53,400 neonates in 1992 (National Institute on Drug Abuse 1996). In addition, it is notable that in 2012, 22.9% of pregnant women entering substance use treatment reported any heroin use, and 28.1% reported any non-heroin opioid misuse (Smith and Lipari 2017). The number of women discharged with a diagnosis of OUD at delivery in the United States increased from 1.2 to 5.6 per 1,000 births annually from 2000 through 2009, correlating with an increase in the diagnosis of neonatal abstinence syndrome (NAS; Patrick et al. 2012).

PHARMACOTHERAPY FOR OPIOID USE DISORDER IN PREGNANCY

Opioid Agonist Medications: Methadone and Buprenorphine

Methadone and buprenorphine have no restrictions on their product labels for use during pregnancy, although they have warnings related to neonatal absence syndrome (neonatal opioid withdrawal syndrome; U.S. Food and Drug Administration 2016), and their use is not considered to be "off label" in that context (Jones et al. 2014). Over the past half-century, significant benefits of these medications have been shown compared with no pharmacological treatment. In contrast to untreated OUD during pregnancy, methadone treatment has been related to more obstetrical care contact, greater fetal growth, lower fetal mortality, lower HIV infection risk, lower preeclampsia risk, and fewer opportunities for fetal exposure to rapid and unpredictable cycles of illicit opioid–induced highs and withdrawal. Under conditions where medication-free and methadone treatment are both available, methadone is associated with longer treatment retention and less relapse (Jones et al. 2008b). Finally, a meta-analysis and systematic review of the literature showed that the relationship between methadone dose and either incidence or severity of neonatal abstinence syndrome is not conclusive (Cleary et al. 2010). Thus, providing appropriate opioid agonist pharmacotherapy during pregnancy may attenuate adverse consequences of nonprescribed opioid use, for mother, fetus, and neonate.

The literature indicates that both methadone and buprenorphine have benefits for the mother, fetus, and newborn. The largest RCT on this topic showed no significant differences in maternal outcomes between the two medications. This study, the Maternal Opioid Treatment: Human Experimental Research (MOTHER) study, provided the most rigorous data to date to support the relative safety and efficacy of methadone as well as the relative safety and efficacy of buprenorphine during pregnancy. In terms of abstinence from opioids, two randomized clinical trials, Pregnancy and Reduction of Opiates: Medication Intervention Safety and Efficacy (PROMISE) and MOTHER, have shown high rates of abstinence from illicit opioids in mothers during the prenatal period. With buprenorphine, 9% (5 of 58) of the MOTHER participants and 0% (0 of 9) of the PROMISE participants tested positive for illicit opioids at delivery. For methadone, 15% (11 of 73) of the MOTHER participants and 0% (0 of 11) of the PROMISE participants tested positive for illicit opioids at delivery. The difference between the buprenorphine and methadone conditions on the substance use measures was not significant in either the MOTHER or PROMISE studies.

In the MOTHER study, approximately 50% of neonates were treated for NAS, and there were no differences in the rates at which the neonates in the buprenorphine (47% [27 of 58]) and methadone (57% [41 of 73]) conditions were treated for NAS, suggesting that the rates at which neonates were exposed to either medication are comparable. The mean total amount of morphine given to MOTHER neonates of buprenorphine-maintained mothers during the course of their NAS treatment was 2.8 mg, whereas in the PROMISE study, an equivalent mean total of 0.47 mg of morphine was administered to the two neonates of buprenorphine-maintained mothers treated for NAS. Finally, it is important to note that the MOTHER study showed that neonates prenatally exposed to buprenorphine had a significantly shorter mean hospital stay and a significantly shorter duration of NAS treatment than did neonates prenatally exposed to methadone (Jones et al. 2005a, 2010b) (Figure 14–1).

Two secondary studies examined the neurobehavioral development of prenatal buprenorphine-exposed neonates using the Neonatal Intensive Care Unit Network Neurobehavioral Scale (NNNS), with both PROMISE (Jones et al. 2005a) and MOTHER (Jones et al. 2010b) results suggesting improved neurobehavioral functioning in buprenorphine-exposed neonates relative to methadone-exposed neonates (Coyle et al. 2012; Jones et al. 2010a). In addition, preliminary analysis suggests that buprenorphine treatment may be more cost-effective than treatment with methadone when savings from costs associated with NAS, preterm birth, and intrauterine growth restriction are taken into account (John et al. 2017).

Opioid Antagonist Medication: Naltrexone

Many features of the opioid antagonist naltrexone make it highly attractive as a treatment for OUD. Therapeutic doses of naltrexone are devoid of misuse potential, produce blockade of the euphoric effects of opioid agonists, have a benign adverse effect profile, and do not result in tolerance developing over time. Naltrexone has been slow to be used by clinicians. As this medication gains acceptance, it is likely that women will become pregnant while receiving it or women will seek this medication as a part of their treatment for OUD during pregnancy. There are presently no published protocols that can provide guid-

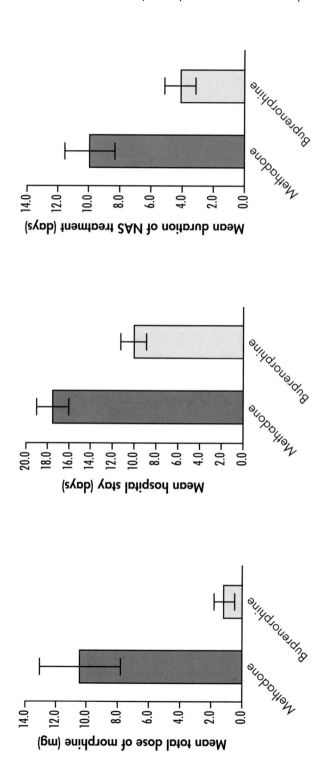

FIGURE 14–1.   **Mean neonatal morphine dose, length of neonatal hospital stay, and duration of treatment for neonatal abstinence syndrome.**

Source.   From Jones HE, Kaltenbach K, Heil SH, et al.: "Neonatal abstinence syndrome after methadone or buprenorphine exposure." New England Journal of Medicine, 363(24):2327, 2010, Figure 2, http://www.nejm.org/doi/full/10.1056/NEJMoa1005359. Copyright © 2010, Massachusetts Medical Society. Reprinted with permission.

ance in these cases, nor are there studies of safety or efficacy for use of naltrexone in pregnancy.

PAIN MANAGEMENT DURING LABOR AND DELIVERY

Pain management during labor and delivery should be provided in the safest and most effective way possible, consistent with the patient's desires. For patients maintained on opioid agonist medication, analgesic needs should be based on the clinical evaluation of the patient and not on the prescribed dose of opioid agonist medication. For both opioid and non-opioid substance-using women, multimodal therapy for postoperative pain management can be beneficial and typically involves some combination of nonsteroidal anti-inflammatory medications (beginning with an intraoperative ketorolac dose, if appropriate), spinal or epidural morphine, and acetaminophen with or without patient-controlled analgesia (PCA) for breakthrough pain. If spinal or epidural morphine is used, then PCA should be provided by demand only, and the patient should be carefully monitored for respiratory depression.

MOTHER-INFANT DYAD

A critical issue that we have failed to address up until this point is the need to weigh the impact of any treatment on mother, fetus, and child. Despite debate regarding whether or not the fetus is a patient separate from the mother, McCullough and Chervenak (2011) have noted: "The pregnant and fetal patients are not separate patients, because beneficence-based obligations to the fetal patient *and* beneficence-based obligations to the pregnant women must *always* be taken into account in clinical ethical obstetric judgment" (p. W3). In addressing the needs of pregnant women with SUDs, treatment should be focused on providing supportive, dyadic-centered newborn services to optimize pregnancy outcomes.

NEONATAL ABSTINENCE SYNDROME

Signs and Symptoms

The number of newborns with NAS increased from 1.2 to 3.4 per 1,000 hospital births per year for the period 2000–2009 in the United States. The most severe NAS requires pharmacological treatment and is characterized by signs and symptoms of central nervous system hyperirritability, gastrointestinal irregularities, respiratory distress, and autonomic symptoms (Kaltenbach et al. 1998). Most infants prenatally exposed to opioids (e.g., heroin, oxycodone, Percocet [acetaminophen and oxycodone], methadone, buprenorphine), will exhibit NAS signs and symptoms, with a high percentage requiring pharmacological intervention.

The severity and presentation of NAS differ on the basis of the specific opioid involved. Withdrawal from heroin does not appear as severe as withdrawal from methadone, but untreated heroin use in pregnant women is associated with a high incidence of fetal demise, prematurity, and intrauterine growth restriction (Glass and Evans 1972; Kandall et al. 1977). Although the incidence of withdrawal requiring treatment is the same for methadone and buprenorphine, the amount of medication needed for treatment and the length of hospital stay are significantly less for buprenorphine-exposed infants compared with methadone-exposed infants (Jones et al. 2010b). Findings from fetal behavior studies suggest that buprenorphine produces less suppression of fetal heart rate and fetal heart rate reactivity and results in a superior biophysical profile after medication dosing than does methadone. However, it is not known to what extent the fetal results lead to any changes after birth. Further, different dosing regimens of methadone and/or buprenorphine may produce different results. The withdrawal associated with oxycodone (e.g., OxyContin, Percocet) also may have unique characteristics, but there have not yet been any studies examining NAS related to this opioid.

Non-opioid substances—notably, benzodiazepines, nicotine, selective serotonin reuptake inhibitors (SSRIs), and alcohol— also can cause behaviors consistent with withdrawal and/or can exacerbate NAS. Cocaine and methamphetamines do not cause withdrawal, but infants prenatally exposed to these substances may exhibit behaviors similar to those of newborns experiencing NAS. Data suggest that withdrawal from prenatal opioid and benzodiazepine use is more severe and more difficult to manage than withdrawal from opioid use alone (Berghella et al. 2003; Seligman et al. 2008). Although the neonatal behavior syndrome associated with SSRI exposure has been found to have self-limiting symptoms that can be managed with supportive care (Moses-Kolko et al. 2005), when SSRIs are used by pregnant women maintained on methadone or buprenorphine, they exacerbate the length of treatment needed for NAS (Jansson et al. 2010; Kaltenbach et al. 2012). Prenatal nicotine exposure has also been found to exacerbate the expression of NAS associated with prenatal opioid exposure (Chisolm et al. 2013).

Treatment

All babies exposed to opioids prenatally should be assessed for withdrawal using a standardized measure (e.g., Finnegan scoring system or Lipsitz tool). When pharmacological treatment is required, the medication most commonly used in the United States is morphine sulfate solution (Sarkar and Donn 2006). If the infant has been exposed to multiple substances, including non-opioids, the treatment of choice is often phenobarbital, in addition to or instead of morphine sulfate. The infant receives escalating doses of the medication until the symptoms are under control and then is weaned from the medication. Most infants who require medication will begin NAS treatment within 2–3 days after birth. The length of treatment is highly variable and on average ranges from several days to several weeks.

In addition to pharmacological treatment, supportive treatment can be most helpful for infants exhibiting signs of withdrawal. Infants should be kept in a quiet, dimly lit room and should be handled gently. Swaddling helps to moderate the infant's agitation, and providing a pacifier may eliminate the baby's frantic attempts to get his or her fingers into the mouth. Some infants are soothed by rocking. Infants may have their own idiosyncratic responses to different techniques, so caregivers should identify what works best for each infant. Rooming-in has been shown to reduce the proportion of babies who need medication to treat NAS compared with separating mother and baby (e.g., Abrahams et al. 2007). On one study, rooming-in reduced admissions to the neonatal intensive care unit (NICU) and led to a shorter NICU length of stay for term infants, increased likelihood of breastfeeding during the hospital stay, and increased odds of the baby being discharged home with the mother (Abrahams et al. 2010).

Postpartum Care

Pregnant and postpartum patients may experience multiple stressors in meeting the developmental needs of a newborn as well as such challenges as rearing older children, lack of an intimate partner relationship, lack of family and/or social support, depression and other psychiatric problems, inadequate housing or homelessness, exposure to violence, and financial difficulties. Any of these issues alone or in combination with an SUD poses risks to successful childrearing. Comprehensive ongoing maternal treatment for OUD that includes addressing other stressors besides opioid and other substance use reduces the chance of an adverse outcome for both mother and child. Otherwise, these factors can hamper the recovering woman's effectiveness as a parent, thus contributing to the risk of relapse to opioid use.

If a mother is successful in treatment, she may be able to regain or retain custody of her children. For the woman whose children have been removed from her home, a goal of treatment and recovery should be reunification of her family. Effective maternal treatment and intervention are cost-effective in the short and long term and become the first and most effective prevention interventions for children.

Breastfeeding and Buprenorphine

Breastfeeding has known advantages for both mother and infant. A mother maintained on buprenorphine should generally be encouraged to breastfeed unless she is using illicit substances to which the infant could be exposed through breast milk and/or she is HIV-positive. Research has indicated that the concentration of buprenorphine in breast milk is similar to maternal serum levels. Infant exposure to buprenorphine from breast milk ingestion is minimal given the poor oral bioavailability of buprenorphine. However, there is some research to suggest that breastfeeding may reduce the symptoms of NAS in infants whose mothers are maintained on buprenorphine, particularly in combination with maternal-child skin-to-skin contact, swaddling, and rooming-in. As such, a joint committee of the American College of Obstetricians and Gynecologists and the American Society of Addiction Medicine concluded that "patient stabilization with opioid-assisted therapy [including buprenorphine] is compatible with breastfeeding" (ACOG Committee on Health Care for Underserved Women and American Society of Addiction Medicine 2012). The World Health Organization (2014) recommended both breastfeeding and rooming-in to reduce NAS severity and to increase maternal-infant bonding.

Long-Term Child Outcomes Following Prenatal Buprenorphine Exposure

A long-term outcome study (K. Kaltenbach, K.E. O'Grady, S.H. Heil, et al., "Prenatal exposure to methadone or buprenorphine: early childhood developmental outcomes," submitted to *Drug and Alcohol Dependence*, 2017) followed 96 children and their mothers who completed the MOTHER study, an RCT of opioid-agonist pharmacotherapy during pregnancy. The study examined child physical growth parameters, temperament, cognition, language abilities, and sensory processing from 0 to 36 months postbirth. Maternal perceptions of parenting stress, home environment, and mother's addiction severity were examined. Changes over time occurred in most outcomes, including expected increases in height, weight, and head circumference and overall gains in cognitive development, language abilities, sensory processing, and temperament. Tests of mean differences between medications over the 3-year period yielded no sustained differences between medications over time. For mothers, significant findings in parenting stress showed increasing difficulties with their children over 36 months, and the home environment outcomes showed a more enriched home environment from 6 to 36 months. Findings indicated that prenatal opioid agonist exposure does not lead to adverse physical and mental development. Further, there were no deleterious effects of buprenorphine relative to methadone or of treatment for NAS relative to no treatment for NAS on growth, cognitive development, language abilities, sensory processing, and temperament.

Behavioral Treatments for Pregnant Women

The same behavioral interventions that have efficacy in nonpregnant patients also appear to be efficacious for pregnant women. For pregnant women enrolled in prenatal care but not enrolled in substance use treatment, those patients who were compliant with four sessions of motivational interviewing (MI) delivered babies with higher average birth weight compared with patients who completed zero to three MI sessions (Jones et al. 2002). In another study, which compared pregnant women enrolled in prenatal care but not substance use treatment, MI combined with behavioral incentives for abstinence and case management improved maternal outcomes of reduced substance use at a rate similar to that found for those pregnant women receiving MI and behavioral incentives alone (Jones et al. 2004).

Pregnant women with OUD undergoing treatment with MI and cognitive-behavioral therapy (CBT) showed decreases in substance use by almost 50% from baseline in promising data from an RCT comparing the intervention to no treatment and usual care treatment (Yonkers et al. 2009). Compared with usual substance use treatment, the Community Reinforcement Approach plus contingency management (CM) and MI provided to pregnant patients with SUDs produced higher levels of treatment utilization and improved abstinence from substance use, with shorter lengths of hospital stays for the neonates (Jones et al. 2011). Cognitive-behavioral treatment also has been shown to be effective in reducing HIV injection drug risk behaviors among methadone-maintained pregnant women (O'Neill et al. 1996). Although there is a lack of RCTs examining the efficacy of cognitive-behavioral treatment for reducing substance use and improving maternal and neonatal outcomes for pregnant women with SUDs, there are numerous programs that have been described in the literature that include aspects of relapse prevention and other cognitive skills–based training among their many components of comprehensive care.

CM systematically delivers reinforcement (rewards such as cash or, more often, gift cards redeemable for goods or services) for a successful target behavior (e.g., providing a psychoactive substance–negative urine sample) or withholds reinforcement when a target behavior is not successful (e.g., urine-positive event) (Higgins et al. 2004). CM has been used widely in the treatment of substance use and is generally considered the single most powerful behavioral intervention for the treatment of SUDs, although its use in the treatment of pregnant women with OUD has been limited. Moreover, there are barriers that have prevented its widespread adoption, including cost of implementation and staff training and the fact that matching rewards to patient preferences is necessary to optimize success.

Other psychosocial treatment approaches may prove useful in the treatment of pregnant women with OUDs. However, it is critical to understand that OUD in pregnant women does not occur in a vacuum. The vast majority of women with OUD have a long history of opioid use prior to the onset of pregnancy. Historically, that opioid has been heroin, although the nonmedical use of prescription analgesics is becoming more prevalent in pregnant women. Thus, a pregnant woman with OUD needs access to multiple health-related services throughout pregnancy and the postpartum period and beyond. This statement is particularly true given her role as a woman in treatment for OUD, parent of an infant and often other children, sometimes a partner but frequently a head of household, and an employee in the workforce. Case management services can provide support and guidance to a pregnant woman and can help her in accessing health services; psychological services, such as treatment for alcohol use and other substance use treatment; and mental health services, as well as other social services.

Conclusion

Though women use opioids at lower rates than do men, they are especially vulnerable to the consequences of opioid use. They have had increasing rates of death due to overdose from prescription opioids and have higher rates of comorbid medical and psychiatric issues. Women, when pregnant, are faced with serious fetal and maternal consequences when using opioids. Comprehensive treatment is especially important when treating women and should include a combination of medication-assisted treatment, psychotherapy (MI, CBT, CM), case management, psychiatric services, and medical treatment. Treatment providers should be sensitive to the needs of women and should approach women in a nonjudgmental way that reduces stigma. BUP/NX or methadone can be used as first-line treatments in women at the same doses as in men, although doses usually need to be increased during pregnancy. Switching from BUP/NX to the buprenorphine mono product during pregnancy is currently considered best practice. Methadone has been the standard of care for pregnant women, but buprenorphine alone also can be used in those women who are or will become pregnant, and buprenorphine is associated with lower levels of NAS in infants compared with methadone. Opioid agonist treatment has been shown to improve outcomes in mothers and infants compared with no pharmacotherapy and can be continued postpartum, including when the woman is breastfeeding, if no other contraindications exist.

Clinical Pearls

- Although rates of opioid use are higher in men than in women, in recent years, rates for prescription overdose death have increased more in women than in men.

- Women are more likely to use prescription opioids than heroin.

- Screening for substance use should be conducted with all pregnant and nonpregnant women in a normalized and nonjudgmental way.

- Women who use substances are more likely than men to have psychiatric comorbidities, and their use can escalate more rapidly ("telescoping").

- First-line treatment for moderate to severe opioid use disorder (OUD) includes buprenorphine-naloxone and methadone. There are no specific dosing adjustments in nonpregnant women, but dose increases are often needed in pregnant women, and pregnant women should transition to the mono product buprenorphine if possible.

- Methadone and buprenorphine are safe and efficacious for OUD in pregnancy with benefits to the mother, fetus, and newborn.

- The MOTHER study showed that newborns prenatally exposed to buprenorphine had a significantly shorter hospital stay and a shorter duration of NAS than did those exposed to methadone.

- The use of buprenorphine is not contraindicated when a woman is breastfeeding.

- When women with OUD are being treated, a range of services should be offered and implemented, including medical treatment, psychiatric treatment, psychotherapy (motivational interviewing, contingency management, cognitive-behavioral therapy), and case management.

- Women with OUD deserve to receive the medication that best meets their clinical treatment needs and goals. No one medication works best for all patients.

CASE 14

You are a BUP/NX prescriber and get a referral to see Kelsea, a 35-year-old woman with an extensive history of childhood and adult trauma and intravenous heroin use. She has spent the last 5 years either in jail or homeless. She was on methadone but lapsed back to heroin and cycled between jail and taking street buprenorphine. She is referred to you by her obstetrician because she is pregnant and taking prescribed buprenorphine mono product. She says she has been sober for 6 months but is now 34 weeks pregnant, is "wicked anxious," and needs a buprenorphine provider to get her to her delivery date with planned caesarian section. You review her medical chart and see she is adherent to obstetric appointments, and urine toxicology screens reveal only prescribed medication.

1. What are the indications for buprenorphine during pregnancy?

2. Should Kelsea go back on methadone?

3. Could she be prescribed buprenorphine?

CASE 14 (CONTINUED)

Kelsea returns after 14 days from her first visit and says she is getting increased cravings for opioids. She says she read this can happen during pregnancy, and she is worried about whether she will need more buprenorphine before or during her surgery. She also wonders how she can manage her anxiety and worry about being a mother going forward.

1. Are there physiological changes of pregnancy that can affect buprenorphine dose?

2. Does Kelsea need to taper off of buprenorphine for the caesarian section?

3. What additional treatments would be helpful for her anxiety and would support her mental health and recovery going forward?

References

Abrahams RR, Kelly SA, Payne S, et al: Rooming-in compared with standard care for newborns of mothers using methadone or heroin. Can Fam Physician 53(10):1722–1730, 2007 17934036

Abrahams RR, MacKay-Dunn MH, Nevmerjitskaia V, et al: An evaluation of rooming-in among substance-exposed newborns in British Columbia. J Obstet Gynaecol Can 32(9):866–871, 2010 21050520

ACOG Committee on Health Care for Underserved Women; American Society of Addiction Medicine: ACOG Committee Opinion No. 524: Opioid abuse, dependence, and addiction in pregnancy. Obstet Gynecol 119(5):1070–1076, 2012 22525931

Ayanga D, Shorter D, Kosten TR: Update on pharmacotherapy for treatment of opioid use disorder. Expert Opin Pharmacother 17(17):2307–2318, 2016 27734745

Back SE, Payne RL, Simpson AN, et al: Gender and prescription opioids: findings from the National Survey on Drug Use and Health. Addict Behav 35(11):1001–1007, 2010 20598809

Berghella V, Lim PJ, Hill MK, et al: Maternal methadone dose and neonatal withdrawal. Am J Obstet Gynecol 189(2):312–317, 2003 14520184

Centers for Disease Control and Prevention: Prescription Painkiller Overdoses. Atlanta, GA, Centers for Disease Control and Prevention, 2013. Available at http://www.cdc.gov/vitalsigns/prescriptionpainkilleroverdoses/. Accessed February 10, 2016.

Centers for Disease Control and Prevention: Prescription Opioid Overdose Data. Atlanta, GA, Centers for Disease Control and Prevention, 2015. Available at http://www.cdc.gov/drugoverdose/data/overdose.html. Accessed February 10, 2016.

Chisolm MS, Fitzsimons H, Leoutsakos JM, et al: A comparison of cigarette smoking profiles in opioid-dependent pregnant patients receiving methadone or buprenorphine. Nicotine Tob Res 15(7):1297–1304, 2013 23288871

Cleary BJ, Donnelly J, Strawbridge J, et al: Methadone dose and neonatal abstinence syndrome-systematic review and meta-analysis. Addiction 105(12):2071–2084, 2010 20840198

Coyle MG, Salisbury AL, Lester BM, et al: Neonatal neurobehavior effects following buprenorphine versus methadone exposure. Addiction 107 (suppl 1):63–73, 2012 23106928

Glass L, Evans HE: Narcotic withdrawal in the newborn. Am Fam Physician 6(1):75–78, 1972 5086893

Graziani M, Nisticò R: Gender differences in pharmacokinetics and pharmacodynamics of methadone substitution therapy. Front Pharmacol 6(6):122, 2015 26106330

Greenfield SF, Back SE, Lawson K, et al: Substance abuse in women. Psychiatr Clin North Am 33(2):339–355, 2010 20385341

Greenfield SF, Sugarman DE, Freid CM, et al: Group therapy for women with substance use disorders: results from the Women's Recovery Group Study. Drug Alcohol Depend 142:245–253, 2014 25042759

Higgins ST, Heil SH, Lussier JP: Clinical implications of reinforcement as a determinant of substance use disorders. Annu Rev Psychol 55:431–461, 2004 14744222

Jansson LM, Dipietro JA, Elko A, Velez M: Infant autonomic functioning and neonatal abstinence syndrome. Drug Alcohol Depend 109(1–3):198–204, 2010 20189732

John CS, Savitsky LM, Fowler J, et al: 777: A cost effectiveness analysis of buprenorphine vs. methadone for maintenance of opioid addiction during pregnancy. Am J Obstet Gynecol 216(1):S449, 2017

Jones HE, Svikis DS, Tran G: Patient compliance and maternal/infant outcomes in pregnant drug-using women. Subst Use Misuse 37(11):1411–1422, 2002 12371578

Jones HE, Svikis D, Rosado J, et al: What if they do not want treatment? Lessons learned from intervention studies of non-treatment-seeking, drug-using pregnant women. Am J Addict 13(4):342–357, 2004 15370933

Jones HE, Johnson RE, Jasinski DR, et al: Buprenorphine versus methadone in the treatment of pregnant opioid-dependent patients: effects on the neonatal abstinence syndrome. Drug Alcohol Depend 79(1):1–10, 2005a 15943939

Jones HE, Fitzgerald H, Johnson RE: Males and females differ in response to opioid agonist medications. Am J Addict 14(3):223–233, 2005b 16019973

Jones HE, O'Grady KE, Malfi D, et al: Methadone maintenance vs. methadone taper during pregnancy: maternal and neonatal outcomes. Am J Addict 17(5):372–386, 2008a 18770079

Jones HE, Martin PR, Heil SH, et al: Treatment of opioid-dependent pregnant women: clinical and research issues. J Subst Abuse Treat 35(3):245–259, 2008b 18248941

Jones HE, O'Grady KE, Johnson RE, et al: Infant neurobehavior following prenatal exposure to methadone or buprenorphine: results from the neonatal intensive care unit network neurobehavioral scale. Subst Use Misuse 45(13):2244–2257, 2010a 20482340

Jones HE, Kaltenbach K, Heil SH, et al: Neonatal abstinence syndrome after methadone or buprenorphine exposure. N Engl J Med 363(24):2320–2331, 2010b 21142534

Jones HE, O'Grady KE, Tuten M: Reinforcement-based treatment improves the maternal treatment and neonatal outcomes of pregnant patients enrolled in comprehensive care treatment. Am J Addict 20(3):196–204, 2011 21477047

Jones HE, Deppen K, Hudak ML, et al: Clinical care for opioid-using pregnant and postpartum women: the role of obstetric providers. Am J Obstet Gynecol 210(4):302–310, 2014 24120973

Kaltenbach K, Berghella V, Finnegan L: Opioid dependence during pregnancy. Effects and management. Obstet Gynecol Clin North Am 25(1):139–151, 1998 9547764

Kaltenbach K, Holbrook AM, Coyle MG, et al: Predicting treatment for neonatal abstinence syndrome in infants born to women maintained on opioid agonist medication. Addiction 107 (suppl 1):45–52, 2012 23106926

Kandall SR, Albin S, Gartner LM, et al: The narcotic-dependent mother: fetal and neonatal consequences. Early Hum Dev 1(2):159–169, 1977 617308

Lund IO, Fischer G, Welle-Strand GK, et al: A comparison of buprenorphine+naloxone to buprenorphine and methadone in the treatment of opioid dependence during pregnancy: maternal and neonatal outcomes. Subst Abuse 7:61–74, 2013 23531704

McCullough LB, Chervenak FA: The fetus as a patient and the ethics of human subjects research: response to commentaries on "An ethically justified framework for clinical investigation to benefit pregnant and fetal patients." Am J Bioethics 11(5):W3–W7, 2011 21534136

Moody DE, Fang WB, Morrison J, et al: Gender differences in pharmacokinetics of maintenance dosed buprenorphine. Drug Alcohol Depend 118(2–3):479–483, 2011 21515002

Moses-Kolko EL, Bogen D, Perel J, et al: Neonatal signs after late in utero exposure to serotonin reuptake inhibitors: literature review and implications for clinical applications. JAMA 293(19):2372–2383, 2005 15900008

National Institute on Drug Abuse: National Pregnancy and Health Survey: Drug Use Among Women Delivering Live Births 1992. Washington, DC, U.S. Department of Health and Human Services, 1996. Available at: www.datafiles.samhsa.gov/study-dataset/national-pregnancy-and-health-survey-drug-use-among-women-delivering-live-births-1992. Accessed September 7, 2017.

National Institute on Drug Abuse: Chart of Evidence-Based Screening Tools for Adults and Adolescents. Bethesda, MD, National Institute on Drug Abuse, 2015. Available at https://www.drugabuse.gov/nidamed-medical-health-professionals/tool-resources-your-practice/screening-assessment-drug-testing-resources/chart-evidence-based-screening-tools-adults. Accessed August 28, 2016.

Ondersma SJ, Svikis DS, Thacker LR, et al: Computer-delivered screening and brief intervention (e-SBI) for postpartum drug use: a randomized trial. J Subst Abuse Treat 46(1):52–59, 2014 24051077

O'Neill K, Baker A, Cooke M, et al: Evaluation of a cognitive-behavioural intervention for pregnant injecting drug users at risk of HIV infection. Addiction 91(8):1115–1125, 1996 8828240

Patrick SW, Schumacher RE, Benneyworth BD, et al: Neonatal abstinence syndrome and associated health care expenditures: United States, 2000–2009. JAMA 307(18):1934–1940, 2012 22546608

Sarkar S, Donn SM: Management of neonatal abstinence syndrome in neonatal intensive care units: a national survey. J Perinatol 26(1):15–17, 2006 16355103

Seligman NS, Salva N, Hayes EJ, et al: Predicting length of treatment for neonatal abstinence syndrome in methadone-exposed neonates. Am J Obstet Gynecol 199(4):396.e1–396.e7, 2008 18928986

Smith K, Lipari R: Women of Childbearing Age and Opioids (The CBHSQ Report Jan 17, 2017). Rockville, MD, Substance Abuse and Mental Health Services Administration, 2017. Available at: www.samhsa.gov/data/sites/default/files/report_2724/ShortReport-2724.html. Accessed: September 7, 2017.

Substance Abuse and Mental Health Services Administration: Substance Abuse Treatment: Addressing the Special Needs of Women. Treatment Improvement Protocol (TIP) Series, No 51. HHS Publ No (SMA) 13-4426. Rockville, MD, Substance Abuse and Mental Health Services Administration, 2009

Substance Abuse and Mental Health Services Administration: Drug Abuse Warning Network, 2011: National Estimates of Drug-Related Emergency Department Visits. HHS Publ No (SMA) 13-4760, DAWN Series D-39. Rockville, MD, Substance Abuse and Mental Health Services Administration, 2013

Substance Abuse and Mental Health Services Administration: Results from the 2013 National Survey on Drug Use and Health: Summary of National Findings, NS-DUH Series H-48, HHS Publ No (SMA) 14-4863. Rockville, MD, Substance Abuse and Mental Health Services Administration, 2014a.

Substance Abuse and Mental Health Services Administration, Center for Behavioral Health Statistics and Quality. The TEDS Report: Gender Differences in Primary Substance of Abuse Across Age Groups. Rockville, MD, Substance Abuse and Mental Health Services Administration, April 3, 2014b

Suarez Ordoñez RM, Cesolari J, Ofelia C, et al: Behavioral health screening and intervention for women in Argentina: a preliminary model for the childbearing years. Int J Womens Health 7(7):635–643, 2015 26203284

U.S. Food and Drug Administration: Neonatal opioid withdrawal syndrome and medication-assisted treatment with methadone and buprenorphine. Silver Spring, MD, U.S. Food and Drug Administration, 2016. Available at: www.fda.gov/drugs/drugsafety/ucm503630.htm. Accessed August 18, 2017.

World Health Organization: Guidelines for the Identification and Management of Substance Use and Substance Use Disorders in Pregnancy. Geneva, World Health Organization, 2014. Available at: http://apps.who.int/iris/bitstream/10665/107130/1/9789241548731_eng.pdf?ua=1. Accessed April 26, 2017.

Yonkers KA, Howell HB, Allen AE, et al: A treatment for substance abusing pregnant women. Arch Women Ment Health 12(4):221–227, 2009 19350369

Zubieta JK, Dannals RF, Frost JJ: Gender and age influences on human brain mu-opioid receptor binding measured by PET. Am J Psychiatry 156(6):842–848, 1999 10360121

15

Comments on the Case Vignettes

John A. Renner Jr., M.D.
Gregory Acampora, M.D.

Case 1

FROM CHAPTER 5, "CLINICAL USE OF BUPRENORPHINE"

Given that Sally is over 18 years old and meets 4 of the 11 criteria for opioid use disorder (OUD; tolerance, withdrawal, unsuccessful attempts to cut down on her opioid use, and continued use despite negative impact on her functioning; see Box 4–1, "DSM-5 Diagnostic Criteria for Opioid Use Disorders"), she meets federal criteria for buprenorphine treatment. Because she meets 4 criteria, her OUD would be rated as moderate (American Psychiatric Association 2013). She would not be eligible for methadone maintenance because she has not been dependent for the required 12 months. Because there is no evidence of another drug or alcohol use disorder or another psychiatric disorder and she has been doing well in college, she would likely be an excellent candidate for office-based treatment and would not likely need the structure of a methadone clinic to do well in her recovery.

Before starting treatment, Sally should be educated about buprenorphine and asked to sign an informed consent form for treatment. It would be important to stress that 1) buprenorphine will cause physiological opioid dependence; 2) withdrawal symptoms will occur if she stops taking the drug abruptly; and

3) although the medication is safe when taken as directed, it can cause death if taken with benzodiazepines or other sedative-hypnotic drugs, including alcohol. A urine toxicology screen for opioids and other common drugs of abuse is a highly recommended element in the initial evaluation of potential buprenorphine patients as well as a urine pregnancy test in women of childbearing age. Sally should be asked to abstain from any opioid use for at least 24 hours before induction. If a monitored induction is indicated, she should plan to spend 2–4 hours in the office on the day of induction. It will be necessary for her to be experiencing some moderate withdrawal symptoms before her initial dose, but she should also be told that the symptoms can be easily controlled once buprenorphine therapy is started. Her history suggests that she will be reliable, so it would be appropriate to write an initial buprenorphine prescription to cover the first 2 or 3 days of induction. An initial sublingual dose of 4 mg buprenorphine/ 1 mg naloxone would be standard, once you have documented a moderate level of opioid withdrawal. If symptoms of precipitated withdrawal occur, additional buprenorphine doses of 2–4 mg (combination formulation with naloxone 0.5–1 mg) should be adequate to control the symptoms. Most individuals with OUD are very familiar with withdrawal and will collaborate with their clinician to avoid this event.

Unfortunately, there are more cases of patients with illicit fentanyl misuse presenting to office-based practices. Buprenorphine induction may be complicated in such cases because of the binding affinity of fentanyl and clearance. In cases where patients are using fentanyl, precipitated withdrawal can occur. In these cases, the patient should not be given additional doses of buprenorphine because this will increase withdrawal symptoms. The patient should be treated symptomatically, and if symptoms are severe enough, the patient may require referral to an inpatient facility. To avoid precipitated withdrawal in these cases, it is recommended to wait at least 24–48 hours after last use of fentanyl and for the patient to be in significant withdrawal (Clinical Opiate Withdrawal Scale [COWS] > 5) before starting buprenorphine/naloxone (BUP/NX).

In most circumstances, no more than 8 mg of buprenorphine would likely be required for the first 24 hours of induction. A target buprenorphine dose range of 12–16 mg/day is reasonable for most patients. However, in younger patients with shorter histories of opioid use disorders, a lower target dose range of 8–12 mg/day may be adequate. The initial goal of treatment should be stabilization, control of craving and withdrawal symptoms, and elimination of illicit drug use. Once stability is achieved, a gradual buprenorphine taper can be initiated. We recommend at least 1 year of treatment before attempting any dose reduction or taper off of BUP/NX, assuming the patient has invested in counseling and mutual support groups and has demonstrated a mature level of coping skills. Before you attempt dose reduction or taper, you need to educate the patient about the high risk of relapse and the value of long-term, if not indefinite, agonist therapy. If the patient requests taper off of BUP/NX, an alternative therapy such as extended-release intramuscular naltrexone (XR-NTX) may be suggested to the patient.

Case 2

FROM CHAPTER 5, "CLINICAL USE OF BUPRENORPHINE"

Converting a patient from methadone to buprenorphine treatment is fairly straightforward. After obtaining a release from the patient, you should contact the methadone clinic to verify the patient's status and negotiate a gradual methadone taper to approximately 30 mg/day. After the patient has been stable on that dosage for at least a week, methadone should be discontinued, and the patient should report to your office 24–36 hours after the last methadone dose, at a time when he is in mild to moderate opioid withdrawal. After you document his withdrawal symptoms with COWS, induction can begin with a dose of 4 mg buprenorphine/1 mg naloxone, following standard induction recommendations. After the first dose of buprenorphine, no further methadone should be taken. Any ongoing symptoms of withdrawal should be handled with additional doses of buprenorphine, up to a total first-day dose of 12 mg buprenorphine/3 mg naloxone. Although most patients do well on an initial total dose of 8 mg/2 mg, this patient has a higher tolerance due to being on long-term methadone treatment, and a higher first-day dose may be important to make the patient feel comfortable. Further increases can be made on subsequent days.

Case 3

FROM CHAPTER 5, "CLINICAL USE OF BUPRENORPHINE"

Any patient requesting transfer from another buprenorphine provider should be assessed carefully. It is important to verify the patient's report by obtaining and documenting a release of information and talking directly with his current prescriber. In some cases, patients may be trying to avoid participation in counseling or other important supportive services; in other cases, they may have family, work, or social obligations that make it difficult to participate in more services. You may choose to establish a minimum level of participation in ancillary treatment or recovery activities for your practice; if you decide to do so, make sure that patients understand your requirements before you accept them into treatment. Weekly group therapy with a skilled addiction counselor and/or regular involvement in Alcoholics Anonymous (AA) or Narcotics Anonymous (NA) is helpful to most—but not all—patients. Similar treatment outcomes can be seen if patients are monitored closely by their prescribing clinician.

Case 3 (Continued)

It is often recommended that patients sign a treatment agreement that describes expectations regarding attendance, urine testing, participation in psychosocial treatment, and rules about the use of other medications as well as expectations for abstinence from all illicit drugs. The occurrence of cocaine use and a missed group therapy session indicate the need to review the patient's status and may require an increase in counseling, a shortening of the time between medication visits, or more frequent urine tests. Although clear rules are important, the clinician should be flexible and approach problems from the perspective that rule violations indicate the need for more intensive treatment, not punishment. Patients should always be given the opportunity to correct problems before any decision is made to terminate care or to refer the patient to a more structured opioid treatment program.

Case 4

FROM CHAPTER 6, "BUPRENORPHINE TREATMENT IN OFFICE-BASED SETTINGS"

Clinicians treating patients with buprenorphine should have a working knowledge of drug testing and interpretation of test results. Most standard drug tests provide very accurate results within a nominal cost structure, and the availability of mass spectroscopy–gas chromatography assures valid confirmation of questionable results. Positive test results for illicit drugs require a meeting with the patient to review the results. If the patient continues to deny use (after confirmatory laboratory tests), we recommend gentle confrontation (*carefronting*) from the perspective of motivational interviewing: comment on the frequency of relapse, the ongoing struggle with the disease of addiction, the difficulty many individuals have admitting problems, and the patient's likely ambivalence about complete sobriety. The best approach to talking to patients about toxicology examinations is to view and treat testing as a *collaboration toward recovery*. Be sure to emphasize your desire to work with the patient to establish a successful recovery program. Clinicians can expect occasional relapses, even in the most motivated patients, and may use these episodes to educate the patient about the nature of the illness and identify weaknesses in the current recovery program. Transfer to a higher level of care should be considered only after clear evidence of recurrent failure in office-based treatment.

Case 5

FROM CHAPTER 6, "BUPRENORPHINE TREATMENT IN OFFICE-BASED SETTINGS"

Some buprenorphine patients may escalate their drinking once their opioid problem is under control or may increase their use of other substances. Discuss with

Henrietta that her drinking is beyond the limits of safe social consumption and that mixing buprenorphine and alcohol or other sedative-hypnotic drugs can be dangerous. The additive risk for respiratory depression is notable in that oral opioids mixed with alcohol are subject to a phenomenon called *dose dumping* (Walden et al. 2007) wherein the release and absorption of the opioid is accelerated. It is likely that Henrietta will need treatment for an alcohol use disorder, including formal alcohol withdrawal treatment. People with OUD are at high risk for other substance use disorders (SUDs), especially with benzodiazepines. The safest recovery necessitates the elimination of all alcohol, tobacco, and illicit drug use; buprenorphine patients, in particular, need to carefully monitor their use of alcohol or prescribed medications with any misuse potential. In this case, Henrietta should be encouraged to join AA, and 12-step facilitation may be a useful therapy approach. If she requires alcohol withdrawal treatment, be sure to refer her to a facility that will permit her to continue taking buprenorphine during hospitalization. If her alcohol use continues, she may be a good candidate for XR-NTX instead of BUP/NX.

Case 5 (Continued)
FROM CHAPTER 10, "PSYCHIATRIC COMORBIDITY"

It is helpful to have office policies regarding the management of intoxicated patients. In this case, the immediate issue is patient and staff safety. If the patient refuses medically supervised alcohol withdrawal treatment, she should not be permitted to drive home intoxicated. However, it is not safe to challenge uncooperative, intoxicated individuals; in rare circumstances, it may be necessary to seek assistance from law enforcement or security personnel to contain the situation. Although this problem is very rare with buprenorphine patients, staff should be educated about the management of belligerent or intoxicated patients. If patients are unable to control inappropriate behavior or cover the cost of treatment, they should be referred to a structured program, most typically a public opioid treatment program, which is better equipped to manage their care. Discussion of nonpayment should be reserved for when the patient is not intoxicated. Information regarding nonpayment should be given to the patient in writing. If transfer of care is necessary, a list of alternatives in the community such as clinics that prescribe BUP/NX or XR-NTX through hospital systems that accept public insurance or public opioid treatment programs should be given to the patient.

Case 6
FROM CHAPTER 7, "PSYCHOSOCIAL AND SUPPORTIVE TREATMENTS"

Martha should be encouraged to seek out a new sponsor who is accepting of medication-assisted therapy (MAT) for addiction. Make sure that she understands that taking buprenorphine as prescribed under medical supervision is not a form of addiction. Also let her know that patients who attempt recovery on their own are less likely to succeed.

Her initial participation in AA was an important element of her success with buprenorphine treatment; having a sponsor and joining a "home group" are good indications that an individual is seriously committed to the AA program. Clinicians should encourage participation in mutual support groups, but patients need to be informed about both the benefits and the risks of such programs. AA's stance on medical treatment is supported in their literature and addressed at www.aa.org, and the organization is supportive of medication taken under physician supervision and of psychotherapy. Unfortunately, some individual AA members strongly discourage any form of psychopharmacology, including methadone and buprenorphine. If Martha is not able to find a more supportive sponsor or AA group, she should be encouraged to explore alternative mutual support programs or be referred for individual or group psychotherapy. Alternatives to AA or NA include such organizations as Rational Recovery, SMART Recovery, Secular Organizations for Sobriety, Women for Sobriety, and Against the Stream Meditation Society.

Case 6 (Continued)

FROM CHAPTER 12, "ACUTE AND CHRONIC PAIN"

Perioperative pain control for a buprenorphine patient builds on the options described in the discussion of Case 12 below. When buprenorphine was first introduced, it was recommended that it be stopped 24–48 hours before surgery, but this procedure was neither practical nor risk reducing, as intended. A more modern understanding of buprenorphine has moved thinking away from "all or none" strategies. For minor planned surgery, the patient may continue on her daily buprenorphine dose and be given supplemental low doses of sublingual buprenorphine (buprenorphine 2 mg/naloxone 0.5 mg) or a short-acting opioid (oxycodone, hydrocodone) every 6–8 hours as needed for 1 or 2 days after surgery. For major surgery, holding the buprenorphine is no longer recommended. Instead, the daily buprenorphine dose should be split and given every 6–8 hours to take advantage of buprenorphine's analgesic properties, and normal anesthesia/pain management should take place during the surgery, with the understanding that higher levels of opioids will be needed during surgery because of the patient's tolerance (opioid debt). Immediately following the surgery, the patient should be maintained on the split buprenorphine dose. An oral or parenteral short-acting opioid analgesic, including patient controlled analgesia (PCA), can be added for pain control depending on the severity of the patient's postoperative pain. If adequate analgesia is not being achieved with split-dose buprenorphine and the short-acting opioid analgesic, hospitalized patients can have their buprenorphine discontinued and can be treated with a long-acting opioid (such as methadone 30–40 mg daily or extended-release morphine 15 mg twice daily for the baseline opioid requirement to avoid withdrawal), with a short-acting opioid analgesic as needed for pain control. Once the acute postsurgical pain has resolved, buprenorphine therapy can be re-induced.

Case 7

From Chapter 9, "Methadone, Naltrexone, and Naloxone"

Some clinicians regularly test for marijuana and treat it like any other illicit substance, and other clinicians ignore it. Given increasing use and the growing pressure for legalization, it is important that all buprenorphine providers think through their position on this issue. Neither methadone nor buprenorphine is a treatment for cannabis use disorder. In most circumstances, issues with other substances, legal and illegal, must be dealt with in counseling.

Although some individuals with an OUD may be able to drink alcohol socially or occasionally smoke marijuana, the most prudent approach is to recommend abstinence from all substances for anyone with an OUD. The high incidence of co-occurring substance use disorders in any person with an OUD makes any other approach very risky. Participation in mutual support groups will reinforce this message in support of total sobriety. This being said, there is no reason to terminate opioid agonist treatment because of occasional marijuana use. However, any patient who is seriously impaired by the misuse of marijuana or any other substances requires referral for a higher level of care.

Case 7 (Continued)

In Carl's case, his misuse of cocaine is the primary area of clinical concern. There is no evidence that a higher methadone dose will resolve the problem. There would be no contraindication to a trial of disulfiram because disulfiram does not interact with methadone, nor does it prolong QTc. Other off-label options to treat his cocaine use disorder would be topiramate, modafinil, or baclofen. Most clinicians would recommend a behavioral approach with reduced take-home medication privileges and increased individual or group counseling. There is very strong evidence to support the efficacy of contingency management to address cocaine misuse problems in patients on methadone maintenance, as is recommended in the Department of Defense/Veterans Health Administration practice guidelines. This would also be an appropriate time to discuss how the patient's marijuana use influences his cocaine use in a manner using motivational interviewing. If the patient is willing to discontinue marijuana, discussing cannabis withdrawal with him so that this does not trigger other drug use should also be considered.

Case 7 (Continued)

There is little evidence to support the efficacy of treatment termination, even after a successful course of methadone maintenance. Relapse rates are as high as 80% within 12 months. A taper should not be considered unless patients are highly motivated and have established a stable drug-free lifestyle with strong supports in the recovery community. Carl needs to be educated about the risks of medication termination, and his feelings about being on long-term MAT should be explored in depth in counseling. Transfer to buprenorphine or XR-NTX may be reasonable alternatives in this case. Carl would be a good candidate for either option, and the decision could be guided by his preferences. All MAT patients should be provided with a naloxone rescue kit, particularly anyone considering or undergoing a taper from methadone or buprenorphine. Individuals are at high risk for relapse and a fatal opioid overdose in the period immediately following taper from opioid agonist therapy.

Case 8

FROM CHAPTER 10, "PSYCHIATRIC COMORBIDITY"

All patients undergoing treatment with buprenorphine should undergo psychiatric screening. If there is concern for comorbid psychiatric problems, a detailed psychiatric evaluation should be completed. In this case, Maria's symptoms are suggestive of posttraumatic stress disorder (PTSD) or borderline personality disorder (BPD) and indicate the need for a more thorough psychiatric evaluation. Should these diagnoses be confirmed, more specialized psychiatric treatment is needed, although this is not a contraindication to buprenorphine treatment. Treatment should include psychotherapy for SUD and for PTSD or BPD. The evidence-based standard therapies for PTSD are prolonged exposure and cognitive processing therapies. These have been found to be effective for patients with dual diagnoses if combined with treatment for SUD. Psychotherapies for SUD such as Seeking Safety, motivational enhancement therapy, or cognitive-behavioral therapy (CBT) for SUD would be appropriate in this case. Seeking Safety was specifically designed to increase coping skills and manage substance use in women with co-occurring substance use disorders and a history of trauma or PTSD. Other options would be dialectical behavior therapy or Skills Training in Affect and Interpersonal Regulation (STAIR) with a clinician who is skilled in working with patient with concurrent SUD, but there have been few research studies to date with the use of these therapies in the dual-diagnosed population.

Case 9

FROM CHAPTER 10, "PSYCHIATRIC COMORBIDITY"

Co-occurring psychiatric disorders are common among individuals with an OUD. In this case, Karen's symptoms of depression and anxiety had been well controlled with antidepressant treatment. Given her stability with buprenorphine and the absence of any recent illicit drug use, it is unlikely that the reoccurrence of these symptoms is drug induced. Clarification of Karen's psychiatric symptomatology before her opioid use and the presence of symptoms during extended periods of sobriety suggest that she has recurrent major depression with associated anxiety. Given the recent increase in her symptoms of depression and anxiety, it would be appropriate to review and adjust her antidepressant medications and consider referring her for psychotherapy.

There is no evidence that any particular antidepressant is more effective in buprenorphine patients, or that there would be any significant drug-drug interactions between buprenorphine and any of the standard antidepressants. If Karen develops a panic disorder, she should be referred for CBT. If her panic symptoms do not respond to the combination of CBT and antidepressant treatment, the addition of a long-acting benzodiazepine such as clonazepam can be explored. This option should not be considered if she has a history of a benzodiazepine use disorder. She needs to be warned of the risk for overdose if buprenorphine is combined with high-dose benzodiazepines or any other sedative-hypnotic drug, including alcohol.

Case 10

FROM CHAPTER 10, "PSYCHIATRIC COMORBIDITY"

During periods of illicit drug use, it is difficult to separate drug-induced depressive symptoms from those secondary to PTSD or to an independent depressive disorder. In this case, the patient's suicidal ideation and homicidal comments necessitate immediate hospitalization, regardless of etiology. He will also require treatment to control opioid withdrawal symptoms and should be considered for long-term opioid agonist treatment. There is a very high risk for relapse following opioid withdrawal treatment, and individuals with serious PTSD are even less likely to remain drug free. Although this veteran meets DSM-5 criteria for OUD, he has been using opioids for only 4 months and thus does not meet criteria for methadone maintenance therapy. Buprenorphine or XR-NTX would be possible options. Once his OUD has stabilized with MAT, he will need to be reassessed to rule out the presence of an independent depressive disorder and referred to the Veterans Health Administration system to initiate treatment for PTSD. If he prefers XR-NTX, that can be initiated after a gradual buprenorphine taper. However, it may be preferable to continue him on buprenorphine until his PTSD symptoms are under good control and he has committed himself to a strong recovery program. There is limited clinical experience managing similar patients on XR-NTX.

Case 11

FROM CHAPTER 11, "MEDICAL COMORBIDITY"

In this case, jaundice is most likely a systemic sign of underlying hepatic illness manifested by an increase in serum bilirubin levels. It is very unlikely that buprenorphine prescribed in routine clinical care causes hepatotoxicity. In the rare cases where liver toxicity is thought to be related to buprenorphine, the dose was supratherapeutic and the medication was injected. Anecdotal reports of jaundice and liver failure exist, with sublingual buprenorphine use in combination with acetaminophen in patients with significant underlying liver disease. Research has documented the safety of sublingual BUP/NX treatment (or methadone treatment) in individuals treated for up to 24 weeks with either medication. Liver enzymes and total bilirubin are rarely elevated in patients receiving buprenorphine. Risk of hepatotoxicity is greater in individuals infected with HIV, hepatitis C virus (HCV), or HIV/HCV co-infection, who may benefit from increased monitoring (Tetrault et al. 2016).

In the case of Rosie, it would be reasonable to continue buprenorphine treatment with increased monitoring of blood work. She will also require additional counseling and other services to help her find housing and to avoid other potential liver toxins such as alcohol. Additionally, she should be screened for HIV, as well as hepatitis A virus (HAV) and hepatitis B virus (HBV), with vaccination for HAV and HBV provided if immunity is not demonstrated. Once her condition has stabilized, she can be considered for HCV treatment with direct-acting antiviral agents that include a combination of protease inhibitors, nonstructural protein 5A (NS5A) inhibitors, and/or NS5B polymerase inhibitors.

Case 12

FROM CHAPTER 12, "ACUTE AND CHRONIC PAIN"

Prescribing buprenorphine can seem complicated in patients with either acute or chronic pain problems. Options for addressing less severe acute pain include use of the following:

- Non-opioid analgesics such as nonsteroidal anti-inflammatory agents and acetaminophen
- Non-opioids such as antidepressants and antiepileptics

- Local anesthetics (e.g., lidocaine)
- Topical anesthetics (e.g., capsaicin, menthols)
- Nonpharmacological treatments (e.g., massage, relaxation, physical therapy)

For moderate to severe pain, consider splitting the daily buprenorphine dose to every 6–8 hours to take advantage of buprenorphine's analgesic properties. In addition, options include the following:

- Prescribing supplemental low doses of sublingual buprenorphine (buprenorphine 2 mg/naloxone 0.5 mg) every 6–8 hours as needed
- Adding a short-acting opioid (e.g., oral oxycodone or hydrocodone or parenteral fentanyl or hydromorphone) to the buprenorphine and titrating to effect

If the pain is prolonged, in many cases, divided buprenorphine doses (sometimes at a slightly higher total dosage than the previous maintenance dosage) will adequately control the pain. Sublingual buprenorphine provides significant analgesia, but the duration of this effect is 6–8 hours; thus, divided doses are required. Adding supplemental full agonists to a stable BUP/NX dose will not precipitate withdrawal, and these drugs can then be safely titrated to effect. Combining buprenorphine with mixed agonist-antagonists such as butorphanol, nalbuphine, or pentazocine should be avoided because the effect is unpredictable. In addition, if the prescriber does not regularly treat pain (e.g., psychiatrists, psychiatry advanced practice registered nurses), then split dosing with buprenorphine can be done, but the other options (adding other opioids or conversion to methadone) should be deferred to other providers such as the primary care physician or pain management specialists. Collaboration with other specialists should also be obtained in unusually complicated cases or whenever the patient fails to respond to the standard treatment options described above.

Case 13

FROM CHAPTER 13, "OPIOID USE BY ADOLESCENTS"

Although many clinicians avoid long-term opioid therapy in adolescents, the relapse rate is very high following medication withdrawal treatment, except for those adolescents who complete an intensive residential program. Tommy has a 3-year history of OUD with two prior episodes of medication withdrawal treatment and is clearly a candidate for long-term buprenorphine therapy. His parents will need support and education to help them understand the benefits of buprenorphine and the high risks associated with drug-free treatment. At 16, Tommy is legally eligible for buprenorphine treatment, although parental consent is required in most states. Family therapy would be beneficial in this case, and ongoing court supervision increases the likelihood that he will follow through with treatment. Treatment goals should include elimination of all illicit drug use. Treatment with buprenorphine for a minimum of 1–2 years is indicated. Alternatively, Tommy could be placed on XR-NTX following a BUP/NX taper after a year of treatment with BUP/NX. A gradual buprenorphine taper or switch to XR-NTX should not be considered until Tommy is stable, is fully invested in a drug-free lifestyle, and has established a network of drug-free peers. Recent research indicates that engendering a sense of belonging, providing role models, and melding recovery with a menu of fun activities results in more participation in recovery structure for adolescents.

Case 14

From Chapter 14, "Women's Health and Pregnancy"

The present recommendations are that pregnant women with active OUD receive MAT because of neonatal risks during withdrawal and the danger of maternal relapse to illicit opioid use following detoxification while pregnant. Although methadone has been used safely for 45 years, buprenorphine MAT is gaining popularity because it is associated with shorter treatment duration of neonatal abstinence syndrome (NAS), less medication needed to treat NAS symptoms, and shorter hospitalizations for neonates. Unfortunately, conversion to buprenorphine has a risk of precipitated withdrawal and can cause fetal distress, so inductions should be completed cautiously. Because this patient is already taking buprenorphine with good response, there is no indication to switch to methadone at this point. As of 2016, human safety data regarding naloxone studies during pregnancy are absent. Several studies reviewing neonatal outcomes when mothers were treated with BUP/NX show no difference from those who were treated with methadone or buprenorphine monotherapy. To date, most authorities recommend pregnant women treated with BUP/NX at conception switch to either buprenorphine monotherapy or methadone.

Case 14 (Continued)

In randomized clinical trials, there was a need for dose increases of both methadone and buprenorphine throughout pregnancy to avoid withdrawal symptoms in expectant mothers. These results correlate with other pharmacokinetic research that shows the need to increase buprenorphine dose during the course of pregnancy in order to maintain therapeutic blood levels. The Maternal Opioid Treatment: Human Experimental Research (MOTHER) study suggested that 2 mg increases were needed 1.1 and 1.3 times in the second and third trimester (Jones et al. 2012).

The question of tapering down or off of buprenorphine before any procedure is addressed elsewhere (see Case 12). There is a greater trend toward maintaining MAT through a procedure and adding an opioid if needed, allowing for the buprenorphine base to remain.

Women with SUD differ than men in that they have higher rates of PTSD, mood disorders, and histories of trauma. They are more likely to use drugs to self-medicate. Therefore, it is important to treat any co-occurring psychiatric issues when treating women with SUD. Treatment can include psychopharmacology with antidepressants and psychotherapy such as exposure therapy or cognitive processing therapy for PTSD plus Seeking Safety or CBT for SUD. It would also be important to explore with the patient what supports she will have after the birth of her child and provide case management if she has struggles with such problems as homelessness, domestic violence, or financial stressors. Following the birth of the child, it will be important to continue to provide OUD treatment with BUP/NX and to reassure Kelsea that breastfeeding is compatible with her buprenorphine treatment.

References

American Psychiatric Association: Diagnostic and Statistical Manual of Mental Disorders, 5th Edition. Arlington, VA, American Psychiatric Association, 2013

Jones HE, Arria AM, Baewert A, et al: Buprenorphine treatment of opioid-dependent pregnant women: a comprehensive review. Addiction 107(suppl):5–27, 2012 23106923

Saxon AJ, Ling W, Hillhouse M, et al: Buprenorphine/naloxone and methadone effects on laboratory indices of liver health: a randomized trial. Drug Alcohol Depend 128(1–2):71–76, 2013 22921476

Tetrault JM, Tate JP, Edelman EJ, et al: Hepatic safety of buprenorphine in HIV-infected and uninfected patients with opioid use disorder: the role of HCV-infection. J Subst Abuse Treat 68:62–67, 2016 27431048

Walden M, Nicholls FA, Smith KJ, Tucker GT: The effect of ethanol on the release of opioids from oral prolonged-release preparations. Drug Dev Ind Pharm 33(10):1101–1111, 2007 17882730

Appendix 1

Useful Web Sites and Recommended Readings

Erin Zerbo, M.D.

Federal Government Web Sites

- **www.samhsa.gov/medication-assisted-treatment:** The Center for Substance Abuse Treatment (CSAT) of the Substance Abuse and Mental Health Services Administration (SAMHSA), U.S. Department of Health and Human Services, maintains this site for patients and health care providers interested in medication-assisted treatment for opioid use disorders. It contains a wealth of information on opioid treatment programs, buprenorphine trainings and waiver management, Medicare and Medicaid coverage, and locations of treatment centers. There are also resources for patient education and a link to the Buprenorphine Treatment Practitioner Locator.
- **https://findtreatment.samhsa.gov:** This is a Behavioral Health Treatment Services Locator for facilities throughout the United States and its territories. Search results can be sorted by type of service, including mental health, substance abuse, Veterans Affairs, and buprenorphine prescribers. It is an invaluable resource for patients seeking treatment.
- **www.drugabuse.gov/nidamed:** The National Institute on Drug Abuse (NIDA), of the National Institutes of Health, created NIDAMED to provide primary care physicians with an effective tool for alcohol and drug screening, but this approach is useful for all health professionals. The site contains NM ASSIST, an online screening tool for alcohol, tobacco, and other drug use; resources on treatment and prevention; information on clin-

ical trials; and resources that can be provided to patients, including youth (grade school through young adult ages).

- **www.getsmartaboutdrugs.gov:** This Web site was created by the U.S. Drug Enforcement Administration (DEA) as a resource on drugs of abuse for parents, educators, and caregivers. Various sections provide information on each drug, overall trends and statistics, the neurobiology of drug use, and ways to get involved.
- **www.samhsa.gov/sbirt:** Screening, Brief Intervention, and Referral to Treatment (SBIRT) is a resource manual created by SAMHSA. It concentrates on early intervention and treatment services for persons with and at risk for substance use disorders, including alcohol, tobacco, and other drugs. The site provides various resources for screening instruments, health care provider and patient information for brief intervention, treatment center locators, reimbursement coding guidelines, and references for publications regarding screening and intervention.
- **www.guideline.gov:** This site is the home page for the National Guideline Clearinghouse, which provides a complete summary of clinical guidelines for the use of buprenorphine in the treatment of opioid use disorders.
- **www.niaaa.nih.gov:** This excellent site, maintained by the National Institute on Alcohol Abuse and Alcoholism, is focused primarily on alcohol-related diseases rather than opioid use disorders or buprenorphine treatment. Information is up to date and well maintained. Useful resources include research articles, specific links for information related to children and youth, and frequently asked questions directed to the general public.
- **http://turnthetiderx.org:** This Web site was started by the U.S. Surgeon General to help educate physicians and patients about safe pain control options. It includes the U.S. Centers for Disease Control Opioid Prescribing Guide as well as resources for alternatives to opioids.

Private Nonprofit Web Sites

Organizational Web Sites

- **http://pcssmat.org** and **http://pcss-o.org:** The Providers' Clinical Support System for Medication-Assisted Treatment (PCSS-MAT) and the Providers' Clinical Support System for Opioid Therapies (PCSS-O) are a collaborative effort led by the American Academy of Addiction Psychiatry in association with the American Society of Addiction Medicine and several other partners. On these Web sites, physicians can either find or become a mentor to other physicians prescribing medication-assisted treatment. Training modules, webinars, and a discussion forum with active participation from current prescribers are also available.

- **www.naabt.org:** The National Alliance of Advocates for Buprenorphine Treatment (NAABT) is a nonprofit organization that serves to educate the public about opioid use disorders and buprenorphine treatment and reduce stigma and discrimination against patients with substance use disorders. In addition to information about buprenorphine, the site includes a patient-physician matching system, information for treatment providers, and online support communities for patients taking buprenorphine.
- **www.csam-asam.org/resources:** The California Society of Addiction Medicine (CSAM) provides practical information for physicians regarding buprenorphine treatment. This very useful site includes clinical tools, presentations, clinical guidelines, training information, and other resources. Clinical forms can be downloaded and edited for the specific requirements of any clinical practice.
- **www.asam.org:** This Web site, run by the American Society of Addiction Medicine (ASAM), provides information on various ASAM activities and public policy initiatives and links to a number of other organizations active in the addiction field. The society's comprehensive ASAM Review Course helps physicians prepare for the board exam in Addiction Medicine.
- **https://amersa.org:** The Association for Medical Education and Research in Substance Abuse (AMERSA) is a nonprofit multidisciplinary professional organization devoted to the development of substance use education, research, clinical care, and policy. The site provides information on AMERSA's journal *Substance Abuse* and annual conference and has an extensive list of helpful resources.
- **www.drugpolicy.org/sites/default/files/aboutmethadone.pdf:** Drug Policy Alliance, a group dedicated to advancing policies and attitudes to reduce the harms of drug misuse and prohibition, created this document, "About Methadone and Buprenorphine," Revised Second Edition, to provide patients with information about methadone and buprenorphine treatment for opioid use disorders. The document is an easy read and covers essential information regarding reasons for treatment, drug interactions, treatment during pregnancy, overdose, detoxification, travel, and contact information for state substance abuse agencies.
- **www.aaap.org/education-training/buprenorphine:** The American Academy of Addiction Psychiatry provides an online training and certification course at this site for physicians interested in office-based opioid addiction treatment with buprenorphine.
- **www.centeronaddiction.org:** The National Center on Addiction and Substance Abuse (CASA) is a nationwide organization that brings together all the professional disciplines needed to study and combat abuse of all substances— alcohol; nicotine; and illegal, prescription, and performance-enhancing drugs—in all sectors of society. This Web site provides information on var-

ious training activities, research reports prepared by CASA, and a range of resources about drug abuse prevention and drug information.

- **www.supportprop.org:** Physicians for Responsible Opioid Prescribing (PROP) is a nonprofit organization whose mission is to "reduce opioid-related morbidity and mortality by promoting cautious and responsible prescribing practices." PROP focuses on prescriber education, consumer education, and advocacy at the state and federal level for more cautious prescribing practices. They encourage members from the community and are not limited to physicians.

- **www.getnaloxonenow.org:** This grant-funded Web site maintained by the National Development & Research Institutes, Inc. (NDRI) offers free on-line training for naloxone administration. Providers can use the "bystander module" to train patients, and the site also provides online training for professional first responders.

- **https://drugfree.org:** Partnership for Drug-Free Kids focuses on community-based efforts to advance effective alcohol and drug policy, prevention, and treatment. This nonprofit organization is an excellent resource for families struggling with a child's substance use disorder, providing support and offering ways to get involved at the local level. The Web site has a news and education section spearheaded by the former organization Join Together. The site also provides links to a number of other helpful resources, such as www.alcoholscreening.org/Home.aspx, www.drugscreening.org, and www.addictionaction.org.

- **www.drugstrategies.com:** Drug Strategies is a nonprofit research institute focusing mostly on adolescents and young adults that promotes "drug abuse prevention, education and treatment." The institute provides resource guides on school drug prevention programs and treatment in the juvenile justice system and has an excellent online directory for teen treatment programs throughout the United States.

- **www.bubblemonkey.com:** Drug Strategies maintains this high-graphic site specifically for teens. Here teens can anonymously find reliable information about drugs and alcohol, take a screening test to see if they may have a problem with substances, read true stories from other teens, ask questions, and get information about where to seek help. Text is available in English and Spanish; sites are specific to cities in California, Colorado, and Massachusetts.

- **www.reclaimingfutures.org:** Reclaiming Futures is an organization that began with a donation from the Robert Wood Johnson Foundation and works to help young people in trouble with drugs, alcohol, and crime. The site describes a six-step model implemented in 10 pilot communities that focuses on coordinated substance abuse treatment for teens in the juvenile justice system. Treatment involves the courts, service providers, community groups, and individual volunteers. This useful site includes results from these communities, names of new communities implementing the model, and resources for individuals interested in juvenile justice.

COMMERCIAL WEB SITES

- **www.suboxone.com:** This site, maintained by the manufacturer of Suboxone, Reckitt Benckiser, contains useful information and resources for patients and physicians, including a ZIP code–based physician locator. There is a link to the Here to Help Program, which offers patients additional support and provides a year of free buprenorphine for patients without prescription drug coverage (each physician can have up to three patients on the program at one time).
- **www.buppractice.com:** This commercial site was developed by Clinical-Tools, Inc. under a contract with NIDA and provides an 8-hour online training for buprenorphine certification. The company also has a forum and a helpful resource center for patient education materials.

Recommended Readings

Alford DP, Compton P, Samet JH: Acute pain management for patients receiving maintenance methadone or buprenorphine therapy. Ann Intern Med 144(2):127–134, 2006 16418412

Ball JC, Ross A: The Effectiveness of Methadone Maintenance Treatment: Patients, Programs, Services, and Outcome. New York, Springer-Verlag, 1991

Baxter LE, Campbell A, DeShields M, et al: Safe methadone induction and stabilization: report of an expert panel. J Addict Med 7(6): 377–386, 2013 24189172

Center for Substance Abuse Treatment: Clinical Guidelines for the Use of Buprenorphine in the Treatment of Opioid Addiction (Treatment Improvement Protocol (TIP) Series 40, DHHS Publ No (SMA) 04-3939). Rockville, MD, Substance Abuse and Mental Health Services Administration, 2004. Available at: www.ncbi.nlm.nih.gov/bookshelf/br.fcgi?book=hssamhsatip&part=A72248. Accessed May 28, 2017.

Center for Substance Abuse Treatment: Medication-Assisted Treatment for Opioid Addiction in Opioid Treatment Programs (Treatment Improvement Protocol (TIP) Series 43, HHS Publ No (SMA) 12-4214). Rockville, MD: Substance Abuse and Mental Health Services Administration, 2005

Cicero TJ, Ellis MS, Surratt HL, et al: The changing face of heroin use in the United States: a retrospective analysis of the past 50 years. JAMA Psychiatry 71(7):821–826, 2014 24871348

Compton WM, Jones CM, Baldwin GT: Relationship between nonmedical prescription-opioid use and heroin use. N Engl J Med 374(2):154–163, 2016 26760086

Cowan A: Buprenorphine: the basic pharmacology revisited. J Addict Med 1(2):68–72, 2007 21768937

Denning P, Little J: Practicing Harm Reduction Psychotherapy: An Alternative Approach to Addictions, 2nd Edition. New York, Guilford, 2011

Dole VP, Nyswander M: A medical treatment for diacetylmorphine (heroin) addiction: a clinical trial with methadone hydrochloride. JAMA 193:646–650, 1965 14321530

Fiellin DA, Moore BA, Sullivan LE, et al: Long-term treatment with buprenorphine/naloxone in primary care: results at 2–5 years. Am J Addict 17(2):116–120, 2008 18393054

Fudala PJ, Bridge TP, Herbert S, et al: Office-based treatment of opiate addiction with a sublingual-tablet formulation of buprenorphine and naloxone. N Engl J Med 349(10):949–958, 2003 12954743

Galanter M, Kleber HD, Brady KT (eds): The American Psychiatric Publishing Textbook of Substance Abuse Treatment, 5th Edition. Washington, DC, American Psychiatric Publishing, 2014

Hser YI, Hoffman V, Grella CE, et al: A 33-year follow-up of narcotics addicts. Arch Gen Psychiatry 58(5):503–508, 2001 11343531

Jones HE, Heil SH, Baewert A, et al: Buprenorphine treatment of opioid-dependent pregnant women: a comprehensive review. Addiction 107 (suppl 1):5–27, 2012 23106923

Kakko J, Svanborg KD, Kreek MJ, et al: 1-year retention and social function after buprenorphine-assisted relapse prevention treatment for heroin dependence in Sweden: a randomised, placebo-controlled trial. Lancet 361(9358):662–668, 2003 12606177

Kalivas PW, Volkow ND: The neural basis of addiction: a pathology of motivation and choice. Am J Psychiatry 162(8):1403–1413, 2005 16055761

Khantzian EJ: Treating Addiction as a Human Process. Northvale, NJ, Jason Aronson, 1999

Kosten TR, George TP: The neurobiology of opioid dependence: implications for treatment. Sci Pract Perspect 1(1):13–20, 2002 18567959

Leschner AI: Science-based views of drug addiction and its treatment. JAMA 282(14):1314–1316, 1999 10527162

Levounis P: Bench to bedside: from the science to the practice of addiction medicine. J Med Toxicol 12(1):50–53, 2016 26553278

Levounis P, Arnaout B, Marienfeld C (eds): Motivational Interviewing for Clinical Practice, 2nd Edition. Arlington, VA, American Psychiatric Association Publishing, 2017

Levounis P, Zerbo EA, Aggarwal R (eds): Pocket Guide to Addiction Assessment and Treatment. Arlington, VA, American Psychiatric Association Publishing, 2016

Ruiz P, Strain E (eds): Lowinson and Ruiz's Substance Abuse: A Comprehensive Textbook, 5th Edition. New York, Lippincott Williams & Wilkins, 2011

Marlatt GA, Gordon JR: Relapse Prevention: Maintenance Strategies in the Treatment of Addictive Behaviors. New York, Guilford, 1985

McCance-Katz EF: Office-based buprenorphine treatment for opioid-dependent patients. Harv Rev Psychiatry 12(6):321–338, 2004 15764468

McLellan AT, Lewis DC, O'Brien CP, et al: Drug dependence, a chronic medical illness: implications for treatment, insurance, and outcomes evaluation. JAMA 284(13):1689–1695, 2000 11015800

Miller WR, Rollnick S: Motivational Interviewing: Helping People Change, 3rd Edition. New York, Guilford, 2012

Moeller KE, Lee KC, Kissack JC: Urine drug screening: practical guide for clinicians. Mayo Clin Proc 83(1):66–76, 2008 18174009

Moran M: Rule governing confidentiality of substance use data updated. Psychiatric News, February 23, 2017

Musto DF: The American Disease: Origins of Narcotic Control, 3rd Edition. New York, Oxford University Press, 1999

Najavits LM: Seeking Safety: A Treatment Manual for PTSD and Substance Abuse. New York, Guilford, 2002

Nunes EV, Levin FR: Treatment of depression in patients with alcohol or other drug dependence: a meta-analysis. JAMA 291(15):1887–1896, 2004 15100209

Nunes EV, Selzer J, Levounis P, et al: Substance Dependence and Co-occurring Psychiatric Disorders: Best Practices for Diagnosis and Clinical Treatment. New York, Civic Research Institute, 2010

Prochaska JO, DiClemente CC: Transtheoretical therapy: towards a more integrative model of change. Psychotherapy: Theory, Research and Practice 19:276–288, 1982

Quinones S: Dreamland: The True Tale of America's Opiate Epidemic. New York, Bloomsbury, 2015

Ries RK, Fiellin DA, Miller SC, et al: Principles of Addiction Medicine, 5th Edition. Philadelphia, PA, Lippincott Williams & Wilkins, 2014

Sees KL, Delucchi KL, Masson C, et al. Methadone maintenance vs 180-day psychosocially enriched detoxification for treatment of opioid dependence: a randomized controlled trial. JAMA 283(10):1303–1310, 2000 10714729

Sordo L, Barrio G, Bravo MJ, et al. Mortality risk during and after opioid substitution treatment: systematic review and meta-analysis of cohort studies. BMJ 357:j1550, 2017 28446428

Substance Abuse and Mental Health Services Administration: The Determinations Report: A Report on the Physician Waiver Program Established by the Drug Addiction Treatment Act of 2000 ("DATA"), March 30, 2006. Rockville, MD, Center for Substance Abuse Treatment, 2006. Available at: www.samhsa.gov/sites/default/files/programs_campaigns/medication_assisted/determinations-report-physician-waiver-program.pdf. Accessed May 28, 2017.

Westreich LM: Helping the Addict You Love: The New Effective Program for Getting the Addict Into Treatment. New York, Fireside, 2007

Woody GE, Poole SA, Subramaniam G, et al: Extended vs short-term buprenorphine-naloxone for treatment of opioid-addicted youth: a randomized trial. JAMA 300(17):2003–2011, 2008 18984887

Volkow ND, Baler RD: Addiction science: Uncovering neurobiological complexity. Neuropharmacology 76(Pt B):235–249, 2014 23688927

Volkow ND, Koob GF, McLellan AT: Neurobiologic advances from the brain disease model of addiction. N Engl J Med 374(4):363–371, 2016 26816013

Zerbo EA, Schlechter A, Desai S, Levounis P (eds): Becoming Mindful: Integrating Mindfulness Into Your Psychiatric Practice. Arlington, VA, American Psychiatric Association Publishing, 2017

Appendix 2

Buprenorphine and Office-Based Treatment of Opioid Use Disorder Supplemental Materials

Beatrice A. Eld

Professional Organizations

American Psychiatric Association (APA): www.psychiatry.org
American Academy of Addiction Psychiatry (AAAP): www.aaap.org
American Osteopathic Academy of Addiction Medicine (AOAAM): www.aoaam.org
American Society of Addiction Medicine (ASAM): www.asam.org

Training and Clinical Mentoring

Providers' Clinical Support System–Medication Assisted Treatment (PCCS-MAT): http://pcssmat.org
Providers' Clinical Support System–Opioid Therapies (PCSS-O): http://pcss-o.org
APA Learning Center: http://education.psychiatry.org (search for "substance use disorders")

PCSS-MAT Resources

CLINICAL GUIDELINES

Available at www.pcssmat.org/opioid-resources/clinical-tools, Clinical Guidances tab:
- Adherence, Diversion and Misuse of Sublingual Buprenorphine
- Buprenorphine Induction

- Clinically Relevant Drug Interactions: Buprenorphine or Methadone With Other Frequently Prescribed Drugs
- Management of Psychiatric Medications in Patients Receiving Buprenorphine/Naloxone
- Monitoring of Liver Function Tests and Hepatitis in Patients Receiving Buprenorphine/Naloxone
- Monitoring of Liver Function Tests in Patients Receiving Naltrexone or Extended-Release Naltrexone
- Off-Label Use of Sublingual Buprenorphine and Buprenorphine/Naloxone for Pain
- Pregnancy and Buprenorphine Treatment
- Psychosocial Aspects of Treatment in Patients Receiving Buprenorphine/Naloxone
- Transfer from Methadone to Buprenorphine
- Treatment of Acute Pain in Patients Receiving Buprenorphine/Naloxone
- Treatment of Opioid Dependent Adolescents and Young Adults Using Sublingual Buprenorphine

PCSS-MAT BROCHURES

- Childbirth, Breastfeeding and Infant Care: Methadone and Buprenorphine: http://pcssmat.org/wp-content/uploads/2013/10/ASAM-WAGBrochure-Opioid-Labor_Final.pdf
- Pregnancy: Methadone and Buprenorphine: http://pcssmat.org/wp-content/uploads/2013/10/WAGBrochure-Opioid-Pregnancy_Final.pdf

PREPARING FOR DEA INSPECTIONS

- How to Prepare for a Visit from the Drug Enforcement Agency (DEA) Regarding Buprenorphine Prescribing: http://pcssmat.org/wp-content/uploads/2014/02/FINAL-How-to-Prepare-for-a-DEA-Inspection.pdf
- Documentation used by DEA agents doing an inspection: http://pcssmat.org/wp-content/uploads/2015/03/DEA-Inspection-References.pdf

Clinical Practice Guidelines

- U.S. Department of Veterans Administration and Department of Defense Clinical Practice Guidelines on the Management of Substance Use Disorder: www.healthquality.va.gov/guidelines/MH/sud
- ASAM National Practice Guideline for the Use of Medications in the Treatment of Addiction Involving Opioid Use: www.asam.org/docs/default-source/practice-support/guidelines-and-consensus-docs/asam-national-practice-guideline-supplement.pdf?sfvrsn=24

- CDC Guideline for Prescribing Opioids for Chronic Pain: www.cdc.gov/drugoverdose/prescribing/guideline.html

Selected Resources of Agencies of the U.S. Government

DEPARTMENT OF HEALTH AND HUMAN SERVICES

- Opioids: The Prescription Drug & Heroin Overdose Epidemic: www.hhs.gov/opioids/index.html

CENTERS FOR DISEASE CONTROL AND PREVENTION

- CDC Guideline for Prescribing Opioids for Chronic Pain: www.cdc.gov/drugoverdose/prescribing/guideline.html
- A Guide to Comprehensive Hepatitis C Counseling and Testing: www.cdc.gov/hepatitis/Resources/Professionals/PDFs/Counselingand Testing.pdf

U.S. SURGEON GENERAL

- Surgeon General's Turn the Tide Rx campaign: http://turnthetiderx.org
- Summary of HHS Agency Resources - https://addiction.surgeongeneral.gov/supplementary-materials/hhs-agency-resources

FOOD AND DRUG ADMINISTRATION: MEDICATION GUIDES AND RISK EVALUATION AND MITIGATION STRATEGIES (REMS)

Suboxone® sublingual film: www.fda.gov/downloads/drugs/drugsafety/post marketdrugsafetyinformationforpatientsandproviders/ucm227949.pdf and www.accessdata.fda.gov/drugsatfda_docs/label/2012/022410s006s007 mg.pdf

Buprenorphine-naloxone sublingual tablet: www.fda.gov/downloads/drugs/drugsafety/postmarketdrugsafetyinformationforpatientsandproviders/ucm191529.pdf

Vivitrol®: www.fda.gov/downloads/Drugs/DrugSafety/UCM206669.pdf

Bunavail®: www.accessdata.fda.gov/drugsatfda_docs/label/2014/205637s000 lbl.pdf

Zubsolv®: www.fda.gov/downloads/Drugs/DrugSafety/UCM362203.pdf

Probuphine® REMS: https://dailymed.nlm.nih.gov/dailymed/drugInfo.cfm?setid=10fd7088-cc4a-4bda-a5e3-a82563540a9a

SUBSTANCE ABUSE AND MENTAL HEALTH SERVICES ADMINISTRATION (SAMHSA)

- Medication-assisted treatment: www.samhsa.gov/medication-assisted-treatment
  - Summary of the Drug Addiction Treatment Act of 2000
  - Buprenorphine waiver management
  - Physician waiver qualifications
  - Waiver application form (notice of intent) for initial waiver and patient limit increase
  - Patient limits
  - Physician clinical discussion WebBoard
- Center for Substance Abuse Treatment: www.samhsa.gov/about-us/who-we-are/offices-centers/csat
- Division of Pharmacologic Therapies: www.samhsa.gov/medication-assisted-treatment/about
- Confidentiality of patient records: www.samhsa.gov/laws-regulations-guidelines/medical-records-privacy-confidentiality
- Regulation: Confidentiality of Substance Use Disorder Patient Records: www.ecfr.gov/cgi-bin/text-idx?c=ec-fr&sid=b7e8d29be4a2b815c404988e29c06a3e&rgn=div5&view=text&node=42:1.0.1.1.2&idno=42

SAMHSA Publications

- Clinical Guidelines for the Use of Buprenorphine in the Treatment of Opioid Addiction (Treatment Improvement Protocol 40) www.ncbi.nlm.nih.gov/books/NBK64245/pdf/Bookshelf_NBK64245.pdf
- Key Substance Use and Mental Health Indicators in the United States: Results from the 2015 National Survey on Drug Use and Health www.samhsa.gov/data/sites/default/files/NSDUH-FFR1-2015/NSDUH-FFR1-2015/NSDUH-FFR1-2015.pdf
- Managing Chronic Pain in Adults With or in Recovery From Substance Use Disorders (TIP 54): https://store.samhsa.gov/shin/content/SMA12-4671/TIP54.pdf
- Medication-Assisted Treatment for Opioid Addiction in Opioid Treatment Programs (TIP 43): https://www.ncbi.nlm.nih.gov/books/NBK64164/pdf/Bookshelf_NBK64164.pdf
- Opioid Overdose Toolkit: Facts for Community Members: http://content.govdelivery.com/accounts/USSAMHSA/bulletins/88c847
- Substance Abuse Treatment for Persons With Co-Occurring Disorders (TIP 42): https://store.samhsa.gov/product/TIP-42-Substance-Abuse-Treatment-for-Persons-With-Co-Occurring-Disorders/SMA13-3992

- What Every Individual Needs to Know About Methadone Maintenance: Introduction to Methadone: http://healthqwest.us/pdfs/Methadone. Brochure.pdf

No-Cost Publications Available From the SAMHSA Store

The following publications are available at https://store.samhsa.gov:
- A Collaborative Approach to the Treatment of Pregnant Women with Opioid Use Disorders
- An Introduction to Extended-Release Injectable Naltrexone for the Treatment of People With Opioid Dependence
- Clinical Use of Extended-Release Injectable Naltrexone in the Treatment of Opioid Use Disorder: A Brief Guide
- Decisions in Recovery: Treatment for Opioid Use Disorder
- Federal Guidelines for Opioid Treatment Programs 2016
- MATx Mobile App to Support Medication-Assisted Treatment of Opioid Use Disorder
- Medication for the Treatment of Alcohol Use Disorder: A Brief Guide
- Medicaid Coverage and Financing of Medications to Treat Alcohol and Opioid Use Disorders
- SAMHSA Opioid Overdose Prevention Toolkit
- Sublingual and Transmucosal Buprenorphine for Opioid Use Disorder: Review and Update
- Pocket Guide: Medication-Assisted Treatment of Opioid Use Disorder
- Medication-Assisted Treatment for Opioid Addiction: Facts for Families and Friends

NATIONAL INSTITUTE ON ALCOHOL ABUSE AND ALCOHOLISM (NIAAA)

- Helping Patients Who Drink Too Much: A Clinician's Guide: https://niaaa.nih.gov/publications/clinical-guides-and-manuals/helping-patients-who-drink-too-much-clinicians-guide
- Alcohol Screening and Brief Intervention for Youth: A Practitioner's Guide: https://niaaa.nih.gov/publications/clinical-guides-and-manuals/alcohol-screening-and-brief-intervention-youth

NATIONAL INSTITUTE ON DRUG ABUSE (NIDA)

- Medications To Treat Opioid Addiction: Research Report Series: www.drugabuse.gov/publications/research-reports/medications-to-treat-opioid-addiction/overview

- Factors Predicting the Transition From Prescription Opioids to Heroin: www.drugabuse.gov/news-events/latest-science/factors-predicting-transition-prescription-opioids-to-heroin
- NIDAMED: Resources for Medical and Health Professionals: www.drug abuse.gov/nidamed-medical-health-professionals
- Monitoring the Future 2016 Survey Results: www.drugabuse.gov/related-topics/trends-statistics/infographics/monitoring-future-2016-survey-results

Federation of State Medical Boards

- Guidelines for the Chronic Use of Opioid Analgesics: www.fsmb.org/ Media/Default/PDF/Advocacy/Opioid%20Guidelines%20As%20 Adopted%20April%202017_FINAL.pdf
- Model Policy on DATA 2000 and Treatment of Opioid Addiction in the Medical Office, April 2013: www.fsmb.org/Media/Default/PDF/FSMB/ Advocacy/2013_model_policy_treatment_opioid_addiction.pdf
- Model Policy on the Use of Opioid Analgesics in the Treatment of Chronic Pain, July 2013: www.fsmb.org/Media/Default/PDF/FSMB/Advocacy/ pain_policy_july2013.pdf

Index

Page numbers printed in **boldface** type refer to tables or figures.